W0042004

Coarticulation
Theory, Data and Techniques

The variation that a speech sound undergoes under the influence of neighbouring sounds has acquired the well-established label 'coarticulation'. The phenomenon of coarticulation has become a central problem in the theory of speech production. Much experimental work has been directed towards discovering its characteristics, its extent and its occurrence across different languages. This book contains eighteen contributions on coarticulation by major researchers. It provides a definitive account of the experimental findings to date, together with discussions of their implications for modelling the process of speech production. Different components of the speech production system (larynx, tongue, jaw, etc.) require different techniques for investigation and a whole section of this book is devoted to a description of the experimental techniques currently used. Other chapters offer a theoretically sophisticated discussion of the implications of coarticulation for the phonology–phonetics interface.

WILLIAM J. HARDCASTLE is Professor of Speech Science and Head of the Department of Speech and Language Sciences at Queen Margaret University College, Edinburgh. He has published a number of books including *Physiology of Speech Production* and *Disorders of Fluency*, and is the co-editor of the *Handbook of Phonetic Sciences*. He has carried out research into the mechanisms of speech production and sensori-motor control in both normal and pathological speech, and his research findings have been published in numerous journals, including the *Journal of Phonetics*, *Journal of Speech and Hearing Research*, *Phonetica*, *Language and Speech*, *European Journal of Disorders of Communication* and *Clinical Linguistics and Phonetics*.

NIGEL HEWLETT is a Senior Lecturer in the Department of Speech and Language Sciences at Queen Margaret University College, Edinburgh. As well as writing chapters for various books, he has published articles in the *Journal of Phonetics*, *Clinical Linguistics and Phonetics* and the *European Journal of Disorders of Communication*, mainly in the areas of child speech development and adult speech disorders.

Coarticulation

Theory, Data and Techniques

EDITED BY

WILLIAM J. HARDCASTLE AND NIGEL HEWLETT

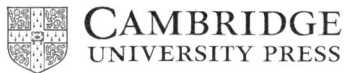

CAMBRIDGE
UNIVERSITY PRESS

CAMBRIDGE UNIVERSITY PRESS
Cambridge, New York, Melbourne, Madrid, Cape Town, Singapore, São Paulo

Cambridge University Press
The Edinburgh Building, Cambridge CB2 2RU, UK

Published in the United States of America by Cambridge University Press, New York

www.cambridge.org
Information on this title: www.cambridge.org/9780521440271

First published 1999
This digitally printed first paperback version 2006

A catalogue record for this publication is available from the British Library

Library of Congress Cataloguing in Publication data

Coarticulation : theory, data, and techniques /
[edited by] William J. Hardcastle and Nigel Hewlett.
    p.   cm.
Includes bibliographical references and index.
ISBN 0 521 44027 0 (hardback)
1. Speech–Physiological aspects.   2. Phonetics.   I. Hardcastle,
William J., 1943–   .   II. Hewlett, Nigel.
QP306.C68   1999
612.7′8–dc21   98-44696   CIP

ISBN-13 978-0-521-44027-1 hardback
ISBN-10 0-521-44027-0 hardback

ISBN-13 978-0-521-02985-8 paperback
ISBN-10 0-521-02985-6 paperback

Contents

List of figures   *page* vii
List of tables   xi
List of contributors   xii
Acknowledgments   xiv

Introduction
William J. Hardcastle and Nigel Hewlett   1

Part I Theories and models

1 The origin of coarticulation
   Barbara Kühnert and Francis Nolan   7

2 Coarticulation models in recent speech production theories
   Edda Farnetani and Daniel Recasens   31

Part II Research results: components of the motor system for speech

3 Velopharyngeal coarticulation
   Michel Chafcouloff and Alain Marchal   69

4 Lingual coarticulation
   Daniel Recasens   80

5 Laryngeal coarticulation
   Philip Hoole, Christer Gobl and Ailbhe Ní Chasaide   105
   Coarticulatory investigations of the devoicing gesture: 107
   Philip Hoole
   Voice source variation in the vowel as a function of consonantal
   context: Christer Gobl and Ailbhe Ní Chasaide   122

v

6   Labial coarticulation
    Edda Farnetani   144

7   Lip and jaw coarticulation
    Janet Fletcher and Jonathan Harrington   164

Part III Wider perspectives

8   Cross-language studies: relating language-particular
    coarticulation patterns to other language-particular facts
    Sharon Manuel   179

9   Implications for phonological theory
    Mary Beckman   199

Part IV Instrumental techniques

10 Palatography
    Fiona Gibbon and Katerina Nicolaidis   229

11 Imaging techniques
    Maureen Stone   246

12 Electromagnetic articulography
    Philip Hoole and Noel Nguyen   260

13 Electromyography
    William J. Hardcastle   270

14 Transducers for investigating velopharyngeal function
    Michel Chafcouloff   284

15 Techniques for investigating laryngeal articulation
    Philip Hoole, Christer Gobl and Ailbhe Ní Chasaide   294
    Investigation of the devoicing gesture: Philip Hoole   294
    Techniques for analysing the voice source: Christer Gobl and
    Ailbhe Ní Chasaide   300

16 Acoustic analysis
    Daniel Recasens   322

    References   337
    Index   383

Figures

2.1 The revised model of vowel undershoot of Moon and
Lindblom (1994). Reprinted with permission; copyright
1994, Acoustical Society of America   *page* 36

2.2 The model of tongue body coarticulation in the production
of retroflex alveolars. Reprinted with permission from
Lindblom (1983); copyright 1983, Springer-Verlag Gmbtt
& Co.   37

2.3 From phonological representation to phonetic representation,
through anticipatory feature-spreading rules as proposed by
Daniloff and Hammarberg (1973). Reprinted with permission
from Keating (1988b). Copyright 1988, Cambridge
University Press   42

2.4 Keating's window model   47

2.5 Representation of three overlapping phonetic gestures.
(Reprinted with permission from Fowler and Saltzman (1993).
Copyright 1993, Kingston Press Services Ltd.   52

2.6 The additive blending model proposed by Munhall and
Löfqvist (1992). Reprinted with permission; copyright 1992,
Academic Press   55

2.7 Anticipatory labial coarticulation   62

4.1 Linguopalatal configurations of maximal disclosure or
constriction for different Catalan consonants   86

4.2 EPG contact displays for Catalan speaker DR   88

4.3 Average F2 data representing C-to-V and V-to-V anticipatory
effects in VCV sequences   95

4.4 F2 coarticulatory effects for the Catalan speaker DR   96

5.1 Typical pattern of laryngeal–oral coordination in aspirated stops 110

5.2   Simplified illustration of relationship between hypothesized
      underlying gestural input and observable behaviour   118
5.3   EE and RA values superimposed for the /p–p(ː)/ and /p–b(ː)/
      contexts in German, French, Swedish and Italian   126
5.4   Oral airflow and speech waveform illustrating contrasting
      intervocalic stops in Swedish and Italian and in German and
      French   128
5.5   Multi-channel recording of the Icelandic word /laʰpa/   130
5.6   L1 relative to L0 for the contexts /p–p(ː)/, /b–p(ː)/, /p–b(ː)/
      and b–b(ː)/ in French, German, Italian and Swedish   131
5.7   The first vowel of the Swedish words /babːa/ and /bapːa/   132
5.8   Averaged EE, RA and RK values   134
5.9   Oral airflow and speech waveform illustrating contrasting
      intervocalic labiodental fricatives in Swedish, Italian and
      French   135
5.10 EE and RA values superimposed for the /p–/ and /b–/ contexts
      in French and German   136
5.11 Spectral (L1 relative to L0) data and source parameters EE, RA
      and FA for the Swedish /a/   138
5.12 Levels of F0 (L0) and F1 (L1) in the vowel following the post-
      aspirated stop in Swedish and German   139
6.1   Tongue and lip profiles for the three high front vowels and the
      high back vowel of Swedish. Reprinted with permission from
      Fant (1973). Copyright 1969, Speech Transmission Laboratory,
      Royal Institute of Technology (KTH), Stockholm and the
      author   145
6.2   The facial muscles involved in the labial articulation for vowels.
      Reprinted with permission from Gentil and Boë (1980).
      Copyright 1980, the authors   150
6.3   The look ahead and the coproduction (or time-locked) models
      of anticipatory labial coarticulation   153
6.4   The two-phase or hybrid model   157
6.5   The movement expansion model of anticipatory labial
      coarticulation proposed by Abry and Lallouache (1995).
      Reprinted with permission; copyright 1995, the authors   160
7.1   Jaw displacement trajectory for a production of [bab]   170
8.1   Examples of phonemic vowels of Ndebele, Shona and
      Sotho   185
8.2   Acoustic effects of following context vowel on the target
      vowels /ɑ/ and /e/ in Ndebele, Shona and Sotho   186

8.3 First and second formants for the middle vowel /ɑ/ in a single token of /pɑpɑpɑ/ and /pɑpɑpi/ from English, Sotho and Ndebele 187

10.1 Electrode distribution on the Reading, Rion and the Kay Palatometer artificial palates. Reprinted with permission from Fletcher (1985, 1988). Copyright 1985 and 1988, American Speech–Language–Hearing Association 231

10.2 Phonetic zoning systems for the Reading and Rion artificial plates 234

10.3 Computer print-out of the /kt/ sequence in the word 'actor' 235

10.4 Computer print-out of velar segments in two different vowel environments 236

10.5 Individual EPG frames from [ɑkɑ] and [iki] at the point of maximum constriction 239

10.6 Calculation of the coarticulatory index (CI) 241

10.7 Multi-channel screen display of [ɑʔtʃɪ] in the word 'starchy' 243

11.1 Depiction of medical sections and terminology used to describe imaged data 248

11.2 View of a subject's head in a CT scanner 249

11.3 CT image of a transverse section of the oropharynx at rest 250

11.4 Artist's rendition of the effects of MRI scanning on hydrogen protons 251

11.5 MRI image of a midsaggital section of the tongue during the production of [ɑ] 252

11.6 Ultrasound image of a coronal section of the tongue at rest. Reprinted from Stone *et al.* (1988). Copyright 1988, Acoustical Society of America 253

11.7 Three-dimensional tongue surface reconstruction of the sound /ʃ/ 254

11.8 Sagittal tongue profiles of [ilɑ] measured from midsaggital ultrasound images 257

11.9 Two tongue movement strategies. Reprinted with permission from Unser and Stone (1992). Copyright 1992, Acoustical Society of America 258

12.1 Rotational axes of magnetometer sensors that lead to a reduction in the induced signal for typical sensor locations on the tongue 262

12.2 Positions of four fleshpoints on the tongue for the German tense–lax vowel pair /eː/ and /ɛ/ in the three consonantal contexts /p/, /t/ and /k/ 268

13.1   Two records of electrical activity recorded with a hooked-wire electrode from the mentalis muscle. Reprinted with permission from Abbs and Watkins (1976). Copyright 1976, Academic Press   277

13.2   Illustration of the smoothing effect of different time constraints on the rectified EMG pattern. Reprinted with permission from Abbs and Watkin (1976). Copyright 1976, Academic Press   281

13.3   A 'motor score' showing schematized results of EMG signals from various different muscles during production of the utterance /əpip/. Reprinted with permission from Honda, Kusakawa and Kakita (1992). Copyright 1992, Academic Press   282

15.1   Example of two-channel transillumination signal for a German sentence ('Lies die Schiffe bitte') containing several voiceless sounds   298

15.2   Simplified schematic representation illustrating the principle of inverse filtering   301

15.3   Modified screen display of an interactive filtering program   306

15.4   The inverse filter output (differential glottal flow) of the Swedish utterance /aˈjøː/   308

15.5   Schematic design of the experimental set-up using the Sondhi tube. Reprinted with permission from Monsen and Engebretson (1977). Copyright 1977, Acoustical Society of America   310

15.6   Schematic diagram of the experimental set-up using miniature pressure transducers; dimensions of the Millar catheter; electrical diagram of the transducer (after Cranen and Boves 1985). Figure 15.6c is reprinted with permission from Cranen and Boves (1985). Copyright 1985, Acoustical Society of America   312

15.7   The LF model   315

15.8   Screen display of an interactive model matching program   316

15.9   The voice source parameters EE, RA, RK and OQ   318

16.1   F2 × F3 values at vowel onset for Swedish CV sequences with voiced and voiceless stops of different place of articulation. Reprinted with permission from Fant (1973). Copyright 1969, Speech Transmission Laboratory, Royal Institute of Technology (KTH), Stockholm and the author   326

16.2   F1, F2 and F3 trajectories. Reprinted with permission from Kewley-Port (1982). Copyright 1982, Acoustical Society of America   328

16.3 Projected CV formant transitions towards F2 and F3 loci for different American English vowels. Reprinted with permission from Kewley-Port (1982). Copyright 1982, Acoustical Society of America 329

16.4 Examples of burst spectra for /b/, /d/ and /g/ in different vowel contexts. Reprinted with permission from Blumstein and Stevens (1979). Copyright 1979, Acoustical Society of America 332

16.5 Spectral differences at the fricative noise of /s/ and /z/ as a function of /i/, /a/ and /u/. Reprinted with permssion from Soli (1981). Copyright 1981, Acoustical Society of America 334

Tables

11.1 Physiological features of the vocal tract that are readily observed, measured and analysed using imaging techniques 247

11.2 Coarticulatory issues well suited to exploration by imaging techniques 255

Contributors

Professor Mary Beckman, Department of Linguistics, Ohio State University, Columbus, Ohio, USA

Dr Michel Chafcouloff, CNRS Institut de Phonétique, Aix-en-Provence, France

Dr Edda Farnetani, Centro di Studio per le richerche di fonetica del CNR, Padua, Italy

Dr Janet Fletcher, Department of Linguistics, University of Melbourne, Australia

Dr Fiona Gibbon, Department of Speech and Language Sciences, Queen Margaret University College, Edinburgh, UK

Christer Gobl, Centre for Language and Communication Studies, Trinity College, University of Dublin, Ireland

Professor William J. Hardcastle, Department of Speech and Language Sciences, Queen Margaret University College, Edinburgh, UK

Dr Jonathan Harrington, Speech, Hearing and Language Research Centre, Macquarie University, Sydney, Australia

Dr Philip Hoole, Institut für Phonetik und Sprachliche Kommunikation, University of Munich, Germany

Dr Barbara Kühnert, Department of Linguistics, University of Cambridge, UK, and Institut für Phonetik und Sprachliche Kommunikation, University of Munich, Germany

Professor Sharon Manuel, Northeastern Univesity, Boston, USA and Research Institute of Electronics, Massachusetts Institute of Technology, Cambridge, Massachusetts, USA

Professor Alain Marchal, CNRS Délégation Régionale de Normandie, Caen, France

Dr Ailbhe Ní Chasaide, Centre for Language and Communication Studies, Trinity College, University of Dublin, Ireland

Dr Noel Nguyen, Laboratoire de Psycholinguistique, University of Geneva, Switzerland

Dr Katerina Nicolaidis, Department of Theoretical and Applied Linguistics, School of English, Aristotle University of Thessaloniki, Thessaloniki, Greece

Dr Francis Nolan, Department of Linguistics, University of Cambridge, UK

Dr Daniel Recasens, CEDI, Institut d'Estudis Catalans, Barcelona, Spain

Dr Maureen Stone, Vocal Tract Visualization Laboratory, University of Maryland School of Medicine, Baltimore, Maryland, USA.

Acknowledgments

The editors would like to acknowledge the contribution of a number of people in the preparation of this book. Andrew Winnard, of Cambridge University Press, has helpfully overseen the various stages of its production. The original manuscript was reviewed by Professor John Ohala, of the University of California at Berkeley; he made numerous valuable suggestions, many of which have been incorporated into the final form of the book. We are grateful to Karen Horton, of the Department of Speech and Language Sciences, Queen Margaret University College, who retyped large sections of the original manuscript. Dr Linda Armstrong, also of the Department of Speech and Language Sciences, performed a vital two weeks' work getting the manuscript into a form fit for submission to the publishers. Lesley Atkin, of Cambridge University Press, has saved the reader of this book from a multitude of errors, discrepancies and inconsistencies and we greatly appreciate her contribution.

All remaining shortcomings are the responsibility of the editors.

Introduction

WILLIAM J. HARDCASTLE and NIGEL HEWLETT

Continuous speech is characterized by great variability in the articulatory and acoustic properties of segments. Sound segments are highly sensitive to context and show considerable influence from neighbouring segments. Such contextual effects are described as being the result of overlapping articulation or *coarticulation*. Coarticulation has been the object of much recent research in speech science and related disciplines.

Coarticulation was the focus of a large-scale research project ACCOR ('Articulatory–acoustic correlations in coarticulatory processes: a cross-language investigation') funded by the EU under the ESPRIT framework. ACCOR ran from 1992–1995 and brought together researchers from different parts of Europe in a unique concerted attempt to tackle the problem of coarticulation from a number of different theoretical perspectives and using a variety of different research methodologies. A cross-language approach was used to differentiate between those aspects of the phenomenon which could be attributed to universal features (due to factors such as inherent characteristics of the speech producing mechanism) and those which are language-specific and which could therefore be related to the phonological rules of the particular language.

The project aimed at a detailed description of the complex coordination between the main phonological systems underlying speech production and the resulting acoustic output. The articulatory dimensions under study were: the respiratory system (producing a flow of air), the laryngeal system (modifying the airflow by the valving mechanism of the vocal folds) and the complex system of supraglottal structures in the mouth and nose, such as the tongue, lip, jaw and soft palate shaping the vocal tract into different resonating cavities. It was possible in ACCOR to investigate specific articulatory processes in the seven languages of the project (English, French, German, Italian,

Irish Gaelic, Swedish, Catalan) with a view to determining how these processes differed according to the different phonological systems. Another aim was to examine the functions of the different motor sub-systems with respect to coarticulation.

This book grew out of the ACCOR project. Most of the authors were original members of the ACCOR consortium and the theoretical perspectives and methodology largely represent the approach used by them.

The book is divided into four sections. Part I contains two chapters which provide the background and history of coarticulation in phonetic theory. Kühnert and Nolan make play with the ambiguity of the word 'origin' in their title, *The origin of coarticulation*, and discuss the origin of the concept of coarticulation in the history of phonetics and the origin of coarticulation in the process of human speech production. Farnetani and Recasens provide a detailed review of alternative contemporary models of coarticulation within phonetic theory in their chapter *Coarticulation models in recent speech production theories.*

The five chapters of Part II are concerned with research findings on coarticulation, and each is focused on a particular aspect of the speech production mechanism. The spreading of nasality from a consonant to a neighbouring vowel was one of the earliest coarticulatory phenomena to be observed and studied systematically. *Velopharyngeal coarticulation*, by Chafcouloff and Marchal, reports on the evidence concerning nasal coarticulation and its theoretical implications. The tongue is a complex, mobile organ which plays a major articulatory role in the production of all vowel sounds and the majority of consonants. In his chapter on *Lingual coarticulation,* Recasens provides a review of empirical findings and theoretical issues and points to important outstanding questions concerning the control processes for lingual coarticulation, such as the question of whether different areas of the tongue (tip, front, back) should be modelled as being quasi-independent of each other. The chapter on *Laryngeal coarticulation*, by Hoole, Gobl and Ní Chasaide, has two parts. Laryngeal vibration has an on/off function in speech and Philip Hoole discusses *Coarticulatory investigations of the devoicing gesture* in the first section of the chapter. Mode of laryngeal vibration is also subject to coarticulatory influence and it is this aspect which is explored in the second section, *Voice source variation in the vowel as a function of consonantal context*, by Gobl and Ní Chasaide. Lip movements, which are relatively accessible to visual inspection, have provided a rich source of data on coarticulation in speech. Farnetani's chapter on *Labial coarticulation* reviews the findings from research in different languages, informed by a description of the muscles involved in the control of lip movement, and explores the implications for competing theoretical models. As Farnetani points out, movements of the lower lip and the jaw are interdependent to a considerable extent. Fletcher and Harrington's chapter, *Lip and jaw coarticulation*, focuses particularly on the coarticulatory influences, involving these structures, upon vowels. They discuss the influence of an adjacent consonant and the influence of another vowel in an adjacent syllable.

We can be reasonably certain that coarticulation is a universal characteristic of human speech production. How particular coarticulatory processes compare across different languages and whether or to what extent coarticulatory processes impinge upon phonological representations are issues explored in Part III. Manuel's chapter, *Relating language-particular coarticulation patterns to other language-particular facts*, focuses on the results of research into non-Indo-European languages. Beckman, in her chapter *Implications for phonological theory*, situates the findings on coarticulation within the issue of the relationship between phonetics and phonology as levels of representation in linguistic theory.

Contemporary phonetics is a mainly experimental science and the development of explanatory models depends crucially on data provided by a number of rather different techniques, from electromyography to acoustic analysis. The details of these techniques may be of less interest to beginning students or to those whose interest in coarticulation lies mainly with its implications for phonological theory. However a discussion of techniques is highly relevant for those intending to undertake empirical research in the area. Part IV contains seven chapters each of which is concerned either with a particular experimental technique or with techniques for investigating coarticulation involving a particular organ of the speech production system. The techniques covered reflect the interests of those involved in the ACCOR project and no claim is made for a completely comprehensive coverage. For techniques not covered here, for example strain gauge and optoelectronic transducers for measuring lip/jaw movements, and electrolaryngography, the reader is referred to other sources such as Abberton and Fourcin (1997), Baken (1998) and Stone (1996).

In practice of course, a particular experimental technique may anyway apply solely, or primarily, to one part of the production mechanism. This is the case with *Palatography* for example, as described by Gibbon and Nicolaidis. Palatography is now a well-established technique for recording the location of, and extent of, lingual contact with the hard palate during speech and it has gathered a comparatively large body of research literature. Direct imaging is probably the ideal method for examining articulatory movements – or it would be, given a system that was sufficiently comprehensive, convenient and risk-free. Stone's chapter, *Imaging techniques,* provides an overview of the advantages and disadvantages of the techniques that are currently available. Hoole and Nguyen's chapter describes *Electromagnetic articulography*, a relatively recent but very promising technique for tracking tongue (and lip) position over time during speech. *Electromyography*, described by Hardcastle, is distinctive in that it is targeted at a stage further back (so to speak) from articulation in speech production, namely that of the neural innervation of articulatory events. Variants of the technique are described in detail together with a discussion of their advantages and disadvantages. Chafcouloff's *Transducers for investigating velopharyngeal function* reviews a variety of techniques available for gaining evidence on the control of velopharyngeal valving. *Techniques for investigating laryngeal articulation*, by Hoole, Gobl and Ní Chasaide, is divided into two sections, which mirror the division of chapter 5 by the same authors. It is the operation of vocal fold abduction in the signalling of a voiceless segment that is the topic of the first section, by Hoole, while the second section, by Gobl and Ní Chasaide, describes techniques for investigating vocal fold vibration itself. The technique with the most extensive history in experimental phonetic research is, of course, that of acoustic analysis and descriptions of acoustic analysis are already plentiful in the literature. Recasens' chapter on *Acoustic analysis* therefore takes a rather different approach from that of the other authors. After briefly surveying variant techniques of analysis and display he discusses applications of acoustic analysis to each of the classes of speech sounds, with special reference to the phenomenon of coarticulation.

Part I
Theories and models

1

The origin of coarticulation

BARBARA KÜHNERT and FRANCIS NOLAN

What is coarticulation, and why does it exist?

The title of this chapter is deliberately ambiguous. *Origin* refers both to the history of the scientific concept of coarticulation and to the question of what causes the phenomena in speech which are known as coarticulation. The history of the concept will be dealt with later, while the reasons why there are phenomena in speech which we can characterize as coarticulation are dealt with explicitly below, as well as implicitly in the discussion of the history of coarticulation. There is even a third sense of 'origin' which is dealt with briefly in this chapter, namely the way in which coarticulation develops as a child learns to speak.

Coarticulation, very broadly, refers to the fact that a phonological segment is not realized identically in all environments, but often apparently varies to become more like an adjacent or nearby segment. The English phoneme /k/, for instance, will be articulated further forward on the palate before a front vowel ([k̟iː] 'key') and further back before a back vowel ([k̠ɔː] 'caw'); and will have a lip position influenced by the following vowel (in particular, with some rounding before the rounded vowel in [k̠ʷɔː] 'caw'). As here, some instances of coarticulation are available to impressionistic observation and constitute an important part of what has traditionally been thought of as allophonic variation. In many other instances, however, the kind of variation which a segment undergoes only becomes apparent from quantitative instrumental investigation, either of the acoustic signal or of speech production itself.

It is essential to the concept of coarticulation that at some level there be invariant, discrete units underlying the variable and continuous activity of speech production. If this were not the case, and, for instance, the mentally stored representation giving rise to a production of the word 'caw' were a fully detailed articulatory plan, then when that word was spoken (in isolation at least) there would be no question of a process of coarticulation – the word would simply correspond to a set of instructions for the time-varying activity of the articulators, and sub-word segments would not exist in any sense, and could therefore not undergo 'coarticulation'.

There are, however, good reasons to assume that the 'componentiality' which characterizes language (sentences made up of words, words made up of morphemes, and so on) extends down at least to the level of phoneme-sized segments. From the point of view of storing and accessing the mental lexicon, it would be massively less efficient if every entry were represented by its own idiosyncratic articulatory (or indeed auditory) properties, rather than in terms of some kind of phonemic code – a finite set of symbols abstracted from phonetic behaviour. Ironically, studies of coarticulation itself, based on the premise of phoneme-sized segments at some level of representation, lend independent support to the premise. For instance such studies have conspicuously not shown, to take a hypothetical example, that the onset of lip rounding is consistently different between the words 'caw' and 'caught' or that the degree of velar fronting is consistently different in each of the words 'key', 'Keith' and 'keen'. If each word were represented holistically and independently, this result would have to be put down to coincidence. Repeated across the lexicon, the coincidence would be huge and extraordinary. On the other hand this kind of regularity across words is predicted by a view in which these sets of words are represented with common sequences of abstract elements, for instance /k/, /ɔː/ in the case of the first set and /k/, /iː/ in the case of the second, and in which the articulatory realization of those sequences is governed by regular principles of integration – that is, by principles of coarticulation.

Accepting the role of segments we may then ask a complementary question: why, if a linguistic system operates in terms of discrete and invariant units (let us say phonemes), are these units not realized discretely and invariantly in speech? After all, there is a medium in which this does happen. When we use a typewriter, each letter is realized on the paper separately from the preceding and following ones, and is realized identically (as near as makes no difference) every time it is typed. English orthography has of course strayed somewhat from a phonemic analysis, but all alphabetic writing systems are in essence a way of representing the phonemic code visually. Why does the speech mechanism not behave like an acoustic typewriter?

One reason is perhaps that we do not have a separate vocal tract for each phoneme, in the way that an old-fashioned typewriter has a separate 'hammer' to produce each letter. Instead, a single vocal tract has to alter its shape to satisfy the requirements of all the sounds in a sequence. The vocal tract is governed by the laws of physics and the constraints of physiology, but (also unlike the typewriter) it is producing its communicative artefact in 'real time'. It cannot move instantaneously from one target configuration to the next. Rather than giving one phoneme an invariant articulation, and then performing a separate and time-consuming transition to the next, it steers a graceful and rapid course through the sequence. The result of this is coarticulation. It is perhaps rather like a slalom skier, whose 'target' is to be to the left and to the right of successive posts, and who minimally satisfies this target with his skis as they zig-zag down the hill, but whose body pursues a more direct course from the top of the hill to the bottom. In the written medium, it is not typing but handwriting which provides the closer analogy to speech. Examine the occurrences of a given letter in any fluent handwriting, and its realizations will vary. Maybe the tail of the 'y' will make a closed loop if a letter follows, but not when it is at the end of a word, and so on. The more fluent the handwriting, the less possible it is to pick out discrete letters, and concomitantly the more each letter's shape will be a product of its environment.

It would be misleading to think of coarticulation in speech as if it were an imperfection in the way language is realized. Speech and language have evolved under the influence of the constraints of the vocal mechanism, and there is no reason to suppose that the relationship between language and the vocal mechanism is not a satisfactory one. The phenomenon of coarticulation may in fact bring advantages beyond the efficient integration of the realizations of successive phonological units.

In particular, the fact that the influence of a segment often extends well beyond its own boundaries means that information about that segment is available to perception longer than would be the case if all cues were confined inside its boundaries. As pointed out by early perceptual theories, the possibility of 'parallel processing' of information for more than one phoneme probably allows speech to be perceived more rapidly than would otherwise be feasible. The possibility that the origin of coarticulation lies not only in the requirements of the articulatory mechanism, but in those of our perceptual system, cannot be discounted.

To recapitulate: the concept of coarticulation entails the hypotheses that at some level speakers make use of a representation in terms of abstract phonological segments, and that there are regular principles governing the articulatory integration of those segments in speech.

Given a coarticulatory standpoint, one way to conceptualize part of the variation in the realization of /k/ in 'caw' and 'key' above is to think in terms of the velar stop having a 'target' place of articulation, which is then modified to facilitate the integration of /k/ with the tongue movement for the following vowel segment. From this perspective coarticulation involves a spatial or configurational modification of the affected segment. Alternatively we can break away from thinking in terms of spatial targets for successive segments, and regard coarticulation as the spreading of a property from one segment to a nearby one. For instance if we concentrate on lip activity in the example above, we noted that the lip rounding always associated with the vowel of 'caw' is also present on the consonant preceding it: [k̠ʷɔː]. In 'key' there is no lip rounding on the velar. From this alternative (temporal rather than spatial) perspective, what matters is when articulatory movements begin and end relative to each other. The rounding of [ɔː] has begun during, or even at the start of, the [k].[1]

It might appear from this example that the spatial/temporal distinction depends on whether or not a property involved in coarticulation is crucial to the identity of the affected segment. A velar stop involves a raising of the tongue dorsum, and it is merely the precise location of that raising which is affected by a following [iː]. On the other hand lip activity is not required for a velar stop, and so, in the word 'caw', the lip movement can be anticipated. It is unlikely, however, that a consistent division can be sustained between 'crucial' properties and other properties of a segment. It may be that the absence of lip rounding on the /k/ of 'key' is just as crucial to the perception of this word as the presence of lip rounding on 'caw' (cf. the 'trough' of rounding found on the fricative in /usu/ sequences – see later). So a simplistic linking of spatial coarticulation to crucial properties, and temporal coarticulation to inessential properties, is not valid.

In fact the very distinction between spatial and temporal coarticulation breaks down as soon as we take a more abstract view of articulation. Recent models of speech production (see later) hypothesize that each segment is associated with an abstract control structure which is in tune with the mechanical properties of the vocal tract, and which defines that segment in terms of dynamic activity of the articulators. In such a view the distinction between space and time becomes less clear. The control structure for [k] would overlap that for [iː] in time in the phonetic plan of an utterance of 'key', but the competing demands of the two would result in a spatial compromise in the resultant articulation. A current hope, therefore, is that a definition of segments not in terms of superficially observable articulatory movements and positions, but in terms of more abstract articulatory control structures, may lead to a more general and unified description of the variety of coarticulatory phenomena.

This section has summarized the origin, in the nature of language and its vocal realization, of the phenomena which are conceived of as coarticulation. We now turn to the origin of the concept of coarticulation in the history of phonetics and its widespread adoption as the basis of a research paradigm.

The historical perspective

The early history

The term 'coarticulation' dates from the 1930s when Menzerath and de Lacerda published *Koartikulation, Steuerung und Lautabgrenzung* (1933). However, the fact that speech sounds influence each other and vary, often substantially, with changes in the adjacent phonetic context had already been known for centuries, while the demonstration that the stream of speech cannot be divided into separate segments corresponding to 'sounds' (or 'letters') coincided with the establishment of experimental phonetics as an independent discipline.

Before experimental techniques were introduced in the study of speech sounds the main tools were 'direct observation' and introspection. Brücke's (1856) and Bell's (1867) insights for German and English, respectively, which laid the foundations for academic phonetics, were based upon such subjective observations. Not surprisingly, early phoneticians shared the assumption that alphabetical letters have corresponding physical realizations in the form of single sounds. The leading idea at the time was that every sound has a static positional (steady state) phase and that different sounds are connected by short transitional glides. The concept of such transitional glides ('Übergangslaute'), which allow the stream of speech to be continuous, was formulated most explicitly by Sievers (1876). For instance, he described the production of a syllable such as 'al' in such a way that there exists neither a pure 'a'-sound nor a pure 'l'-sound during the linking movement of the tongue but a continuous series of transitional sounds which as a whole were referred to as a 'glide'. For an overview of early phonetics, see Tillmann (1994).

There were, however, some indications in the early literature that the classical view might not capture the whole story. Sievers (1876) himself acknowledged the possibility that, in certain sound combinations, articulators which are not involved in the current sound production might anticipate their upcoming configuration as long as it does not compete with the requirements of the present sound. Examples are the rounding of the lips during the production of /k/ in /ku/ or the preparation of the tongue position for the vowel during the consonant in syllables such as /mi/. And from a more theoretical perspective, Paul (1898: 48) wrote: 'A genuine dissection of the word into its elements is not only very difficult, it is almost impossible. The word does not correspond to a sequence of a specific number of independent sounds, each of which could be represented by a sign of the alphabet, but it is, in fact, always a continuous row of an infinite number of sounds . . .'[2]

Historically, phonetics moved towards experimental research during the last quarter of the nineteenth century. 'Kymography' allowed the mechanical recording of time-varying signals, including the acoustic signal, air flow and (via rubber pressure-sensitive bulbs in the mouth) tongue movements (for detailed descriptions of a number of such devices, see Scripture 1902). Initially, instruments were introduced into the discipline in order to find objective measurements of what had been more or less taken for granted: individual speech events. As soon as technical means had been adopted for investigating spoken language, however, the premonitions just mentioned were confirmed and attempts to impose strict linguistic boundaries on articulatory events or the speech signal proved problematic.

Rousselot (1897–1901) was the first who made use of the newly available apparatus for the study of speech. On the one hand, Rousselot still shared the opinion that the obtained speech curves could, and should, be divided into separate sounds. As Tillmann (1994) points out, this assumption led in some instances to a rather questionable methodology. In most recording sessions, more than one speech curve was recorded, such as tracings of the lips, and the nasal and oral air flow. If segment boundaries could not be clearly located by comparing the different curves it was assumed that, in fact, a 'recording error' had occurred and the kymograms were then replaced. On the other hand, Rousselot clearly recognized that at a given point in time there is a superposition of several influences on the movements of the articulators, stressing that the study of sounds in isolation should be replaced by the study of sounds in context.

Rousselot's vast collection of data is full of various examples of phenomena which were later studied extensively within the coarticulation paradigm of phonetic research. For instance, in his analysis of consonant clusters, he observed that if two consonants are produced by two independent articulators, as in /pla/ or /fla/, they are prepared together and the movements uttering them may be simultaneous – a notion confirmed by Stetson (1951). In a related sense, he reported that in some CV sequences the tongue might take the appropriate position for the vowel at the beginning of the preceding consonant. Traces of the lips and the tongue during /ba/ and /bi/ or /za/ and /zi/ productions showed that the tongue lies much higher during the articulation of the consonant when preceding the vowel /i/ than when preceding /a/. On the basis of such evidence Menzerath and de Lacerda (1933) formulated their principle of 'Koartikulation' some 30 years later. Furthermore, Rousselot (1897–1901: 947) pointed out that the lip rounding for the vowel /u/ in a VCV sequence may already start during the first vowel, noting that 'the second of two vowels is the most influential one, as can be seen in *a tu* in the utterance *il a tourné*. At the middle of the *a* the lips start to raise due to the requirements for the production of the *u*'.[3]

Scripture (1902) gives a broad and systematic survey of the experimental research carried out around the turn of the century. In many instances results like the ones outlined above are described, i.e. observations of parallel articulatory activity and modifications of one sound by another. The most noteworthy result for the concept of coarticulation comes from a study by Lacotte (in Scripture 1902: 372; for a history of early investigations in lingual coarticulation, see Hardcastle 1981). Lacotte found that a vowel may influence not only the preceding consonant but also the vowel before the consonant. Records of /eli/ and /ela/ or /ebi/ and /eba/ showed that the articulatory setting for /e/ was different according to the second vowel in the sequence. The tongue rose higher and nearer to the /i/ in /eli/ or /ebi/ than in tokens in which the last sound constituted an /a/. Essentially, this anticipates the form of vowel-to-vowel coarticulation which was postulated by Öhman (1966) and which became influential in the development of some coarticulation theories.

On the basis of this and other studies presented in his book, Scripture (1902) presumed that the character of any movement depends on other movements occurring at the same time and that in speech there are hardly any static postures of the articulators. 'The tongue is never still and never occupies exactly the same position for any period of time' (p. 325). Thus, for the first time the understanding of speech as a sequence of single elements linked by fast transitions was rejected. 'Speech cannot be considered as made up of separate elements placed side by side like letters. In the flow of speech it is just as arbitrary a matter to consider certain portions to be separate sounds as to mark off by a line where a hill begins and a plain ends' (p. 446). On the same grounds, Scripture rejected the division of speech into any higher units, such as the syllable, which would correspond to divisions of a landscape into hill-blocks and valley-blocks.

Thus, although early experimental phoneticians did not have any coherent concept of coarticulation, they were well aware of its existence. The use of the terminology in the field, however, was still rather vague. The terms 'assimilation' and/or 'adaptation' have been loosely applied to all sorts of phenomena, ranging from the treatment of historical sound changes to the articulatory mechanisms described previously.

Jones (1932) introduced a distinction between 'similitude' and 'assimilation', depending on whether two sounds influence each other in such a way that they become more alike but do not change their phonemic identity (similitude – as for instance when the normally voiced /l/ phoneme of English is partially devoiced in [pl̥iːz] 'please'), or whether they influence each other in such a way that one is replaced by another phoneme (assimilation – as when /s/ changes to /ʃ/ in 'horse-shoe'). Jones' concept of similitude therefore covers only some cases which previously had been subsumed under the notion of assimilation, but does include the major part of what was later studied under the heading of coarticulation. The formulation of similitude was, though, still rather static in nature, and seems not far removed from Wickelgren's theory of context-sensitive allophones (1969; see later) which implies that numerous fixed variants of a phoneme are available to the speaker for use when required by the context. The distinction between similitude and assimilation is also reminiscent of Keating's (1990b) distinction between phonological and phonetic coarticulation.

The term 'coarticulation' as such, and perhaps the most explicit rejection of the old view of positional sounds, was put forward by Menzerath and de Lacerda (1933). By means of kymograms including air flow measurements they investigated the production of a series of German labial consonant and vowel sequences. Failing to find stable articulatory positions, Menzerath and de Lacerda proposed that articulation is governed by two major principles, 'Koartikulation' and 'Steuerung'.

'Koartikulation' (or 'Synkinese') indicates that articulators already prepare for following sounds during the production of a preceding segment. Moreover, as proposed afterwards, it was hypothesized that this preparatory activity begins as early as possible. The evidence for the concept of coarticulation was primarily based upon the observation that the articulatory movements for the vowel in tokens such as /ma/ or /pu/ began at the same time as the movements for the initial consonant. Thus, although 'Koartikulation' was postulated as a general organisational principle of articulatory control, its experimental validation was, strictly speaking, restricted to anticipatory labial interactions between consonants and vowels in syllable-initial position.

'Steuerung' (steering, control), on the other hand, is somewhat more difficult to apply to today's understanding of coarticulation. The process was essentially limited to immediately adjacent sounds which involve the same articulator. For instance, the lip movements of vowel articulations were said to be completely controlled ('gesteuert') by the following consonant in syllables such as /am/ or /ap/. The final consonant indicates the direction of the articulatory movement during the vocalic portion. The point in time in which the 'Steuerung' starts was supposed to be dependent upon other sounds which, in turn, precede the vowel during longer utterances. In a more general sense, then, 'Steuerung' seems to apply to the deviation of an articulator in its articulatory target in one sound due to the presence of a different target in another sound.

Thus, for Menzerath and de Lacerda the structure of any utterance is a complex interweaving of simultaneous movements, i.e. 'all articulation is coarticulation'. Somewhat paradoxically, however, they surmised that the complicated combination of articulatory action exists for the sole purpose of producing speech sounds which are acoustically (and perceptually) distinct units. The articulation associated with certain sounds is not separable,[4] but the sounds themselves are.[5] In other words, the problem of segmentation was pushed from one level of speech to another (see Tillmann and Mansell 1980 for discussion).

In the same way as Menzerath and de Lacerda can be regarded as having introduced the concept of coarticulation in phonetic research, Stetson's (1951) approach to the investigation of speech can be regarded as laying the theoretical basis for the redefined notion of coproduction (see later). He was the first to apply methods and concepts from the study of skilled movement to the analysis of speech production, in work which later gained new significance in the context of Action Theory (Fowler *et al.* 1980) and, relatedly, Articulatory Phonology (Browman and Goldstein 1986, 1989) and Task Dynamics (Saltzman and Munhall 1989).

Stetson argued that it is the coordination of the articulatory movements involved in speech production which is of major importance, and this coordination is best studied by looking at different phonetic modifications, specifically those caused by changes of rate and of stress. On these grounds, he defined an allophone, rather unusually, as the variation 'of the phoneme pattern due to rate versus stress' (p. 193). More generally, and prefiguring the concept of coproduction, he stated, 'all generalizations on the reciprocal influence of sounds, like assimilation or prevision or law of economy, must finally be referred to the skilled movements involved' (p.122).

Considering the syllable to be the fundamental unit of speech production, Stetson investigated the coordination of speech sounds primarily with respect to their function within syllable groups. A particular concern was the role and interaction of syllable final ('arresting') and syllable initial ('releasing') consonants. His data showed that if a syllable is constantly repeated with a gradually increasing speaking rate, such as /tas tas tas/, its structure will change abruptly at one moment in time, i.e. resulting in /sta sta sta/. Similar jumps in syllable composition were later taken to be a major source of evidence for the existence of coordinative structures in speech (cf. Kelso *et al.* 1986).

Moreover, Stetson observed that articulatory movements can be present although acoustically they might be covered completely. For example, in slow productions of the nonsense syllable /ispda/ the three intervocalic consonants were kept distinct, articulatorily as well as acoustically. However, in fast productions of the same syllable the two tongue tip movements merged into one, and the lip movement for /p/, although still clearly visible in the kymogram, was overlapped in time by the integrated tongue tip movement for the alveolars, and according to Stetson there was no closure phase for the bilabial evident in the acoustic signal. The manifestation of hidden gestures of this kind was to be of central importance in Browman and Goldstein's Articulatory Phonology (1990d), in particular for the discussion about the relationship between coarticulation/coproduction and casual assimilations.

The coarticulatory research paradigm: models and experiments

Since the late 1960s the experimental investigation of coarticulation has developed into a major area of research. With the detailed investigation of coarticulatory effects it became apparent that the influential interval of a speech sound varies considerably, potentially extending quite far. In particular, studies of anticipatory labial coarticulation demonstrated that the articulatory rounding gesture, associated with the vowel /u/, is initiated up to as many as four to six segments before the actual target vowel, regardless of syllable or word boundaries (Benguerel and Cowan 1974; Sussman and Westbury 1981). Coarticulation, therefore, appeared to be more than the pure consequence of physiological limitations and inertial effects of the speech organs, as had been proposed in some previous accounts.[6]

For example, the first version of Lindblom's target undershoot model (1963a) posited that a string of phonetic segments is realized by a string of commands which in running speech are issued at very short temporal intervals. As the articulators are restricted in the speed with which they can move from one articulatory target to the other, they may not always complete a given response before the command for the next articulatory configuration arrives. In other words, the articulators fail to reach ('undershoot') their targets and respond to more than one input signal simultaneously.

This approach, though, cannot fully account for more extended temporal influences. Much of the phenomenon of coarticulation, therefore, has been regarded as a more active process which occurs at some higher level. For that reason, the key attraction of coarticulation research lay in the hope that by revealing the systematic coarticulatory patterns it would be possible to discover the (universal) underlying units of the speech production process as well as the mechanisms linking them and, in this way, to clarify the mismatch between mental and physical events. Almost every articulatory subsystem was investigated in a variety of studies using a number of different techniques. However, given the large amount of variation observed, it was difficult to impose an unambiguous pattern, and an increasing number of models were developed.

This section will summarize some of the major models but the following is neither a complete survey nor a thoroughgoing critique. Critical reviews of models of coarticulation are available in Kent and Minifie (1977), Sharf and Ohde (1981, who include an excellent comparison between data and models available prior to 1981), Fowler (1980, 1985), Kent (1983) and Farnetani (1990). Detailed experimental results referring to the different articulatory sub-systems can be found in the following chapters, and the most recent theories are discussed in more detail in chapter two.

The publication which most clearly heralded the growing interest in coarticulation was that of Kozhevnikov and Chistovich (1965), whose major concern was the development of a general model of articulatory timing. The largest unit of speech production was assumed to be the syntagma and, within the syntagma, the basic articulatory input unit was assumed to be the articulatory syllable, which consisted of a vowel and any number of consecutive consonants that preceded it.

The concept of the articulatory syllable was derived from recordings of lip movements in Russian speakers which revealed that the lip protrusion for the vowel /u/ began simultaneously with the first consonant when either one or two consonants preceded the vowel. The same result emerged when a conventional syllable or word boundary fell between the two consonants. Thus, the temporal extent of anticipatory coarticulation was taken as an indication of the size of the articulatory syllable. Provided that the consonants did not involve contradictory movements, all the articulatory actions connected with one articulatory syllable were supposed to start at its beginning. As a corollary, this view implies that, when possible, a vowel is initiated as soon as a preceding vowel is terminated.

Subsequent studies showed, as in fact Rousselot had shown before them, that coarticulatory effects occur not only within such restricted forms. In his classic spectrographic study on Swedish, Öhman (1966) showed that two vowels interact with each other across intervening stops. Vowel-to-vowel coarticulation has since been reported in both acoustic (Fowler 1981b, Recasens 1989) and articulatory studies (Carney and Moll 1971; Kent and Moll 1972b; Kiritani *et al.* 1977).

Öhman developed a VCV model of coarticulation which shares with Kozhevnikov and Chistovich (1965) the assumption that vowels play some special role in the speech production process. In Öhman's account, the vowel and consonant articulations are considered to be largely independent of each other at the level of neural instructions. Vowels are produced by relatively slow diphthongal movements of the tongue body on which the articulatory gestures for the consonants are superimposed. Vowels therefore coarticulate with each other across the medial consonant(s), while consonant–vowel effects depend on the degree of tongue involvement in the production of the consonant(s) (but see Gay 1977 for some complicating evidence). The idea that vowels and consonants have several quite distinct properties was adapted by Perkell (1969) and, later, implemented in a larger theoretical framework by Fowler (1980, 1981b).

Wickelgren (1969, 1972) put forward an alternative theory which moved coarticulation away from the speech apparatus up to a more central level of speech motor control. According to this account, language users do not have a set of phoneme-like segments as the immediate phonetic constituents of words, but an inventory of context-sensitive allophones. These stored allophones are understood to be versions of segments which are specifically defined according to the potential left and right context in which they are able to occur, i.e. '. . . each allophone is essentially an ordered triple of immediately adjacent phonemes in the phonemic spelling of the word' (1972: 239). For the string 'pin', for example, the context-sensitive elements would be: $_\#p_i$, $_pi_n$, $_in_\#$ (# indicates a word boundary).

Crucially, however, the theory has difficulty with coarticulatory influences that extend beyond adjacent sounds, and with effects caused by prosodic properties. Although it might be possible to cope with such problems in part by specifying all additional contexts in which a phoneme could undergo changes, this procedure would increase the number of allophones exponentially. Most criticisms of Wickelgren's theory, therefore, revolved around the high number of elements that would need to be stored (MacNeilage 1970; Halwes and Jenkins 1971; Kent 1983). The approach also misses generalizations, such as the nasalization of all English vowels preceding a nasal consonant (Kent and Minifie 1977), and at the same time is too rich in information (Fowler 1985). In the present example it is just the nasality which is shared by the vowel but not, for instance, the place of articulation. Even more problematically, different sounds are influenced by different properties of their neighbours; oral consonants preceding a nasal do not become nasalized. Wickelgren's allophone lists conflict with fundamental assumptions about the speech production process, namely that the integration of segments is rule-governed and productive. In a sense, the classical conception of coarticulation disappears in Wickelgren's approach.

Another view which focuses on segment-specific properties is Bladon and Al-Bamerni's (1976) concept of 'coarticulation resistance' (CR). Their spectrographic investigation of the extrinsic allophones of /l/ in British received pronunciation showed that the influence of adjacent vowels on F2, and the influence of adjacent voiceless plosives on the amount of voicelessness in the laterals, decreased from clear [l] to dark [ɫ] to dark syllabic [ɫ̩].

They hypothesized that each extrinsic allophone is stored with a different numerical value of CR to which the speech production mechanism has access. Anticipatory and carryover coarticulation is allowed to spread freely until it is inhibited by a high CR specification on some segment. The CR value was supposed to be determined by a variety of factors – universal, language-specific, context-sensitive, and, possibly, speaker-specific.

Further research indeed suggested that coarticulation phenomena seem to be sensitive to all these factors. However, to trace them back to a different underlying CR value might not constitute a very compelling phonetic explanation, as Kent and Minifie (1977) remark: 'CR values seem to be little more than summary numbers that represent the contributions of many unknown, or poorly known, effects. The CR values do not themselves generate predictions' (p. 120). Moreover, it is also not clear whether a single CR value suffices to describe the overall behaviour of a segment. For example, in the utterance 'feel things', the tongue body configuration of [ɬ] would presumably be resistant to adjacent coarticulatory forces (see above), but the tip would be free to adopt the following dental place of articulation. Perhaps a segment would end up needing a CR value for each phonetic dimension (see Nolan 1983).

'Coarticulation resistance' is therefore now used in a more general sense to refer to the widespread observation that coarticulation is gradual and varies between segments. For example, Bladon and Nolan (1977) reported from a video-fluorographic study of English alveolars that the tongue tip position increased in variability in the order /t,d,n,l/ when the sounds occurred next to /s/ or /z/, while the fricatives themselves were not affected. This overall pattern of contextual sensitivity appears to be a rather robust effect since it has been documented in other languages, such as Italian (Farnetani 1990), Swedish (Engstrand 1989) and German (Kühnert *et al.* 1991). A completely satisfactory account of the order of alveolar variation, however, is yet to be elaborated. One plausible suggestion adduces acoustic distinctiveness, i.e. /l/ and /n/ can be produced with more variability without losing essential acoustic properties, but this hypothesis has never been strictly tested (see Hoole 1993a).

Recasens' articulatory model of lingual coarticulation (1984b, 1987, 1989), which is related to Öhman's model (1966), connects the notion of coarticulatory resistance with a sound's degree of tongue dorsum elevation. On the basis of electropalatographic and acoustic studies of Catalan and Spanish VCV and VCVCV sequences, Recasens posits that the temporal extent and the strength of vowel-to-vowel coarticulation varies inversely with the degree of tongue dorsum raising required for the intervening consonants, i.e. the larger the contact between the tongue and the palate, the less the coarticulatory modifications. The production of the alveolo-palatal nasal /ɲ/, for example, was shown to reduce vowel interactions more than a medial alveolar /n/ (Recasens 1984b).

The approach further suggests that sounds which block coarticulation are the least affected by other sounds while, at the same time, affecting other sounds the most (see Farnetani 1990). For instance, Kiritani and Sawashima (1987) reported from an X-ray microbeam study that the influence of the second vowel appears later in the first vowel of a VCV token when that is a high front /i/ than when it is an /a/. Additionally, /i/ left more prominent traces on the medial consonant than /a/. Similar coarticulatory hierarchies between vowels were observed by Butcher and Weiher (1976) and Hoole, Gfroerer and Tillmann (1990) for German (but note Farnetani, Vagges and Magno-Caldognetto 1985 for some ambiguous evidence).

A different line of thought with a long history refers to distinctive features (e.g. Jakobson, Fant and Halle 1952). Feature-based models (Moll and Daniloff 1971; Daniloff and Hammarberg 1973; Benguerel and Cowan 1974)[7] were initiated by the articulatory computer model developed by Henke (1966). This model starts with a segmental input in which each segment is connected to a set of phonetic features which, in turn, are transferred together to some articulatory (phonemic) goal. Only contrasting properties are specified at the level of phonological input and irrelevant value entries are left empty. For example, in English, in which nasalization is not contrastive for vowels, no vowel is assumed to have a specification for the feature [+/− nasal]. A forward-looking device below the phonological component is then assumed to scan the features of future segments and to copy them onto more immediate segments as long as their goals are not incompatible. Thus, 'forward effects are due entirely to a higher level look ahead or anticipation' (Henke 1966: 47).

Support for the feature-spreading account came primarily from studies showing that anticipatory labial coarticulation started as early as the first consonant preceding a rounded vowel (see Benguerel and Cowan 1974, for partial evidence, Lubker 1981), and showing that velopharyngeal opening was anticipated in a string of vowels before a nasal consonant (Moll and Daniloff 1971). However, the same sub-systems were soon cited as yielding counter-evidence, leading to an ongoing discussion about apparently conflicting results (Gay 1978a; Bell-Berti and Harris 1979, 1981, 1982; Lubker 1981; Sussmann and Westbury 1981; Lubker and Gay 1982, among others).

One controversy concerned the occurrence of 'troughs'. For instance, labial movement or EMG (electromyography) recordings of sequences such as /usu/ show a diminution of rounding during the consonant (Gay 1978a; Engstrand

1981; Perkell 1986). Such data are a problem for 'look-ahead' models since there is no reason to assume a rounding specification for a non-labial consonant and hence the rounding should spread over an entire non-labial string. Explanations for 'troughs' varied considerably. While Gay (1978a) interpreted his results to be in agreement with a syllable-sized production unit, Kozhevnikov and Chistovich (1965) and Engstrand (1981) suggested that acoustic and/or aerodynamic constraints on the intervocalic consonants contribute to troughs. In particular a rounding gesture might interfere with the optimal acoustic conditions for /s/, and therefore the lips exhibit some active retraction. Perkell's (1986) data pointed to a complex of factors which may underlie the reduction of rounding and were only partially consistent with Engstrand's proposals, indicating that its relative importance may vary for different subjects and different languages.

Perkell's study also suggested that alveolar consonants, previously assumed to be neutral with respect to lip rounding, may in fact have their own specific protrusion gesture. More explicit evidence came from an EMG and optoelectrical investigation by Gelfer, Bell-Berti and Harris (1989) who examined the inherent lip activity for /s/ and /t/. Even in /isi/ and /iti/ some consonant related lip rounding could be registered. As Gelfer *et al.* point out, some of the (apparently) conflicting results concerning labial coarticulation might stem from disregarding such subtle alveolar properties (see Bell-Berti and Krakow 1991 for similar arguments concerning vowel production and velum height). Importantly, such results illustrate that any feature-spreading account depends on the *a priori* assumptions made about the feature specifications. Moreover the absence of a feature specification for a sound at an abstract level cannot be taken to imply that the relevant articulator is wholly neutral in the production of the sound. This makes the experimental investigation of coarticulatory effects a delicate matter. (Other general points of discussion of early feature-coding models have been discussed in Kent and Minifie 1977; Sharf and Ohde 1981 or Fowler 1980, 1985.)

Recently, Keating (1988a, 1990b) has proposed a refined approach to coarticulation which preserves the conception of a segmental feature input. For Keating, coarticulation can either be phonological or phonetic in character. Coarticulation at the phonological level is caused by rules of feature spreading along the lines discussed in recent developments in nonlinear phonology (Goldsmith 1990). Phonological assimilation should result in static effects, where successive segments share a certain attribute fully.

On the other hand, phonetic coarticulation effects are typically more gradual in time and space and may affect portions of segments to varying degrees. Keating proposes that phonetic realization involves a conversion of features or feature combinations into spatio-temporal targets. These targets, however, are not understood as fixed configurations (as in the early formulation of an invariant articulatory target model by MacNeilage 1970). Rather, for a given articulatory or acoustic dimension every feature of a segment is associated with a range of values, called a 'window', which represents its overall contextual variability. The wider the window, the greater the permitted coarticulatory variation. Phonetic coarticulation is the result of finding the most efficient pathway through the windows of successive segments. In fact the window model of coarticulation is reminiscent of the original concept of coarticulation resistance (Bladon and Al-Bamerni 1976, and above), and of Nolan's (1983: 119–20) quantitative formalization of it, in which the notional 'costs' of alternative transitions between segments are calculated on the basis of their CR values. A window is more or less the spatial expression of the degree of coarticulatory resistance of a particular phonetic dimension.

Keating's model, especially the details of phonetic implementation patterns, still has to be evaluated in many respects, but, in principle, her concept can handle many coarticulation data more adequately than early feature-spreading approaches which were not able to account for any finer, intersegmental variations of articulatory accommodation. For example, in Keating's account individual English vowels are associated with different windows for velum height, which are relatively wide, but not as wide as possible since the velum is not allowed to lower maximally. In contrast, nasal and oral consonants, which possess either low or high velum positions, are associated with narrow windows. The contours through assumed windows of this kind, then, are compatible with the observation that the velum rises slightly for a vowel between two nasals (Kent, Carney and Severeid 1974), and similar assumptions about the allowed range of lip protrusion of vowels and alveolar consonants could account for the occurrence of troughs in /usu/ or /utu/ tokens.

Like its predecessors, however, Keating's account still embodies the fundamental assumption that there exists some process in which abstract (i.e. non-physical, discrete and timeless) units are converted into the complex, continuous and time-bound realizations evident in the speech event (see Fowler 1990, 1992; Boyce, Krakow and Bell-Berti 1991a). This disparity between phonological descriptions and actual utterances, and hence the notion of coarticulation, is challenged by proponents of 'coproduction' theories (Fowler 1980, 1992; Fowler *et al.* 1980; Bell-Berti and Harris 1981, 1982; Kelso, Saltzman and Tuller 1986; Browman and Goldstein 1986, 1989; Saltzman and Munhall 1989; Fowler and Saltzman 1993). There has been a long debate in the literature which focused on the philosophical differences between what have been called 'translation' or 'extrinsic timing' theories, and 'intrinsic timing' or 'coproduction' theories, and the arguments will not be repeated here (see Hammarberg 1976, 1982; Fowler 1980, 1983b, Fowler *et al.* 1980; Nolan 1982; Parker and Walsh 1985, among others).

Broadly speaking, in coproduction accounts the hypothesis of underlying invariance and the reality of surface variability are reconciled by redefining the primitives of the speech production process as dynamically specified units. Based on the concept of coordinative structures (see Fowler *et al.* 1980; Kelso, Saltzman and Tuller 1986) these underlying units are supposed to be functionally defined control structures, called 'gestures', which represent and generate particular speech-relevant goals and implicitly contain information on articulatory movement in space over time. Such gestures are, for example, the formation of a bilabial closure, or an alveolar near-closing gesture which permits frication for the production of alveolar fricatives. In the case of labial closure, for instance, the jaw, upper lip and lower lip movements are constrained by the coordinative structure to achieve closure regardless of the phonetic context. Crucially this view suggests that, during speech production, a gesture does not change in its essential properties, but rather that it is its temporal overlap with other gestures which results in the variability observable in the vocal tract activity associated with that gesture. Thus coproduction implies that at a given point in time the influences of gestures associated with several adjacent or near-adjacent segments show their traces in the articulatory and acoustic continua. For instance, in a bilabial consonant and vowel sequence the formation of the closure will be influenced by the demands of the following vowel since both gestures share the jaw as an articulating component (for details of the transformation and the blending procedures of abstract gestural primitives into vocal tract actions, see Saltzman and Munhall 1989 and Fowler and Saltzman 1993). In this framework, therefore, coarticulation is rather straightforwardly the consequence of the inherent kinematic properties of the production mechanism and is considered to be merely a general cooperative process of movement coordination.

Besides the conflicting results which were reported in the literature (see references above) a major point of criticism raised against coproduction models is that they lean too heavily on the inherent kinematic properties of the production process, thus neglecting the importance of acoustic salience and perceptual distinctiveness. Lindblom (1990), for example, stresses that speech production is always a 'tug-of-war' between production-oriented factors on the one hand and output-oriented constraints on the other. Production constraints reflect the motor system's tendency towards 'low-cost' behaviour, and output constraints reflect the speaker's response to the requirements of the communicative situation. In addition, doubts have been raised over the role of coordinative structures in speech production, and the assumption that the input to the physical speech mechanism is a contrastive phonological representation (see, for example, the discussions in Nolan 1982; Kent 1983, 1986; Shaffer 1984). Along these lines, Holst and Nolan (1995) and Nolan, Holst and Kühnert (1996) have claimed to show that although coproduction is capable of accounting for many of the observed forms when [s] accommodates to a following [ʃ], there are some forms which can only be accounted for if a process of phonological assimilation has taken place in the representation that is input to the speech mechanism. This view, in its separation of a more phonological and a more phonetic source of observed coarticulatory effects, is similar to the ideas of Keating discussed above.

Consistent with the coproduction view is Bell-Berti and Harris' (1979, 1981, 1982) time-locked or frame model of coarticulation. The model asserts that the component gestures of a phonetic segment begin at relatively time-invariant intervals before the phonetic target itself is achieved. Anticipatory coarticulation is therefore temporally limited and does not extend very far backward in time before the gesture becomes acoustically dominant. Thus, in contrast to feature-spreading approaches, the length of the preceding string of phones and their conflicting or non-conflicting featural specifications are irrelevant (apart from some cases in which an intervocalic consonant duration is very short). The findings in favour of this concept were again primarily derived from investigation of anticipatory labial and velar coarticulation which either showed that the EMG activity of the orbicularis oris associated with lip rounding was initiated at a fixed interval before the onset of a rounded vowel (Bell-Berti and Harris 1979, 1982), or that the lowering of the velum started invariantly relative to the onset of nasal murmur in a nasal consonant production (Bell-Berti and Harris 1981).

The 'hybrid model' of coarticulation, which was put forward by Perkell and Chiang (1986) using their data on lip rounding and some preliminary observations on the temporal patterning of velum lowering by Bladon and Al-Bamerni (1982), constitutes a compromise between the assumptions made by the featural look-ahead mechanism and the time-locked theory. According to this model, the anticipation of a gesture is characterized by two components. For example, in the case of anticipatory lip rounding in English there is first an initial slow phase of rounding which starts as soon as possible, specifically at the acoustic offset of a preceding unrounded vowel. Secondly, there is a more prominent rapid phase (identified by an acceleration maximum in the rounding gesture) which is supposed to be time-locked to the acoustic onset of the rounded vowel. Thus, as the intervocalic consonant string increases, the duration of the first phase increases with it while the duration of the second phase remains constant.

However, in a more recent investigation of the timing of upper lip protrusion Perkell and Matthies (1992) concluded, following the work outlined above by Gelfer, Bell-Berti and Harris (1989), that at least some protrusion effects are probably consonant-specific, and, therefore, qualified some of the original evidence which was taken as support for the hybrid model. The outcome of the study nevertheless did not support a purely time-locked coarticulation pattern, but rather suggested that coarticulatory strategies are based on competing constraints which are both kinematic and acoustic in nature, and that the balance between the constraints may vary from speaker to speaker. This raises a more general question: how does variation in coarticulation between speakers arise?

Acquisition and variation

In recent years attention has increasingly been paid to children's acquisition of coarticulatory behaviour. It is thus now possible to say something about the ontogenetic origin of coarticulation in individuals, although a far from clear general picture emerges. It may be that coarticulatory strategies are essentially idiosyncratic, with each individual free to develop a personal solution to the integration of successive segments. These alternative solutions would be expected to persist into adulthood, and evidence of coarticulatory variation in adults is briefly reviewed later in this section.

It is clear from a number of acoustic investigations (e.g. Kent and Forner 1980) and articulatory measurements (e.g. Sharkey and Folkins 1985) that children are much more variable in their phonetic patterns than adults. With respect to the effect of coarticulation on the variability in children's utterances two differing positions can be broadly distinguished. One account holds that children show the tendency to produce speech rather more segmentally than adults (Kent 1983; Katz, Kripke and Tallal 1991). This is thought to reflect an acquisition process in which the motor skill of temporal sound sequencing is acquired first, while the finer details of the temporal coordination of the articulators develop later. As a corollary, coarticulation is likely to be less prominent for young children. In contrast, an alternative approach to speech development suggests that children's productions might be characterized by more, rather than less, coarticulation (Nittrouer and Whalen 1989; Nittrouer, Studdert-Kennedy and McGowan 1989). By this view, which is consistent with the gestural approach of Browman and Goldstein (1986), children are assumed to rely to a larger extent on syllable-based speech production units and only gradually to narrow their minimal domain of articulatory organization. Thus, the spatio-temporal overlap of gestures is more prominent at early ages and diminishes through a process of differentiation.

Studies investigating the extent and degree of coarticulation in child productions have thus far yielded inconsistent results which appear to depend crucially upon the articulatory sub-system under consideration. The most divided picture arises with respect to anticipatory lingual coarticulation. For example, Nittrouer, Studdert-Kennedy and McGowan (1989) presented evidence from a fricative study with eight adults and eight children at each of the ages three, four, five and seven years that young children organize their speech over a wider temporal domain. F2 estimates and centroid frequency values showed a gradual, age-related decline of the influence of the vowels /i/ and /u/ on the preceding /s/ or /ʃ/. In an attempt to replicate this outcome with ten adults and ten three-, five- and eight-year olds, however, no age-dependent differences could be detected by Katz, Kripke and Tallal (1991). On the other hand greater coarticulation for adults was observed by Kent (1983), who looked at the influence of a following consonant on a preceding vowel. Finally, Serano and Lieberman (1987), looking at the influence on a velar stop by a subsequent vowel in /ki/ and /ka/ syllables of five adults and fourteen children between the ages of three and seven, found consistent coarticulatory effects for adults in the form of different predominant spectral peaks in the consonant. However, their measurements varied greatly between individual children, with some of them displaying adult-like patterns while others did not show any traces of lingual coarticulation. Significantly, the differences among the child speakers did not correlate with age.

More agreement can be found in the literature with regard to anticipatory lip rounding before /u/. The studies by Nittrouer, Studdert-Kennedy and McGowan (1989) and Katz, Kripke and Tallal (1991), as well as an investigation by Serano *et al.* (1987), all indicate that labial coarticulation in the speech of English children is roughly similar to that of adult subjects (but see Repp 1986b). Conversely, for Swedish, which has a more complex lip rounding contrast than English, Abelin, Landberg and Persson (1980) reported that adults adopt a look-ahead strategy while the children's labial coarticulation appeared to be time-locked, i.e. the temporal extent of anticipation became more prominent with age. This difference between the languages is compatible with the more general observation that labial coarticulation is highly influenced by language-specific factors (Lubker and Gay 1982). Thus, in Swedish, in which labial anticipation is constrained by several linguistic and, hence, perceptual factors, the details of possible coarticulation are refined during maturation, while this is not necessary for English.

However, studies of nasal coarticulation using English subjects, which in terms of its linguistic contrast and in terms of being a rather 'sluggish' articulation behaves in a similar way to labial coarticulation, again showed outcomes which are at variance with each other. Thompson and Hixon's (1979) nasal airflow measurements at the mid-point of the first vowel in /ini/ showed a greater proportion of anticipatory nasalisation with increasing age. Flege (1988), comparing the time of velopharyngeal opening and closing during the vowel in /dVn/ and /nVd/ sequences of adults and children aged five and ten years, observed that both groups of speakers nasalized most vowels with no difference in the extent and degree of nasalization.

In view of the results, it becomes obvious that it is premature to derive any general statements about the acquisitional process of coarticulation. The results testify to a general point which is best summarized in Repp's (1986b) words. 'The various patterns of results . . . suggest that phenomena commonly lumped together under the heading of 'coarticulation' may have diverse origins and hence different roles in speech development. Some forms of coarticulation are an indication of advanced speech production skills, whereas others may be a sign of articulatory immaturity, and yet others are neither because they simply cannot be avoided. Therefore, it is probably not wise to draw conclusions about a general process called coarticulation from the study of a single effect. Indeed, such a general process may not exist' (p. 1634).

Speaker-specific behaviour can not only be observed during the process of speech acquisition, but to a certain extent also in the coarticulation strategies of adult speakers. Nolan (1983, 1985) argues for the view that coarticulatory strategies are potentially idiosyncratic, and presents between-speaker variation in the coarticulation of English /l/ and /r/ with following vowels.

Lubker and Gay (1982) examined upper lip movement and EMG activity of four labial muscles in speakers of Swedish and American English. In addition to language-specific differences, they observed different coarticulatory effects for speakers within one language. Among the five Swedish subjects, three seemed to use a look-ahead mechanism, i.e. they adjusted the onset of labial movement to the time available. In contrast, the onset of lip rounding for the other speakers remained essentially constant prior to the acoustic vowel onset and, hence, their behaviour is in accord with the frame model.

Perkell and Matthies (1992) examined upper lip movements using a strain-gauge cantilever system, and included minimal pairs to control for the possibility (mentioned above) of consonant-inherent protrusion effects. The subjects in this investigation were carefully preselected; only speakers without pronounced regional dialect were chosen who primarily used lip protrusion, as opposed to lip closure, in uttering words containing the vowel /u/. Nevertheless, 'there was a lot of variation in the shape and timing of /u/ protrusion trajectories: on a token-to-token basis within each utterance, between utterances, and across subjects' (1992: 2917). The overall outcome of the study did not support, as with most studies, the predictions of any model in a straightforward way. Rather, the authors suggested that the initiation of anticipatory lip rounding is determined by three competing constraints, reflecting elements of both the dynamic properties of coproduction and the perceptually motivated requirements of feature-spreading models. Broadly speaking, the three constraints were (i) end the protrusion movement during the voiced part of /u/, (ii) use a preferred gesture duration, and (iii) begin the protrusion movement when permitted. Thus, variations in the degrees to which the constraints were expressed accounted for differences between the subjects (and, in addition, for inter-individual variations).

These and other studies indicate that speakers seem indeed to have some freedom in coarticulatory behaviour which is beyond that attributable to anatomical differences. Thus far, however, individual differences have been little investigated, and have rarely been taken into account in the formulation of theories. On the one hand, due to methodological limitations the use of a large number of subjects is still rare in most speech production experiments. Thus, truly quantitative statements about coarticulatory effects are yet difficult to derive. A statistical case study by Forrest, Weismer and Adams (1990) shows clearly that care has to be taken in generalizing results from a small number of speakers.

On the other hand, the high variability found in the data makes it difficult to differentiate between effects which should be considered as being idiosyncratic and effects which simply reflect the allowed range of variation for the phenomenon. For example, while, from a classical point of view, the outcome of Lubker and Gay's study (1982) could be considered as representing two fundamentally different organizational strategies for integrating segments, the refined experiment by Perkell and Matthies (1992) rather suggests that the various forces are present at any moment in time for any speaker. That is, they are an integral part of producing and coarticulating segments and speakers only vary in the emphasis they put on the different forces or even fluctuate between them.

It may be hoped that further attention to the development of coarticulation in children, and to the variation exhibited by mature speakers, will contribute to a better overall understanding of the process of speech production.

Conclusion

This chapter has considered three senses of the 'origin' of coarticulation: the reason it exists in speech; its history as a scientific construct; and its ontogenetic development in language acquisition. It was noted in the first section of this chapter that coarticulation presupposes the existence at some level of discrete phonological units. Most obviously, the phenomena described as coarticulation are the result of the integration of those units in the continuously flowing activity of the vocal mechanism, which is ill-suited to abrupt changes of configuration. But, additionally, it is quite possible that coarticulation is favoured for perceptual reasons: putting it crudely, the longer a phonetic property persists, the more chance it has of being spotted.

Historically, the advent of instrumental techniques in the nineteenth century led to a crisis in the conceptualization of speech. No longer was it tenable to visualize speech as the concatenation of 'letters', because physical records stubbornly resisted attempts at strict segmentation. Gradually, from perspectives as diverse as phonology, acoustics and the study of skilled motor activity, the foundations were laid for the concept of coarticulation. At first, coarticulation was mainly an attempt to come to terms with recalcitrant instrumental data which failed to confirm researchers' preconceptions about the nature of speech, but subsequently it became recognized as a phenomenon central to the study of speech production, and in particular from the 1960s onwards became the catalyst for an impressive variety of experiments and theorizing in speech motor control. Throughout, there has been a productive tension between approaches which were more dynamically or more phonologically oriented. In some of the most influential recent work, for instance in 'Articulatory Phonology', the phenomenon of coarticulation has led to a re-evaluation of such distinctions, and to the attempt to use inherently dynamic units as phonological primes.

Studies of children have not led to a definitive picture of whether coarticulation is greater, less or basically the same in childhood. It may be that the emergence of clear trends are confounded by inter-individual differences, which would be compatible with the view that each language learner has to work out, within the constraints of his or her individual vocal tract, a solution to the integration of phonetic segments. This view is supported by indications that coarticulatory behaviour is quite variable even between adult speakers of the same language variety.

Coarticulation, then, bears on issues such as the control of the skilled activity of speech production, the relation between phonological systems and their realization, and the borderline between what is shared in the social code of language and what is individual. The systematic study of coarticulation is central to the development of experimental phonetics and speech science.

Notes

1 In this example the influence is mainly of the vowel on the preceding consonant, and we have instances of what has been termed 'anticipatory' or 'right-to-left' or 'backward' coarticulation, as opposed to 'perseverative' or 'left-to-right' or 'forward' or 'carryover' coarticulation (when an earlier segment influences a later one). Both the direction and extent of coarticulatory effects have been regarded as crucial in testing hypotheses about coarticulation, as will emerge later in this chapter.

2 'Eine wirkliche Zerlegung des Wortes in seine Elemente ist nicht bloss sehr schwierig, sie ist geradezu unmöglich. Das Wort ist nicht eine Aneinandersetzung einer bestimmten Anzahl selbständiger Laute, von denen jeder durch ein Zeichen des Alphabetes ausgedrückt werden könnte, sondern es ist im Grunde immer eine kontinuierliche Reihe von unendlich vielen Lauten (. . .)'.

3 'Entre les deux voyelles, la plus influente est la seconde, comme cela se montre très bien pour *a tu* dans *il a tourné*. Dès le milieu de l'*a*, la ligne des lèvres s'élève à la sollicitation de l'*u*.'

4 'Artikulatorisch-konstante Laute gibt es nicht' (Menzerath and de Lacerda 1933: 61).

5 'Die Sprachlaute sind trennbar' (Menzerath and de Lacerda 1933: 60).

6 Mechano-inertial limitations certainly play some role, especially for some part of carryover influences (see Daniloff and Hammarberg 1973 and Fowler 1980 for discussion).

7 Early feature-coding proposals differ somewhat in the details of their implementation and the way they treat carryover coarticulation; however, they all share the main mechanisms which are exemplified in Henke's approach (1966).

2

Coarticulation models in recent speech production theories

EDDA FARNETANI and DANIEL RECASENS

Introduction

A crucial problem of speech production theories is the dichotomy between the representational and the physical aspects of speech. The former is described as a system of abstract, invariant, discrete units (the phonemes), the latter as a complex of variable, continuous, overlapping patterns of articulatory movements resulting in a variable acoustic signal, a mixture of continuous and discrete events (Fant 1968). There is general agreement in the literature that the variability and unsegmentability of the speech signal is due in great part to the universal phenomenon of coarticulation, i.e. the pervasive, systematic, reciprocal influences among contiguous and often non-contiguous speech segments. This explains why coarticulation has a central place in all recent phonetic theories.

The aim of coarticulation theories is to explain coarticulation, i.e. account for its origin, nature and function, while coarticulation models are expected to predict the details of the process bridging the invariant and discrete units of representation to articulation and acoustics. Coarticulation theories are also expected to explain how listeners overcome coarticulatory variability and recover the underlying message.

As for production, the differences among the various theories of coarticulation may concern the *nature* of the underlying units of speech, the *stage* at which coarticulatory variations emerge within the speech production process, *what* is modified by coarticulation and *why*. According to some theories coarticulatory variations occur at the level of the speech plan and thus modify the units of the plan itself, whilst other theories attribute contextual variations to the speech production system so that high level invariance is preserved. But there are divergences in the reasons why the act of speaking introduces coarticulatory variations: are these to be attributed to the inertia of speech organs and/or to the principle of economy or to the way the speech units are temporally organized?

Two aspects of coarticulation, one mainly temporal and the other mainly spatial, appear to be crucial for testing the predictions of the models, hence the validity of the various theories:

(1)   The *temporal domain of coarticulation,* i.e. how far and in which direction coarticulation can extend in time when the coarticulatory movements are free to expand, that is when the articulators engaged in the production of the key segment are not subject to competing demands for the production of adjacent segments;

(2)   the *outcome of gestural conflict,* i.e. what happens when competing articulatory and coarticulatory demands are imposed on the same articulatory structures. Some models predict that coarticulation will be blocked in these cases; according to others, conflict is resolved by allowing coarticulatory changes to different degrees, depending on the different constraints imposed on the competing gestures.

Another fundamental question concerns interlanguage differences in coarticulation. It has been shown that differences across languages in inventory size and/or phoneme distribution, or in the articulatory details of speech sounds transcribed with the same phonemic symbols affect the degree and the temporal extent of coarticulation. The theoretical accounts for interlanguage differences are various: the issue is developed in detail elsewhere in this volume.

Moreover, it is well known that the spatio-temporal extent of coarticulation does not depend only on the articulatory characteristics of the key segment and of its immediate environment. Experimental research continues to uncover a number of factors that affect the degree and/or temporal extent of contextual variability in a significant way. The most relevant are:

(a)   the linguistic suprasegmental structure such as stress (Benguerel and Cowan 1974; Harris 1971; Fowler 1981b, Tuller, Harris and Kelso 1982) and prosodic boundaries (Bladon and Al-Bamerni 1976; Hardcastle 1985; Abry and Lallouache 1991a, 1991b)

(b)   speech rate (Lindblom 1963a, Hardcastle 1985)

(c)   speaking style (Lindblom and Lindgren 1985; Krull 1989; Moon and Lindblom 1994, among others)

None of the models we are going to review deals with all the variables listed above but undoubtedly the validation of a theory or model will eventually depend also on its ability to account for these factors.

On the side of perception of coarticulated speech, there is experimental evidence that coarticulatory influences are perceived and that listeners can correctly identify the intended segment by normalizing the percept as a function of context, i.e. by factoring out the contextual influences. This is shown in a number of identification, discrimination and reaction-time experiments (e.g. Mann and Repp 1980; Martin and Bunnell 1981; Repp and Mann 1982; Whalen 1981, 1989; Fowler and Smith 1986; Ohala and Feder 1994). What exactly *normalization* means is an object of debate: do listeners use the acoustic information for recovering the invariant coarticulated gestures as propounded by the theory of direct perception (Fowler 1986; Fowler and Smith 1986) or is the sound itself and its acoustic structure the object of perception, as propounded by a number of other speech scientists (Diehl 1986; Ohala 1986)?

It is possible to draw a parallel between this issue and the so-called *motor equivalence* studies. It has been shown that speakers themselves can reduce coarticulatory variability by means of compensatory manoeuvres (Lindblom 1967; Edwards 1985; Farnetani and Faber 1992; Perkell *et al.* 1993, among others, and see Recasens, this volume, chapter 4). What is the function of compensatory movements? Do they attempt to preserve invariance at the level of articulatory targets, or rather at the acoustic level? This issue, which can be re-worded as 'what is the goal of the speaker?', besides being fundamental for production theories, is also intimately related to the theories of perception of coarticulated speech, since the goal of the speaker is presumably the object of perception.

The relation between coarticulation and perception is not the subject of the present chapter. However, from this brief summary of current debates on coarticulation, it becomes clear that, while the testing of theories by analysis and modelling of the spatio-temporal domain of coarticulation is fundamental, it is only one aspect of the issue: experiments on the behaviour of speakers and listeners such as those mentioned above, i.e. compensation and normalization, will also be crucial tests for coarticulation theories.

This review will describe, compare and comment on the most influential coarticulation theories and models, and will address in detail the issues of anticipatory coarticulation, and of gestural conflict and coarticulation resistance.

Current theories and models
Coarticulation within the theory of Adaptive Variability
Speech does not need to be invariant
At the core of the theory of adaptive variability developed by Lindblom (1983, 1989, 1990) are the concepts that the fundamental function of speech is successful communication and that the speech mechanism,

like other biological mechanisms, tends to economy of effort. As a consequence the acoustic form of speech, rather than being invariant, will always be the result of the interaction between the listener-oriented requirement of successful communication and the speaker-oriented requirement of speech economy. Adaptive variability means that speakers are able to adapt their production to the demands of the communicative situation, i.e. to perceptual demands. When the communicative situation requires a high degree of phonetic precision, speakers are able to over-articulate; when this is not needed, speakers tend to under-articulate and economize energy. In the latter situation, listeners can recover the intended message by using signal independent information (i.e. top–down information) which helps interpret the information conveyed by a more or less poor speech signal. The full range of phonetic possibilities is represented by Lindblom as a continuum from hyper- to hypo-speech (Lindblom 1990).

Within this framework, coarticulation plays a fundamental role: perceptually the hyper- to hypo-speech continuum is manifested as a gradual decrease in phonetic contrast, and articulatorily as a gradual increase in coarticulation. So, coarticulation instantiates one of the two principles that govern speech production, i.e. the principle of economy.

Vowel reduction and coarticulation: the duration-dependent undershoot model

The first version of the model (Lindblom 1963a) is based on acoustic research on vowel reduction in Swedish. In this study Lindblom showed, first that the process of vowel reduction is not categorical but continuous, and second that it is not a process towards vowel centralization,[1] but rather the effect of consonant–vowel coarticulation. He found that in CVC syllables the formant frequencies during the vowel vary as a function of vowel duration and of the consonantal context: as duration decreases, the formants tend to undershoot the acoustic target value (an ideal invariant acoustic configuration represented by the asymptotic values towards which the formant frequencies aim) and to be displaced towards the values of the consonant context; undershoot tends to be larger in the contexts exhibiting sizeable consonant–vowel transitions (i.e. large locus–nucleus distances[2]). The direction of the formant movement and its dependence on the consonant–vowel distance clearly indicated that vowel reduction is the result of consonant-to-vowel coarticulation.

Lindblom's account of the relation between target undershoot and duration was that undershoot is the automatic response of the motor system to an increase in rate of motor commands. The commands are invariable but when they are issued at short temporal intervals, the articulators do not have sufficient time to complete the response before the next signal arrives and thus have to respond to different commands simultaneously. This induces both vowel shortening and reduced displacement of formants.

Subsequent research showed that the response to high rate commands does not automatically result in reduced movements (Kuehn and Moll 1976; Gay 1978b) and that reduction can occur also at slow rates (Nord 1986). This indicated that duration is not the only determinant of reduction. Extensive research on context-dependent undershoot in different speech styles (Lindblom and Lindgren 1985; Krull 1989; Lindblom *et al.* 1992) showed that the degree of undershoot varies across styles, indicating that speakers can functionally adapt their production to communicative and sociolinguistic demands. This is the core of Lindblom's theory of Adaptive Variability described above.

Coarticulation and speech style

In the recent, revised model of vowel undershoot (Moon and Lindblom 1994), vowel duration is still the main factor but variables associated with speech style can substantially modify the amount of formant undershoot. The model is based on an acoustic study of American English stressed vowels produced in clear speech style and in citation forms (i.e. over-articulated versus normal speech). The results on vowel durations and F2 frequencies indicate that in clear speech the vowels tend to be longer and less reduced than in citation forms and, in the cases where the durations overlap in the two styles, clear speech exhibits a smaller amount of undershoot. A second finding is that clear speech is in most cases characterized by higher formant velocities than citation forms. This means that, for a given duration, the amount of context-dependent undershoot depends on the velocity of the articulatory movements, i.e. it decreases as velocity increases. In the revised model (where the speech motor mechanism is seen as a second-order mechanical system) the amount of undershoot is predicted by three variables reflecting the strategies available to speakers under different circumstances: duration, input force, and stiffness (the time constant of the system). Thus, in speech, an increase in articulatory force and/or an increase in speed of the system response to commands contribute to increase the movement velocity, and hence to decrease the amount of context-dependent undershoot. The relations among these variables are illustrated in figure 2.1 (from Moon and Lindblom 1994). Duration on the abscissa represents the duration of the input force; displacement on the ordinate represents the excursion of the articulator movement, high displacement means a small amount of target undershoot. It can

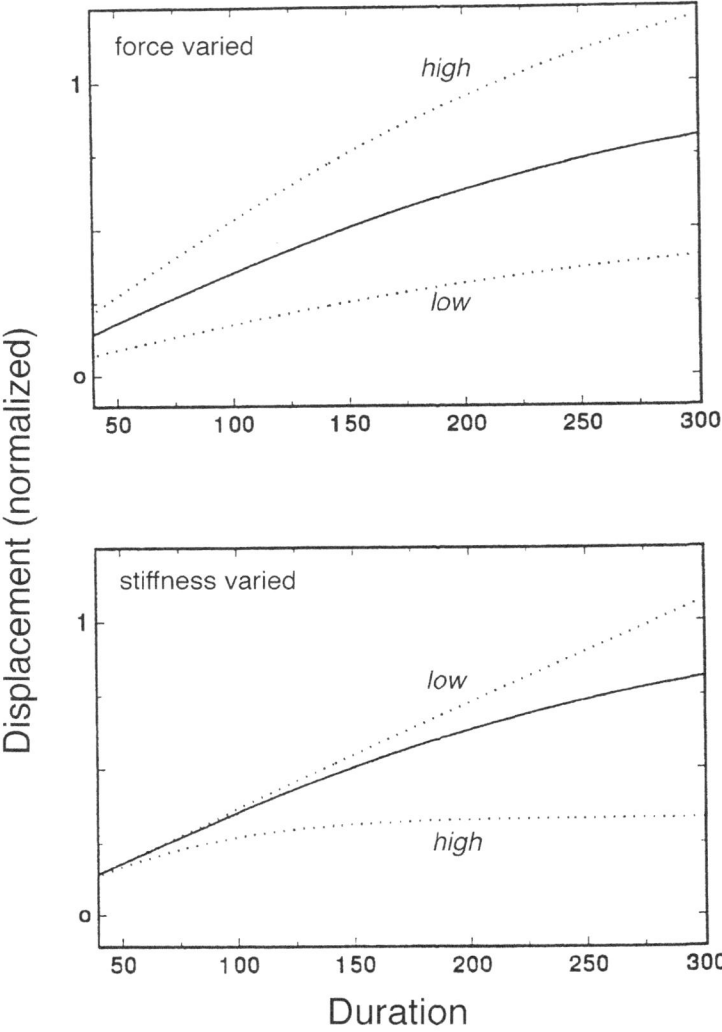

Figure 2.1   The revised model of vowel undershoot of Moon and Lindblom (1994). Movement displacement (ordinate) is a function of input force duration (abscissa) and can increase or decrease as a function of input force (top panel) and stiffness of the system (bottom panel). See text for expansion.

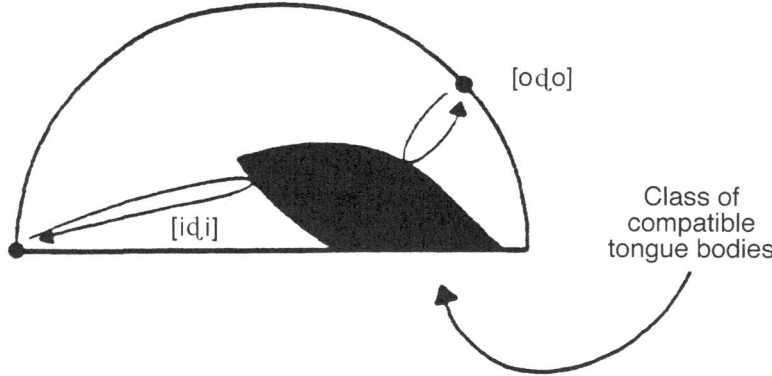

Figure 2.2   The model of tongue body coarticulation in the production of retroflex alveolars in the contexts of vowels /i/ and /o/ (filled circles). The black area contains all the tongue body contours compatible with the apical closure. The V-to-C and C-to-V trajectories reflect the minimum displacement constraints. The amount of coarticulatory effects are represented by the differences between tongue body configurations in the two contexts (from Lindblom 1983).

be seen that displacement is positively related to duration but can increase or decrease as a function of the amount of input force (top panel) or system stiffness (bottom panel).

An explanatory model of vowel-to-consonant coarticulation

In the parametric model of Lindblom, Pauli and Sundberg (1975) it is shown that V-to-C coarticulation results from a low-cost production strategy. The model is based on the analysis of VCV symmetric sequences with dental or retroflex apical stops, and vowels /i/or /o/. The model explores the reciprocal interactions between tongue tip parameters (elevation and protrusion/retraction) and tongue body parameters (position and shape) when the vocalic context is changed. Evaluation of the model is done by defining a procedure for deriving the formant values from the articulatory parameters, and by comparing the output of the model with the acoustic characteristics of natural VCV sequences, until the best match is reached. The authors show that the best match between the output of the model and natural utterances is a tongue configuration always compatible with the apical closure but characterized by a minimal displacement from the adjacent vowels. In other words, among a number of tongue body configurations compatible with the achievement of the tongue tip target, the tongue body always tends to take those requiring the least movements (see figure 2.2).

The predictions of the model are based on two kinds of constraints: first, the constraints associated with the position of the apical occlusion reduce the degrees of freedom of the tongue body (tongue tip extensibility/retractability constraints); second, the configuration of the tongue body is determined by that of the adjacent vowel, which further reduces the degrees of freedom of the system (constraints minimizing the tongue body movements, i.e. the principle of economy). The latter constraints determine the presence of coarticulation, the former its amount. Either set of constraints may be more or less severe and this is the source of the quantitative variations in coarticulation that we may expect across consonants, subjects and communicative situation.

The 'locus equation' as a measure of coarticulation
Krull (1987) was the first to use Lindblom's 'locus equations' (Lindblom 1963b) to quantify coarticulatory effects in CV syllables. For a given consonant in a variety of vocalic contexts, the locus equation reflects the relation between the formant values at the onset of CV transitions (at the consonant loci) and those at the mid-points of the following vowels, i.e. the extent to which the locus of a given consonant varies as a function of the following vowel nucleus. When such values are plotted against each other, their relation is expressed by the slope of the regression line (i.e. by the regression coefficient), which is an index of vowel-dependent variations of consonantal loci.

Using locus equations Krull showed that labial-consonant loci undergo larger coarticulatory effects than dental-consonant loci and that coarticulation is larger in spontaneous speech than in words read in isolation (Krull 1987; 1989). Since then, locus equations have been widely used for quantifying coarticulation (Duez 1992; Sussman, Hoemeke and McCaffrey 1992; Crowther 1994; Molis *et al.* 1994). A parallel approach (quantification of coarticulation through regression analysis) has been taken in articulatory studies of lingual consonants and vowels in different styles (Farnetani 1991; Farnetani and Recasens 1993).

Öhman's vowel-to-vowel coarticulation model
Öhman's model (Öhman 1966, 1967) is based on acoustic and articulatory analysis of Swedish VCV utterances produced in isolation, and on acoustic analysis of comparable utterances in American English and Russian. The major and most influential finding of Öhman's study is that in sequences V_1CV_2 where C is a stop consonant, the values of V_1C and CV_2 second formant transitions depend not only on C and the adjacent V but also on the identity of the transconsonantal vowel. Such coarticulatory effects, observed

for Swedish and American English in all the VCV sequences with intervocalic stops, indicated that vowels must be produced continuously, that is, the production of VCV utterances does not involve three linearly ordered successive gestures but rather a vowel-to-vowel diphthongal gesture on which the consonantal gesture is superimposed. The effects of a vowel on transconsonantal transitions are referred to as vowel-to-vowel coarticulatory effects. As for Russian, the VCV utterances consisted of various vowels with intervocalic palatalized /b/, /d/, /g/ and their unpalatalized (i.e. velarized) variants. The second formant data indicated that for all the consonants analysed, the variations of V_1C transitions as a function of the identity of V_2 were much smaller than those observed in American English and Swedish, and probably not above chance.

In the physiological model proposed by Öhman to account for his data, the tongue is viewed as a system of articulators executing invariant neural instructions from three independent articulatory channels: the apical (for apical consonants), the dorsal (for palatal and velar consonants) and the tongue body channel (for vowels). The variable vocal-tract shapes characterizing intervocalic consonants in different vocalic contexts are the results of the simultaneous individual motions of the three articulators. The model accounts for the different coarticulatory patterns of alveolar and velar consonants shown in the X-ray tracings for a Swedish subject: for alveolars, only the unconstricted part of the tongue (the tongue body) is modified by the adjacent vowels, while the constriction place remains invariant. Instead, for velars, the constriction place itself is modified and during closure the tongue moves continuously from V_1 to V_2: this is because independent vocalic and consonantal commands activate simultaneously adjacent tongue regions and 'the dynamic response of the tongue to a compound instruction is a complex summation of the responses to each of the components of the instruction' (Öhman 1966: 166). This implies that independent vocalic and consonantal commands on adjacent tongue regions never conflict, although the gestural trajectory from V_1 to V_2 may deviate due to the consonant command. Finally, the absence of V-to-V coarticulation in Russian is explained as a consequence of the interaction between two simultaneous and conflicting vowel commands on the tongue body during the consonants (for example, for palatalized consonants, the [i]-like command for palatalization, and the command for the adjacent vowel): coarticulation is blocked because during the consonant, 'the consonant gesture somehow overrules the vowel gesture if the latter is antagonistic to the former' (Öhman 1966: 167).

The numerical model of coarticulation developed for VCV utterances with intervocalic stops (Öhman 1967) is an algorithm predicting the appropriate vocal-tract shapes under various conditions from two kinds of information: the idealized target shape of the consonant, and a coarticulation function derived from the vocalic context.

Comments

Öhman's model has in common with Lindblom's the idea that coarticulatory variability does not originate from variations at the level of motor commands. In both models the instructions to the articulators are invariant but for Öhman the presence of coarticulation in VCV utterances results from the cooccurrence of consonantal and vocalic instructions, whilst for Lindblom it results from economy constraints tending to minimize the articulator displacements from a segment to the following one. Öhman's model, where the tongue body movements are organized from one vowel to the next, offers a more comprehensive account of transconsonantal effects (in both the anticipatory and the carryover direction) than Lindblom's, where the movements are organized from a target to the next, i.e. from V_1 to C and from C to V_2.

Coarticulation within featural phonology
Standard generative phonology
The position taken by standard generative phonology (Chomsky and Halle, *The Sound Pattern of English*, 1968, hereafter *SPE*) provides a clear-cut distinction between coarticulation and other context-dependent changes, such as assimilations. Coarticulation is defined as 'the transitions between a vowel and an adjacent consonant, the adjustments in the vocal tract shape made in anticipation of a subsequent motion etc.' (*SPE*: 295), while assimilations involve operations on phonological features (the minimal classificatory constituents of a phoneme), and are accounted for by phonological rules, mapping lexical representation onto phonetic representation. The speech events so represented are those controlled by the speaker and perceived by the listener, and are language-specific. Coarticulatory variations, instead, originate from the physical properties of speech, and are determined by universal rules.

The theory of feature spreading
The 'feature-spreading' theory, proposed by Daniloff and Hammarberg (1973) and Hammarberg (1976) is a clear departure from the view that coarticulatory variations originate from the speech production mechanism and are governed by universal rules. According to Hammarberg (1976) a purely physiological account of coarticulation would entail a sharp dichotomy between intent and execution, whereby mental processes would be

unaware of the capacities of the speech mechanism or the articulators would be unable to carry out the commands as specified. Such extreme dualism can be overcome if coarticulation is assigned to the phonological component and viewed as a spreading of features across segments before the commands are issued to the speech mechanism. This way the articulators will just have to execute high-level instructions.

This new account of coarticulation was supported by a number of experimental results which contradicted the idea that coarticulation is the product of inertia. The studies of Daniloff and Moll (1968) on labial coarticulation and of Moll and Daniloff (1971) on velar coarticulation revealed that the lowering of the velum in anticipation of a nasal consonant and the rounding of lips in anticipation of a rounded vowel can start two, three or even four segments before the influencing one. These patterns clearly indicated that anticipatory coarticulation cannot be the product of inertia, but rather a deliberate spread of features. Also spatial adjustments made in anticipation of subsequent segments are to be viewed as deliberate feature-spreading processes (Daniloff and Hammarberg 1973). One example is the English voiced alveolar stop, which becomes dental when followed by a dental fricative (as in the word *width)*. According to the authors, such 'accommodations' have the purpose of smoothing out and minimizing transitional sounds which might otherwise occur between individual segments. These spatial adjustments, however, are not to be considered inescapable and universal phenomena: in languages like Russian, for instance, the degree of accommodation between sounds seems to be minimal, which results in the introduction of transitional vocoids between adjacent consonantal and vocalic segments. The idea of the universality of coarticulatory patterns had also been challenged by Ladefoged (1967), who observed differences between French and English in the coarticulation of velar stops with front and back vowels.

Daniloff and Hammarberg (1973) and Hammarberg (1976) propose that all anticipatory (or right-to-left) coarticulation processes be accounted for in the grammar of a language by phonological feature-spreading rules, in principle not different from other assimilatory rules. Instead, most of the carryover (or left-to-right) processes are viewed by the authors as a passive result of the inertia of the articulatory system.

The look-ahead model

Daniloff and Hammarberg (1973) borrowed Henke's articulatory model (Henke 1966) to account for the extent of anticipatory coarticulation. Another well known model considered by the authors was the 'articulatory syllable' model proposed by Kozhevnikov and Chistovich (1965). The model

	S1	S2	S3		S1	S2	S3
F	0	0	+		+	+	+
G	+	0	−	--->	+	−	−
H	0	−	+		−	−	+

Figure 2.3   From phonological representation (left) to phonetic representation (right), through anticipatory feature-spreading rules as proposed by Daniloff and Hammarberg (1973). From Keating (1988b).

was based on durational relations among acoustic segments and on articulatory data on labial and lingual coarticulation in Russian, which suggested that the C_nV-type syllable is both a unit of rhythm and a unit of articulation. According to that model, the commands for a vowel are issued simultaneously with those for all the consonants preceding the vowel, hence a high degree of coarticulation is predicted within C_nV syllables, while little or no coarticulation is expected within other syllable types. Therefore, the Kozhevnikov and Chistovich model would fail to predict anticipatory coarticulation within VC syllables, in contradiction with the data of Moll and Daniloff (1971), showing that velar coarticulation extended from a nasal consonant across two preceding vowels.

Unlike the articulatory syllable model, Henke's model does not impose top–down boundaries to anticipatory coarticulation. Input segments are specified for articulatory targets in terms of binary features (+ or −). Unspecified features are given the 0 value. Phonological rules assign a feature of a segment to all the preceding segments unspecified for that feature. The feature-spreading mechanism is a look-ahead scanning device. Figure 2.3 (from Keating 1988b) shows the operation of the look-ahead mechanism over a sequence of three segments (S1, S2, S3) defined by three features (F, G, H).

It can be seen in the figure that no segment is left unspecified in the output phonetic representation (right-hand patterns) and that the anticipatory feature spreading is blocked only by specified segments (e.g. the spreading of feature G from S3 is blocked by S1, specified as + for that feature).

Comments

We can summarize the criticism of the 'feature-spreading' account of coarticulation by considering three important tenets of the theory:

(1)   The assumption that the look-ahead mechanism assigns the coarticulated feature to all preceding unspecified segments and therefore

coarticulation extends in time as a function of the number or duration of these segments. The studies of Benguerel and Cowan (1974), Lubker (1981) and of Sussman and Westbury (1981) are consistent with the look-ahead hypothesis. Studies on anticipatory velar movements by Ushijima and Sawashima (1972) for Japanese and by Benguerel *et al.* (1977a) for French are only in partial agreement: their data indicate that the temporal extent of velar lowering in anticipation of a nasal segment is rather restricted and does not begin earlier in sequences of three than in sequences of two preceding segments. Other studies fully contradict the look-ahead model and show that the onset time of lip rounding and velar lowering is constant (Bell-Berti and Harris 1979, 1981, 1982) (see below for further discussion).

(2)   The assumption that anticipatory coarticulation is blocked by segments specified for a feature that contradicts the spreading feature. Many data in the literature show that coarticulatory movements tend to start *during* rather than *after* the contradictorily specified segment, especially when few neutral segments intervene (e.g. Benguerel and Cowan 1974; Sussman and Westbury 1981, for lip rounding). Moreover, all the studies on lingual coarticulation in VCV sequences indicate that V_1 is influenced by V_2 even if it is specified for contrastive features with respect to V_2, e.g. /a/ is usually influenced by transconsonantal /i/ (see Butcher and Weiher 1976, for German; Farnetani, Vagges and Magno-Caldognetto 1985, for Italian; Magen 1989, for American English).

(3)   The assumption that unspecified segments acquire the spreading feature. Data show that phonologically unspecified segments may not completely acquire the coarticulating feature, i.e. they can be non-neutral articulatorily and therefore they can be affected only to a certain degree by the influencing segment. For example, Bell-Berti and Harris (1981) showed that in American English the velum lowers during oral vowels produced in an oral context; Engstrand showed that in Swedish lip protrusion decreases during /s/ in /usu/ sequences (Engstrand 1981) and that the tongue body lowers during /p/ in /ipi/ sequences (Engstrand 1983). Such findings (and others reported below) indicate that supposedly unspecified segments may nonetheless be specified for articulatory positions.

Altogether these data indicate that a coarticulatory model based on the spreading of binary features fails to account for the graded nature of coarticulation and for its temporal changes during the segments.

The 'coarticulation resistance' model (Bladon and Al-Bamerni 1976) and the 'window' model (Keating 1985b, 1988a, 1988b, 1990a) overcome some of the inadequacies of the feature-spreading model in two different ways: the former proposes that specification in terms of binary features be accompanied by a graded coarticulatory resistance specification, the latter proposes that coarticulation be accounted for by two distinct components of the grammar, the phonological and the phonetic component.

The 'coarticulation resistance' model

The notion of coarticulatory resistance was introduced by Bladon and Al-Bamerni (1976) in an acoustic study of coarticulation in /l/ allophones in English (clear versus dark versus syllabic /l/). The study analyses the steady state frequencies of F1 and F2 in the target allophones and in a number of vowels. The results indicate that the V-to-C coarticulatory effects decrease gradually from clear to dark to syllabic /l/ and vary systematically also as a function of boundary type. These graded differences could not be accounted for by binary feature analysis which would block coarticulation in the dark (i.e. velarized) allophones, specified as [+ back]. The authors propose that all the observed coarticulatory variations be accounted for in phonology by a rule assigning a coarticulatory resistance (CR) coefficient to the feature specification of each allophone and each boundary condition. According to the authors, CR coefficients are not necessarily universal, they can be language- and dialect-specific and thus account for interlanguage differences as well as for the differences in nasality between British and American English. According to the authors, the CR coefficients would be in line with the phonetic specifications in terms of numerical feature values proposed in *SPE*. A subsequent cineradiographic experiment (Bladon and Nolan 1977) showed that English apical consonants (e.g. /l/, /n/) become laminal in the context of laminal /s/, /z/ while laminal fricatives never become apical in an apical context. The data are accounted for by attaching to /s/ and /z/ feature specification a CR coefficient higher than that applied to apical consonants.

The window model

The 'window' model of coarticulation, elaborated by Keating (1985b, 1988a, 1988b, 1990a) accounts both for the continuous changes in space and time observed in speech, and for intersegment and interlanguage differences in coarticulation.

The phonological and the phonetic component of the grammar

Keating agrees that binary features and phonological rules cannot account for the graded nature of coarticulation but disagrees that such graded

variations should be ascribed to phonetic universals as automatic consequences of the speech production mechanism, since they may differ across languages (Keating 1985b). In particular she shows that contextual variations in
vowel duration as a function of whether the following consonant is voiced or
voiceless – an effect traditionally thought to be universal – are relevant and
systematic in English and unsystematic or even absent in Polish and Czech.
Therefore each language must specify these phonetic facts in its grammar. Her
proposal is that all graded contextual variations, both those assumed to be
phonological and those assumed to be universal and physically determined,
be accounted for by the phonetic component of the grammar.

Keating's model is based on two assumptions which are a substantial
departure from the feature-spreading model: (i) phonological underspecification may persist into the phonetic representation, (ii) phonetic
underspecification is not a categorical but a continuous notion. The phonological representation is in terms of binary features. Unspecified features
may be specified by rule or may remain unspecified. The phonological rules
by which segments acquire a feature are various and may differ across languages: there are fill-in rules such as that specifying /ʃ/ as [+ high] (for artic-
ulatory/aerodynamic reasons), context-sensitive rules such as that specifying
Russian /x/ as [− back] before high vowels (see figure 2.4) and finally there
may be assimilation rules like those proposed in the feature-spreading model
(see below).

The windows

The output of phonological rules is interpreted in space and time by
the phonetic implementation rules which provide a continuous (articulatory
or acoustic) representation over time. For each articulatory or acoustic dimension, the feature value is associated with a range of values, called a *window.*
Windows have their own duration and a width representing all the possible
physical values that a target can take, i.e. the range of variability within a
target. The window width depends first of all on the output of the phonological component: if features are specified, the associated window will be narrow
and allow little contextual variation; if features are left unspecified, their corresponding windows will be wide and allow large contextual variation. The
exact width of a window is derived for each language from information on the
maximum amount of contextual variability observed in speech: all intermediate degrees between maximally narrow and maximally wide windows are then
possible. By allowing windows to vary continuously in width, the model can
represent the phonologically unspecified segments that offer some resistance
to coarticulation, i.e. are associated with articulatory targets (see above for

experimental data). In Keating's model such segments are represented by wide, but not maximal windows, and can be defined phonetically 'not quite unspecified' (Keating 1988a: 22).

The contours

If the window represents the range of possible variability within a segment for a given physical dimension, the path or contour which connects the windows represents actual trajectories over time, i.e. the physical values over time in a specific context. Paths are interpolation functions between windows and are constrained by the requirements of smoothness and minimal articulatory effort (in agreement with the economy principle proposed by Lindblom). Even if trajectories connect one window to the next, cross-segmental coarticulatory effects are possible because windows associated with features left unspecified are wide and 'invisible' as targets; they therefore contribute nothing to the contour and allow direct interpolation between non-adjacent windows. Thus the model can account for V-to-V coarticulation and for anticipatory nasalization across any number of unspecified consonants. Specified segments, on the other hand, make their own contribution to the path, and do not allow interpolations across their windows. Figure 2.4 illustrates the phonological and the phonetic components of the model.

The example is a VCV utterance, where the two vowels are specified for [+ high] and [+ low]. The consonant, unspecified at the lexical level (top panel), can be specified by phonological fill-in rules (panel 2 from top), or by context-sensitive rules (panel 3 from top), or may remain unspecified (bottom). In the first case the specified feature generates narrow windows in all contexts and V-to-V interpolation is not possible. In the second case the window is narrow before the high vowel, but wide before the low vowel. In the third case the unspecified feature generates wide windows and V-to-V interpolation is possible in all contexts.

An important difference between Keating's model and other target-and-connection models proposed in the literature (e.g. Lindblom 1963a, MacNeilage 1970, among others) is that Keating's targets are not points in the phonetic space, subject to undershoot or overshoot but regions, themselves defined by the limits of all possible variations. We must remark that Lindblom, Pauli and Sundberg (1975) (see above and figure 2.2) had proposed a model similar to Keating's for tongue body coarticulation during apical stop production: the various tongue body contours compatible with the apical closure form in fact a region within which all coarticulatory variations take place.

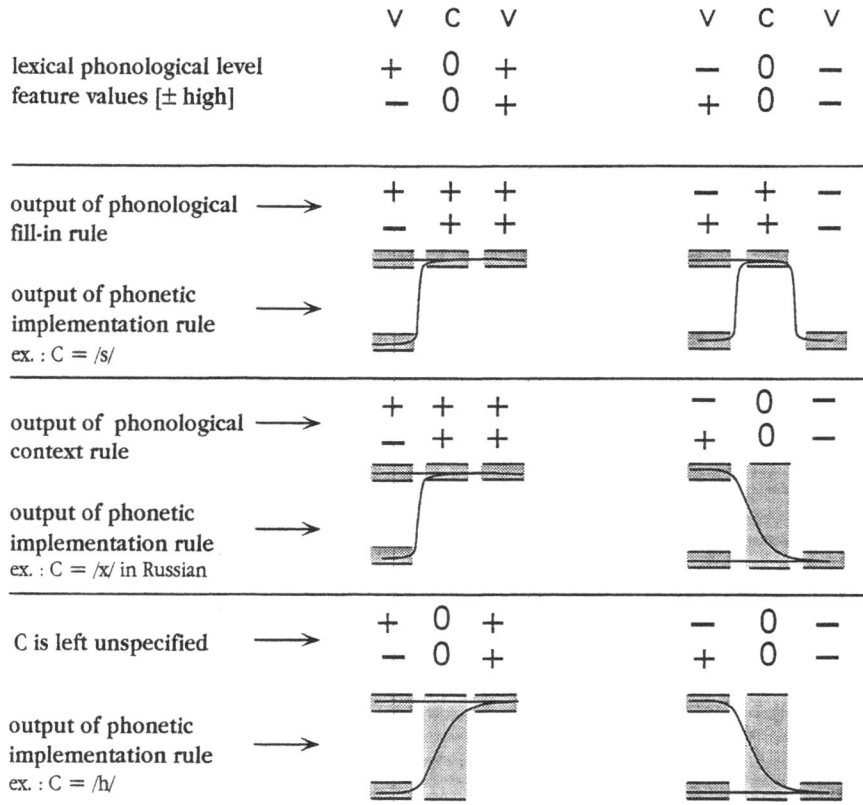

Figure 2.4   Keating's window model: from phonological representation (top panel) to phonetic parametric representation (articulatory or acoustic), through phonological specification rules plus phonetic implementation rules (panels 2 and 3 from top) or through implementation rules only (bottom panel).

Cross-language differences in coarticulation

According to Keating, interlanguage differences in coarticulation may be phonological or phonetic: the former occur when phonological assimilatory rules operate in one language and not in another, the latter occur when different languages give a different interpretation to a feature left unspecified. Speech analysis helps determine which processes are phonological and which phonetic. If phonological assimilation rules assign a contextual feature to a segment, its associated window will be narrow before that context and the contour will have a plateau-like shape (like that observed in figure 2.4, second case, a low vowel followed by C + V both specified as [+ high]).

In a language where assimilation rules do not operate, the key feature remains unspecified and the trajectories will be provided solely by interpolation between the preceding and the following context (as in the third example of figure 2.4).

In a study of nasalization, Cohn (1990) compared the nasal air-flow contour of English nasalized vowels with the contour of nasal vowels in French and of nasalized vowels in Sundanese. In French, vowel nasality is inherently phonological, while in Sundanese it is described as the output of a phonological spreading rule. Cohn found that in the nasalized vowels of Sundanese the flow patterns have plateau-like shapes very similar to the French patterns, while in English the shapes of the contours describe smooth trajectories from the [− nasal] to the [+ nasal] segments. The categorical versus the gradient quality of nasalization in Sundanese versus English indicated that nasalization is indeed phonological in Sundanese and phonetic in English. Similar differences between patterns of anticipatory lip rounding were observed by Boyce (1990) between Turkish and English, suggesting that the process may be phonological in Turkish and phonetic in English. Within Keating's line of research for defining a process as phonological or phonetic, is the acoustic study of vowel allophony in Marshallese (Choi 1992), which shows, through cross-context comparisons, that Marshallese vowels are unspecified for the feature front/back, so that the allophonic variants (traditionally thought to be phonological) result from phonetic rules.

Languages may also differ in coarticulation because the phonetic rules can interpret phonological underspecification in different ways, allowing the windows to be more or less wide. In this case the interlanguage differences are only quantitative. 'Window width is to some extent an idiosyncratic aspect that languages specify about the phonetics of their sounds and features' (Keating 1988a: 22).

Comments

The novelty of Keating's theory, relating the phonological representation and the physical reality of speech through the mediation of the phonetic component of the grammar, has stimulated a number of studies which have contributed to a better understanding of coarticulatory processes. Within her line of research, the studies of Huffman (1990) and Cohn (1990) have contributed to improvements in the implementation theory and that of Choi (1992) has contributed to refining the interpolation functions in order to account for the asymmetries observed between anticipatory and carryover coarticulation.

A serious criticism to Keating's theory comes from Browman and

Goldstein (1993), who argue that the description of speech in two separate domains, requiring two distinct types of representation related to each other only by implementation rules, renders the phonological and the phonetic levels quite distant from each other: 'it becomes very easy to view phonetic and phonological (physical and cognitive) structures as essentially independent of one another, with no interaction or mutual constraint' (Browman and Goldstein 1993: 53). In particular, Boyce, Krakow and Bell-Berti (1991b) point to the difficulty of reconciling phonological unspecified features with specific articulatory positions, which are viewed by Keating as language-specific interpretations of underspecification. For instance, data on tongue body coarticulation (e.g. Engstrand 1989, for Swedish; Farnetani 1991, for Italian) seem to speak against Keating's proposal. These studies show that there are relevant differences in V-to-C coarticulatory effects on tongue dorsum across various consonant types all unspecified for the features high and back: e.g. labial,[3] dental and alveolar consonants (excluding /s/ specified as [+high] in Keating's model) and that in both languages the degree of resistance to vowel effects tends to increase from /l/ to /d/ to /t/ (/p/ shows the lowest degree of resistance). These cross-consonant differences and cross-language similarities indicate that the various degrees of coarticulation resistance, rather than being derived from language-idiosyncratic interpretations of phonological underspecification, must result from consonant-specific production constraints going beyond language peculiarities.

Another problem concerns the effects of speech style or rate on the degree of coarticulation. In a recent neural network model of speech production proposed by Guenther (1994), targets are seen as regions laid out in orosensory coordinates, very much like Keating's windows and these regions are allowed to increase or decrease in size as a function of rate and accuracy in pronunciation. The present version of the model conceives windows as invariable in size. But if the windows associated with specified features are allowed to shrink in duration and stretch in width in order to account for informal or casual speech then the relation between phonological feature specification and window width at the level of acoustic or articulatory representation might weaken further.

Manuel's criticism of Keating's theory (Manuel 1987, 1990) addresses the topic of whether coarticulatory variations should be accounted for in the grammar of a language owing to the fact that they differ quantitatively across languages (i.e. are not universal). Manuel reports data on vowel-to-vowel coarticulation in different languages (Manuel and Krakow 1984; Manuel 1987), showing that coarticulatory variations in vowels tend to be large in languages with a small inventory size and smaller in more crowded inventories. She proposes that cross-language quantitative differences in coarticulation be regulated by *output constraints,* which restrict coarticulatory variations in languages where a crowded vowel space might lead to acoustic overlap and perceptual confusion, i.e. they delimit the areas in the phonetic space within which coarticulatory variations can take place (see chapter 8 of this volume). Clumeck (1976) had proposed a similar principle to account for the restricted extent of anticipatory nasalization in Swedish, as compared to other languages with less crowded vowel inventories. According to Manuel, if these constraints are known for each phoneme and each language on the basis of inventory size and phoneme distribution then no language-particular rules are needed, since the amount of coarticulation should be to some extent predictable. Following Manuel's reasoning, the coarticulatory patterns of vowels in Marshallese (Choi 1992) could also be predicted from its inventory: this language has four vowel phonemes, all distributed along the high/low dimension, thus output constraints would allow minimal coarticulation along the vertical dimension and maximal coarticulation along the front/back dimension, and this is what occurs.[4] Manuel (1987) recognized, however, in line with Bladon and Al-Bamerni (1976), that language-specific coarticulation patterns may also be totally unrelated to phonemic constraints. Data on velar coarticulation (Ushijima and Sawashima 1972, for Japanese; Farnetani 1986b, for Italian) indicate that anticipatory nasalization has a limited extent in these two languages, even if they have a restricted number of oral vowels and no nasal vowels in their inventories. Similarly, the study of Solé and Ohala (1991) shows that in Spanish the extent of anticipatory velar lowering is more restricted than in American English, which has a much more crowded vowel inventory than Spanish.

Altogether, the studies just reviewed suggest that cross-language similarities and cross-language differences in coarticulation are related to different kinds of constraints: production constraints, which seem to operate both within and across languages (as shown above from the tongue body coarticulatory data in Italian and Swedish), constraints deriving from language-specific phonological structure (in agreement with Manuel) but also, in agreement with Keating, language-particular constraints, unrelated to production or phonology and therefore unpredictable. These constraints seem to have the role of preserving the exact phonetic quality expected and accepted in a given language or dialect (Farnetani 1990).

Coarticulation as coproduction and an outline of new models

The coproduction theory and articulatory phonology represent, to date, the most successful effort to bridge the gap between the cognitive and the physical aspects of language. The coproduction theory has been elaborated through collaborative work of psychologists and linguists, starting from Fowler (1977, 1980, 1985), Fowler *et al.* (1980) and Bell-Berti and Harris (1981). In conjunction with the new theory, Kelso, Saltzman and Tuller (1986), Saltzman and Munhall (1989) and Saltzman (1991) have developed a computational model of linguistic structures, the task-dynamic model, whose aim is to account for kinematics of articulators in speech. Input to the model are the phonetic gestures, the dynamically defined units of articulatory phonology proposed by Browman and Goldstein (1986, 1989, 1990a, 1990b, 1992).

The dynamic nature of phonological units

Fowler (1977, 1980) takes a position against the speech production theories that posit phonological features as input to the speech programme and against the view that coarticulation is a phonological feature-spreading process. According to Fowler, the dichotomy between the level of representation and that of production lies in the different nature of the descriptive entities pertaining to the two levels: in all featural theories the units of representation are abstract, static and timeless and need a translation process which transforms them into substantially different entities, i.e. into articulatory movements. In this translation process, the speech plan supplies the spatial targets and a central clock specifies when the articulators have to move. An alternative proposal, which overcomes the dichotomy and gets rid of a time program separated from the plan, is to modify the phonological units of the plan: the plan must specify the act to be executed, hence the phonological units must be planned actions, i.e. dynamically specified phonetic gestures, with an intrinsic temporal dimension (Fowler 1980; Fowler *et al.* 1980; Browman and Goldstein 1986, 1989).

In order to account for coarticulation, the spreading-feature theory posits assimilatory rules by which features are exchanged or modified before being translated into targets. In the coproduction theory it is proposed that gestures are not modified when actualized in speech. Their intrinsic temporal structure allows gestures to overlap in time so gestures are not altered by the context but coproduced with the context.

According to Browman and Goldstein (1993), the new accounts of coarticulation which introduce phonetic implementation rules in addition to phonological spreading rules, e.g. Keating (1985b, 1990a), do not succeed in overcoming the dichotomy between the cognitive and the physical aspects of speech as they are still viewed as different domains, with distinct types of representation, rather than two levels of description of the same system.

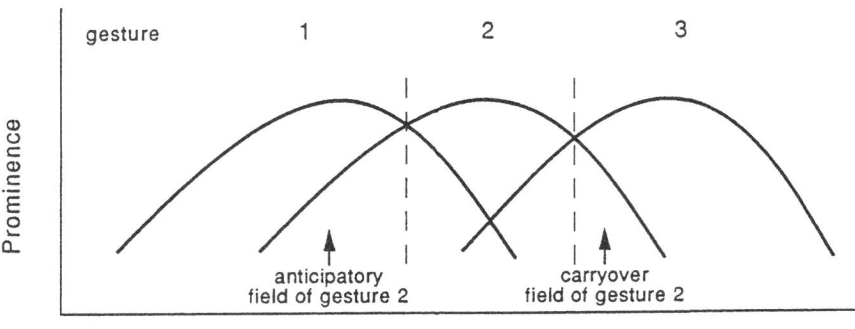

Figure 2.5   Representation of three overlapping phonetic gestures (from Fowler and Saltzman 1993). See text for details.

The gestures and their spatio-temporal organization

Figure 2.5, from Fowler and Saltzman (1993) illustrates how gestures are coproduced in speech. The activation of a gesture increases and decreases smoothly in time and so does its influence on the vocal tract shape and on the acoustic signal. In the figure, the vertical lines delimit a temporal interval (possibly corresponding to an acoustic segment) during which gesture 2 is prominent, i.e. has the maximal influence on the vocal tract shape, while the overlapping gestures 1 and 3 have a much weaker influence. Before this interval, the influence of gesture 1 predominates and the weaker influence of the following gesture gives rise to anticipatory coarticulation; analogously, after the interval of dominance of gesture 2, its influence determines the so-called carryover coarticulation. Thus both anticipatory and carryover effects are accounted for by the same principle of gesture overlap.

Gestures are implemented in speech by coordinative structures, i.e. by transient functional dependencies among the articulators contributing to the gestural goal: for instance, in the production of a bilabial stop, a functional link is established between upper lip, lower lip and jaw, so that a decrease in contribution of one articulator to the lip-closure gesture is automatically compensated for by an increase in the contribution of another. So the compensatory manoeuvres observed in speech stem from the coordination among independent articulators in achieving a gestural goal (Fowler 1977; Saltzman and Munhall 1989).

The overlap between gestures reflects their temporal coordination which is expressed in the model as intergestural phasing (i.e. the onset of a gesture occurs at a specified phase of the cycle of the preceding active gesture). The phasing between gestures is controlled at the plan level: an increase in gestural overlap has the consequence of decreasing the measured segmental durations and of increasing the amount of coarticulatory effects. Quantitative changes in intergestural overlap can account for coarticulatory differences between slow and fast speech (Saltzman and Munhall 1989), for some of the effects of stress on the articulatory and acoustic characteristics of vowels (de Jong, Beckman and Edwards 1993) and for the effects of the number of syllables within a foot on vowel durations (Fowler 1977, 1981a).

The observed movement kinematics (displacement, velocity) is determined by the dynamic parameters that specify the gestures (i.e. force, stiffness). Also these parameters can undergo graded changes. In particular it is proposed that most of the so-called 'connected speech processes', e.g. vowel reduction, place assimilation and segment deletions are not due to categorical changes of the underlying gestures but to graded modifications, such as a decrease in gestural magnitude and an increase in temporal overlap (Browman and Goldstein 1990b, 1992; Farnetani 1997, for an overview of connected speech processes).

According to gestural phonology, cross-language differences in coarticulation (be they related or not to the inventory size and phoneme distribution) are consequences of the different gestural set-up in various languages, i.e. differences in the parameters that specify the dynamics of gestures and in those that specify their phasing relations. The language-specific gestural set-up is learned during speech development by tuning gestures and their organization to language-particular values (Browman and Goldstein 1989).

Spatial coarticulation: coarticulation resistance and intergestural blending

According to Fowler and Saltzman (1993) the amount of articulatory variability induced by coproduction depends on the degree to which the temporally overlapping gestures share articulators. A case of minimal gestural interference is the production of /VbV/ sequences, where the vocalic and the consonantal constriction gestures involve two independent articulators, the tongue body and the lips respectively, and a common articulator, the jaw. Here, coproduction of the vocalic and the consonantal gestural goals takes place with minimal spatial perturbations as the engagement of the shared articulator in the two competing goals is compensated for by the tongue and/or the lips (see above). Instead, coproduction induces relevant spatial perturbations if all articulators are shared by the overlapping gestures. This occurs, for example, in the production of /VgV/ utterances, where the vocalic and the consonantal gestures share both the tongue body and the jaw: the main effect of this interference is the variation of the consonant place of constriction as a function of the adjacent vowel (see discussion of Öhman's model above). The general idea of the coproduction theory is that gestures *blend* their influence on the common articulator, with various possible outcomes (Browman and Goldstein 1989; Fowler and Saltzman 1993).

In a sequence of two identical gestures, the outcome of their temporal overlap is a composite movement, reflecting the sum of the influences of the two gestures. This is shown in a study of laryngeal abduction/adduction movements monitored by transillumination (Munhall and Löfqvist 1992). In sequences of two voiceless consonants, two distinct glottal abduction movements were observed at slow speaking rates, while single movements of various shapes were found at moderate and fast rates. The study shows that all the various movement patterns can be simulated by summing up two distinct underlying gestures overlapping to different degrees, as seen in figure 2.6.

The figure displays the hypothesized gestural score for two distinct abduction gestures of different amplitude arranged in order of decreasing overlap (left-hand series, top to bottom) and the corresponding movements resulting from summation of the underlying gestures (right-hand series). Notice that little or no overlap between the two gestures generates two distinct glottal movements (bottom panels); the outcome of a larger gestural overlap is a single glottal movement which decreases in duration and increases in amplitude as overlap increases (mid to top panels).

The gestural summation hypothesis can account for a number of observations in the coarticulation literature, for example, the patterns of velum lowering during a vowel in CVN sequences appear to be the result of the sum of the velar lowering for the vowel and the velar lowering for the following nasal (Bell-Berti and Krakow 1991). Gestural summation could also account for the differences in tongue tip/blade contact, observed with EPG (electropalatography), in singleton versus geminated lingual consonants (Farnetani 1990), and in singleton /n/ and /t/ or /d/ versus /nt/ and /nd/ clusters (Farnetani and Busă 1994). In both studies the geminates and clusters were produced with a single tongue movement whose amplitude (in terms of extent of the contact area) was significantly larger than in singleton consonants, independently of the vocalic context.

When gestures impose conflicting demands on the same articulatory structures, gestural conflict can be resolved at the plan level, by delaying the onset of the competing gesture so that the ongoing goal can be achieved. In this case the ongoing configuration will be minimally perturbed and the movement to the next goal will be quite fast (Bell-Berti and Harris 1981).

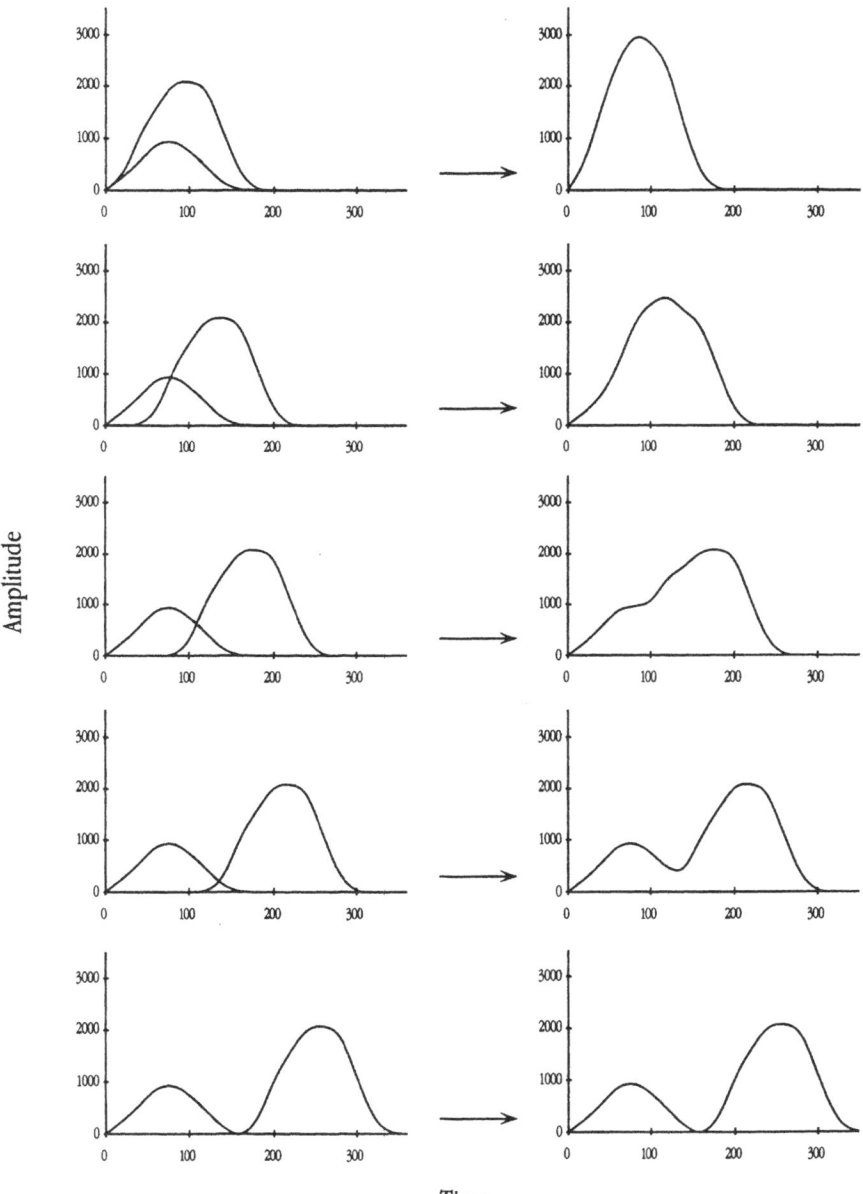

Figure 2.6   The additive blending model proposed by Munhall and Löfqvist (1992) for laryngeal gestures. The left-hand graphs of each pair show two laryngeal gestures gradually decreasing in overlap (top to bottom), the right-hand graphs show the output articulator movements resulting from gestural summation.

Alternatively, according to Saltzman and Munhall (1989) and Fowler and Saltzman (1993) no changes may be needed at the plan level and the articulatory consequences of gestural overlap 'would be shaped by the manner in which the coarticulating gesture blends its influence on the vocal tract with those of an ongoing one' (Fowler and Saltzman 1993:180). This means that the outcome of blending varies according to the gestures involved and depends in great part on the degree of resistance to coarticulation associated with the ongoing gesture.

As seen above, the notion of coarticulatory resistance was proposed by Bladon and Al-Bamerni (1976) to account for different degrees of spatial coarticulatory variations. Later studies (Bladon and Nolan 1977; Recasens 1984b, 1987; Farnetani and Recasens 1993) indicated that segments with a high degree of coarticulation resistance not only exhibit little coarticulatory variability but also induce strong coarticulatory effects on neighbouring segments. This appears to demonstrate that conflicting gestures *can* overlap: if they could not, no coarticulatory variations would be observed either in the highly resistant segment or in the weaker segment. Fowler and Saltzman (1993) propose the concept of *blending strength* to capture the relation between coarticulatory resistance and coarticulatory aggression: all the components of a given gesture have their own characteristic degree of blending strength, associated with the specific demands placed on the vocal tract so that when overlap occurs between a stronger and weaker gesture, the stronger tends to suppress the influence of the weaker and to exert greater influence on the common articulator; on the other hand, when overlap occurs between competing gestures of similar degree of blending strength, its outcome tends to be an averaging of the two influences.

Fowler and Saltzman's proposal implies that various outcomes are possible when two gestures are blended, from configurations mainly reflecting the influence of one gesture, to intermediate configurations reflecting both components of the coproduced gestures. The latter seem to occur notably between vowels, which are characterized by a moderate degree of blending strength.[5] Gestural blending is a general notion that applies to each of the articulators shared by two gestures. For example, in the production of alveolar consonants in VCV sequences, the tongue blade is controlled by the consonantal gesture alone but the jaw and the tongue body are controlled simultaneously by the consonantal and the overlapping vocalic gestures, which impose competing demands on them. Then, the observed coarticulatory V-to-C effects on the tongue body and the jaw reflect a blending of the influences of the overlapping V and C gestures, exactly like the blending of influences on the main articulator in the /VgV/ sequences mentioned above.

Comments

In order to account for the various degrees of resistance to coarticulation, the phonetic literature has used the notion 'constraints', which can be related to 'the demands placed on the vocal tract' proposed by Fowler and Saltzman (1993:180). According to Sussman and Westbury (1981), the term 'constraints' reflects resistance to coarticulation due to two possible factors: (a) aerodynamic requirements for the production of the ongoing segment (e.g. velar lowering for a nasal consonant does not occur during a preceding /s/ even if in itself it does not contradict the tongue movements for the formation of an /s/-like configuration); (b) antagonism proper, such as lip rounding versus lip spreading: according to the authors this kind of conflict does not preclude the onset of the lip-rounding neuromotor commands during /i/ because this can actively counteract the lip-spreading command. While, on the one hand, gestural phonology can account for the second type of constraints, by allowing antagonistic gestures to overlap, on the other hand, it is difficult to see how it can account for coarticulation resistance due to the aerodynamic requirement that an /s/-like lingual configuration generates the intended friction noise, unless the theory incorporates some sort of aerodynamic constraints.

In Recasens' review of lingual coarticulation (see chapter 4 of this volume) the different degrees of coarticulatory resistance observed in various studies on C-to-V and V-to-C effects are accounted for by *articulatory constraints* of different degree and different nature, functional and/or physical – the latter due to mechanical coupling between tongue regions (see also earlier for our account of the V-to-C coarticulatory patterns in Swedish and Italian). The data reviewed by Recasens show that production constraints are higher in the tongue regions directly involved in the formation of the constriction than in other regions and higher in laminodorsal consonants and in trills than in laminal fricatives than in apical stops, laterals, nasals and taps; for vowels, they seem to be higher in high/front vowels than in back and in low vowels. It is also shown that the degree of constraints associated with a gesture can account for the directionality and the temporal extent of coarticulation, i.e. coarticulatory anticipation depends heavily on the strength of the carryover effects of the preceding segment and vice versa. The high production constraints associated with trills (Recasens 1991b) are counter-evidence to the hypothesis that resistance to coarticulation varies inversely with gestural sonority. As for clusters, it appears that the gestural blending hypothesis accounts for some but not for all of the outcomes of gestural interference: the review shows that in Catalan, blending occurs in /ʃ/ + /s/ sequences and can be avoided if articulator velocity is sufficient to produce the consonants at different places, as occurs in /rð/ clusters. This indicates that blending can be avoided by increasing articulator velocity (in agreement with Bell-Berti and Harris 1981). We should note that in Recasens' review, gestural blending is intended in the strict sense used by Browman and Goldstein (1989) to account for changes in consonant place of articulation.

Anticipatory extent of coarticulation
The coproduction model versus the look-ahead model
According to the coproduction theory, gestures have their own intrinsic duration. Hence the temporal extent of anticipatory coarticulation must be constant for a given gesture. Bell-Berti and Harris (1979, 1981, 1982) on the basis of experimental data on lip rounding and velar lowering, proposed the 'frame' model of anticipatory coarticulation (also referred to as the time-locked model): the onset of a movement of an articulator is independent of the preceding phone string length but begins at a fixed time before the acoustic onset of the segment with which it is associated. A number of other studies are instead consistent with the look-ahead model (see above). The cross-language study of Lubker and Gay (1982) on anticipatory labial coarticulation in English and Swedish shows that Swedish subjects use longer, more ample and less variable lip protrusion movements than English subjects; according to the authors, this is due to the perceptual importance of lip protrusion in Swedish, where lip rounding is contrastive; the relation between protrusion duration and the number of consonants indicates that three of the five Swedish speakers use a look-ahead strategy, and two a time-locked strategy. As noted earlier, two studies on velar movements (Ushijima and Sawashima 1972; Benguerel *et al.* 1977a) are in only partial agreement with the look-ahead hypothesis. These studies are based on timing measurements (like most of the studies on anticipatory coarticulation) and on observations of movement profiles as well. The study of Benguerel *et al.* (1977a) is of particular interest: the authors observed a clear velar lowering in oral open vowels in non-nasal context and, in sequences of oral vowels and nasal consonants, they could distinguish two patterns of velar movements: a lowering movement associated with the vowels (always beginning with the first vowel in the sequence), followed by a more rapid velar descent for the nasal, which caused the opening of the velar port and whose temporal extent was rather limited. Apparently this finding passed unnoticed: similar composite anticipatory movements were later observed in a number of other studies, starting with Al-Bamerni and Bladon (1982) and were given a totally different interpretation.

The hybrid model

Al-Bamerni and Bladon (1982), in a study of velar coarticulation in English, observed that speakers used two production strategies, a single velar opening gesture (one-stage pattern) and a two-stage gesture whose onset was aligned with the first non-nasal vowel and whose higher velocity stage was coordinated with the oral closing gesture of the nasal consonant. Perkell and Chiang (1986) were the first to observe two-stage patterns in lip rounding movements, which converged with Al-Bamerni and Bladon's observations: in /iC$_n$u/ utterances the onset of lip protrusion was temporally linked to the offset of /i/ (as predicted by the look-ahead model) but the onset of the second phase of the movement (detectable from the point of maximum acceleration) was linked to /u/ (as predicted by the time-locked model). The authors proposed a third model of anticipatory coarticulation, the hybrid model, a compromise between the look-ahead and the time-locked. Perkell's lip protrusion data on three English subjects (Perkell 1990) confirmed the preliminary observations of Perkell and Chiang, showing that two of the subjects used the two-stage hybrid strategy.

Boyce *et al.* (1990) give a different account of the hybrid movement profiles: they argue that the early onset of anticipatory movements cannot be attributed to a look-ahead anticipatory strategy unless it is shown that the phonologically unspecified segments preceding the key segment do not themselves have a target position for lips or velum. The data of Bell-Berti and Krakow (1991) on velar lowering show, through comparisons between vowels in nasal and oral context, that the velum lowers during vowels in oral context.[6] Accordingly, the early onset of velar lowering in the two-stage patterns is associated with a velar target position for the oral vowels, while the second stage, temporally quite stable, is associated with production of the nasal consonant. This interpretation is compatible with that given by Benguerel *et al.* (1977a) for French (see above). Therefore the two-stage patterns do not reflect the mixed anticipatory strategy proposed in the hybrid model, but two independent velar-lowering gestures, a vocalic gesture followed by a consonantal gesture; these may be more or less blended (summed) together and thus give rise to various patterns of movements, as a function of the duration of the vocalic sequence and of speech rate (see above). The velar coarticulation data for American English of Solé (1992) are in disagreement with Bell-Berti and Krakow's study. The American English speakers in Solé's study do not show any velar lowering during high and low vowels in oral context; the systematic onset of velar lowering at the beginning of the vowels preceding a nasal consonant cannot therefore be interpreted as a gesture associated with the vowels but rather as the result of a phonological nasalization rule, specific to American English.

The latest study on lip protrusion of Perkell and Matthies (1992) acknowledges that the early onset of anticipatory coarticulation is due, in part, to a consonant specific lip-protrusion gesture. Lip gestures associated with consonants were in fact observed in /iC$_n$i/ utterances and were mostly due to consonant /s/. However, in /iC$_n$u/ utterances the correlations between the rounding movement interval and the duration of consonants were found to be significant also in utterances without /s/. Moreover, also the second-stage movement, i.e. the interval from the point of maximum acceleration to the acoustic onset of /u/ was not fixed as would be predicted by the hybrid model but tended to vary as a function of consonant duration (although the low values of the correlation coefficient R^2 – from 0.09 to 0.35 – indicate that the factor of consonant duration accounts for a rather small proportion of the variance). The conclusion of this study is that the timing and the kinematics of the lip protrusion gesture are the simultaneous expression of competing constraints, that of using a preferred gestural kinematics independently of the number of consonants (as in the time-locked model) and that of beginning the protrusion gesture as soon as it is allowed by the constraint that the preceding /i/ is unrounded (as in the look-ahead model). The one or the other constraint can prevail in different subjects and even within subjects across repetitions.

The movement expansion model

A new model of anticipatory coarticulation has been recently proposed by Abry and Lallouache (1995) for labial coarticulation in French. Preliminary results on lip kinematics (Abry and Lallouache 1991a, 1991b) in /iC$_5$y/ sequences of two words, with word boundary after C$_3$, indicated that the shape of lip movement was quite stable in the session where the subject had realized the word boundary, while in the session where the phrase had been produced as a whole (and at faster rate) the lip profiles were extremely variable and exhibited both one-stage and two-stage patterns. A detailed analysis of the stable profiles indicated that there is a first phase characterized by no movement (against the predictions of the look-ahead model) followed by a protrusion movement, whose duration is proportional to that of the consonantal interval (against the predictions of the coproduction and the hybrid model).

The corpus analysed for one subject by Lallouache and Abry (1992) and for three subjects by Abry and Lallouache (1995) consists of /iC$_n$y/ utterances with a varying number of consonants, as well as /iy/ utterances, with no consonants in between. The parameters were all the kinematic points and intervals proposed by Perkell, as well as measures of the protrusion amplitude. The overall results can be summarized as follows. First, the protrusion gesture is a one-phase movement; second, the maximum protrusion time tends to occur around the rounded vowel, i.e. the protrusion movements do not have a plateau-like shape; third, the protrusion interval as well as maximum acceleration and maximum velocity intervals correlate with the duration of consonants (the dispersion of data is much less than in Perkell and Matthies' study). Most importantly, the relation between these variables is better described by a hyperbolic function than by a linear function. This is because the protrusion movement tends to expand in longer consonant intervals but cannot be compressed in shorter intervals. In /iC_1y/ as well as in no-consonant /iy/ sequences the protrusion duration remains fixed at around 140–150 ms, indicating that the protrusion gesture heavily modifies the upper lip configuration of vowel /i/. Another finding is that there is much greater movement stability in shorter than in longer consonantal sequences. The temporal expansion of the movement does not mean that protrusion movement is linked to the unrounded vowel: it can start before, within or after it. The new model is speaker dependent and general at the same time: the amount of temporal expansion is in fact speaker specific, while the constraints on temporal compression are the same for every subject analysed (see chapter 6 for more details).

Summary and comments

The graphs in figure 2.7 illustrate the predictions of the look-ahead, the coproduction and the hybrid models, as applied to labial coarticulation. In the graphs V_1 is [− round], V_2 [+ round] and the number of unspecified consonants varies from four (left), to two (middle), to zero (right).

The first two rows show the patterns of anticipatory movements as predicted by featural phonology in terms of Keating's window model, where coarticulation may result either from language-specific phonological rules (manifested in the plateau-like patterns of the first row) or from phonetic interpolation (as shown, in the second row, by the trajectories directly linking the specified V_1 and V_2 across the unspecified segments). In the third row are the patterns predicted by the coproduction model: these patterns result from underlying competing vocalic gestures, whose spatio-temporal overlap increases as the temporal distance between the two vowels decreases. At the bottom is the pattern predicted by the hybrid model, where the duration of the protrusion movement, starting at the point of maximum acceleration, should remain invariant in the shorter sequences. The studies just reviewed (for both labial and velar coarticulation) indicate that, at large temporal distances between the two specified segments (left-hand panels), all the profiles predicted by the different models can occur in speech (see earlier for the

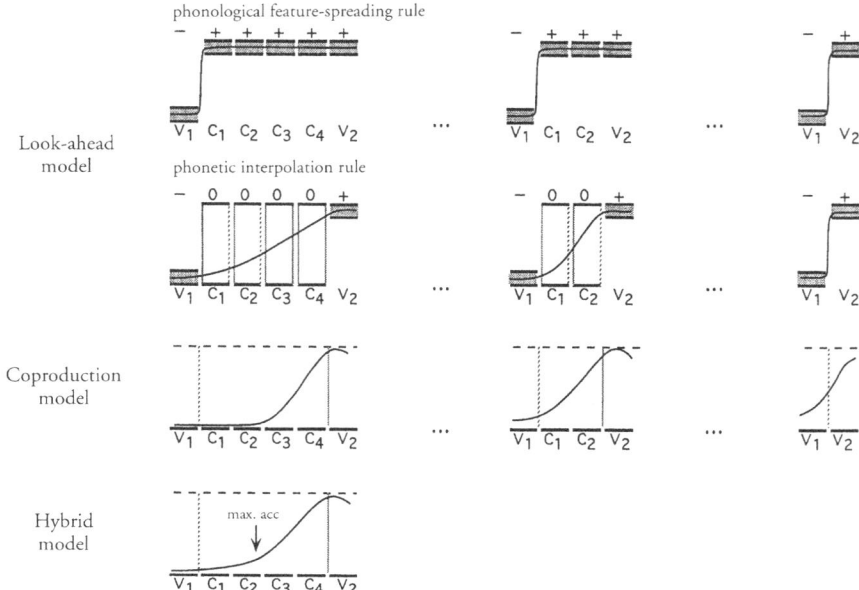

Figure 2.7   Anticipatory labial coarticulation: the predictions of the look-ahead model in terms of phonological feature-spreading rules and of phonetic rules of implementation and interpolation (first and second row respectively), the predictions of the coproduction model (third row) and of the hybrid model (bottom). From left to right: the [− *Round*] and the [+ *Round*] vowels are separated by four, two and zero consonants.

plateau patterns), even if very long interpolation patterns compatible with those of row two are not shown in the studies supporting the look-ahead model (as remarked above, the majority of these studies have analysed the timing rather than the trajectories of anticipatory movements). Moreover, the latest data on labial coarticulation (Abry and Lallouache 1995) show new movement patterns, incompatible with any of these three models. As things stand, none of the models in its strong version can account for the observed data, but models that allow expansion of the coarticulatory movements over long temporal intervals seem to offer a better account of the data than models preventing such expansion.

It can be seen that at shorter temporal intervals (e.g. in the two-consonant patterns shown in the central panels) the movement profiles are much more similar across the models. As the temporal interval decreases further (one consonant or no consonants between the vowels), the predictions are again quite different (see the right-hand panels). Feature-based models predict rapid transition movements between adjacent segments specified for contrastive features (rows one and two), while the coproduction model (row three) predicts an increase in gestural blending, resulting in an increase in anticipation of the protrusion movement within the unrounded vowel and a decrease in the movement displacement either in V_1 or V_2 or both. In other words, the observed movement from V_1 to V_2 is not temporally compressed at the shortest inter-vowel distances. Unfortunately, very few data on vowel sequences are available in the coarticulation literature: in their study of lip rounding in French, Benguerel and Cowan (1974) observed an increase in movement velocity between adjacent unrounded and rounded vowels as compared to VCV sequences and this seems to be consistent with the look-ahead hypothesis. The more systematic data of Abry and Lallouache, on the other hand, indicate that the protrusion movement does not differ, either in duration or velocity in V_1CV_2 sequences as compared to V_1V_2 sequences, and that its onset occurs within the unrounded vowel or even before it, in the shortest V_1V_2 sequences. From these data it appears that at short V_1V_2 distances the coproduction model accounts for the data better than other models. The data on velar coarticulation of Ushijima and Sawashima (1972) may also be compatible with this hypothesis.

To sum up, although some of the discrepancies among the results of the various studies can be attributed to different experimental methodologies and/or to individual differences in the speech rate or style, the overall data indicate that each of the models succeeds only partially in accounting for speakers' behaviour.

Conclusion and perspectives

The last thirty years of theoretical and experimental research have enormously improved our knowledge of the articulatory organization and the acoustic structure of speech, and have been a rich source of novel and challenging ideas. In the introduction we raised some fundamental issues which the different theories had to confront: what is coarticulation? why is it there? and how does it operate? The review shows that the core of the different answers, the real focus of debate, is the nature of the underlying cognitive units of speech, i.e. features versus gestures (and this, as mentioned in the introduction, is also the centre of the debate on the goal of the speaker).

Gestural phonology, whose dynamic units are allowed to *overlap* in time, gives an immediate and transparent account of coarticulatory variations as well as of variations due to stress, position, rate and speaking style. Phonetic gestures are lawfully reflected in the acoustic structure of speech, from which they are recovered by listeners.

According to featural phonology, the underlying units (be they specified by articulatory or by acoustic features) are timeless and cannot overlap. So coarticulation has a different origin and, according to Keating, it stems from phonetic *underspecification* and consequently cannot occur between specified segments, unless specification itself is allowed to be modulated.

Lindblom's theory is based on acoustic features, modelled as acoustic targets: coarticulation stems from *minimum displacement constraints* of the articulatory mechanism, i.e. from the principle of economy, which is at the basis of coarticulatory variations both in the movements connecting successive targets (as occurs for tongue body movements during the production of apical consonants) and in the targets themselves (i.e. duration-dependent target undershoot) when an articulator has to respond simultaneously to different, overlapping commands, as occurs in rapid, casual speech. For Lindblom the goal of the speaker is acoustic/perceptual and itself regulates production. Lindblom's hyper–hypo theory gives an elegant account of the relation between coarticulation, timing and speech style. Although the points of departure are completely different, the predictions of Lindblom's model on the relation between duration and target undershoot are compatible with those of gestural phonology on the relation between the amount of blending and the temporal distance separating the competing gestures.

We believe that analysis of the two aspects of coarticulation brought up in the introduction (i.e. anticipatory extent of coarticulation and gestural conflict) is still a valid test for inferring whether the underlying units are features or gestures. However, the models against which the data are to be confronted require improvements and changes. On the other hand, we cannot dismiss the provoking conclusion of Perkell and Matthies (1992) that speakers are subject to two coexisting and competing constraints: that of preserving their preferred gestural routines and that of breaking them up, by allowing movement onsets to be triggered by the relaxation of constraints associated with the ongoing segments. We can then ask if there can be a rationale behind these two competing production modes, i.e. when the one or the other emerges or tends to prevail (although Perkell and Matthies' data seem to be a random mixture of the two modes): the problem may be open to future research.

These years of experimental research have also led to the overturning of some of the tenets of traditional phonetics, e.g. of the binomial that equated graded changes with universal aspects of speech, and categorical changes with language-specific aspects. Today there is general agreement that graded spatio-temporal coarticulatory variations can also be language-specific. A related issue concerns connected speech processes, traditionally thought to be categorical (i.e. phonological): Lindblom (1963a) was the first to demonstrate the continuous nature of vowel reduction. Browman and Goldstein (1989) go further and propose that the majority of such processes are continuous and, like coarticulatory processes, do not imply changes in the categorical underlying units. This challenging hypothesis has stimulated a great deal of recent research on connected speech processes as well as on rate and boundary effects (see Farnetani 1997; and Künhert and Nolan, in this volume) and we can envisage that articulatory, acoustic and perceptual experiments on continuous speech and different speech styles will be among the main themes of research over the next years.

Acknowledgments

Our thanks to Michael Studdert-Kennedy and Bill Hardcastle for insightful comments and suggestions. This work was supported in part by ESPRIT/ACCOR, WG 7098.

Notes

1 Categorical vowel reduction refers to the phonological change of unstressed vowels to the neutral vowel schwa; continuous (or phonetic) vowel reduction has been traditionally regarded as vowel centralization, i.e. a tendency of vowel formants to shift towards a more central position within the acoustic vowel space. For ample reviews of the literature on vowel reduction see Fourakis (1991), Moon and Lindblom (1994).
2 The locus of a voiced stop followed by a vowel is defined by Lindblom as being at the first glottal pulse of the vowel, i.e. onset of the CV acoustic transition.
3 Only the Italian set of consonants included the labial /p/.
4 Multiple regression analysis indicated that the contribution of vowel category (high, mid and low) to formant variation was maximal for Fl and minimal for F2, whilst the effects of consonantal context (secondary articulations) were much higher on F2 than on Fl (Choi 1992: 37–39).
5 According to the authors, blending strength varies inversely with gestural sonority, a proposal compatible with Lindblom's concept of coarticulatory adaptability, which is maximal in vowels and minimal in lingual fricatives, in line with phonotactically based sonority categories (Lindblom 1983).
6 Velar lowering in American English low vowels in oral context had been observed in a number of other studies, e.g. in Clumeck (1976).

Part II
Research results: components of the motor system for speech

3

Velopharyngeal coarticulation

MICHEL CHAFCOULOFF and ALAIN MARCHAL

Introduction

Among the motor sub-systems for speech, the nasal sub-system plays an important part in speech communication, as the degree of oral–nasal coupling is partly responsible for the auditory quality of the human voice. Consequently, the knowledge of its coarticulatory effects in relation to the overall oral system has important implications in both theoretical and clinical research where the assessment of nasality is a crucial problem. There is much to be learned from studies dealing with defective coarticulatory patterns which result in excessive nasalization, distortion or substitution of sounds. Moreover, most speech production models that have been proposed so far are incomplete in that they often fail to take into account the interactions of the respiratory, phonatory and vocal tract components of the speech-producing mechanism. An examination of the coarticulatory relationship between the various sub-systems should allow assessment of the relevance of recently proposed theories on coarticulation and provide useful information for the development of a more complete speech production model.

In this chapter, the main physiological, acoustic and perceptual findings concerning the coarticulatory effects of nasality will be reviewed, with particular attention to its directional effects and its extent. Lastly, some suggestions for future research will be made in domains which, in our opinion, have not been sufficiently explored.

Coarticulatory effects of nasality

The study of nasal coarticulatory effects, or to put it differently, the spreading of the nasal feature onto adjacent segments, has involved the examination of two types of influence: a contextual effect, the influence of the nasal sound on other segment(s) and a directional effect, the direction and extent of nasality to other segment(s).

Influence of nasal sounds

Physiological evidence

Until the end of the eighteenth century, phonetic research had been of a qualitative nature and consequently few data were available concerning the influence of nasal sounds. With the introduction of the graphic method in the second part of the nineteenth century, evidence was obtained from the observation of kymographic records, that contextual evidence was working both ways, i.e. nasal consonants on vowel(s) and vice versa. From the examination of nasal tracings, Weeks (1893, cited in Scripture 1902) showed that in the English word 'banana', the last two vowels were strongly nasalized as a consequence of the presence of the neighbouring consonant /n/. In the beginning of the twentieth century, substantial information was gained concerning nasalization in other languages. For a review of this work, see Scripture (1902).

Later, X-ray cineradiography confirmed that nasal consonants had a contextual effect on vowel production. In the early 1960s, it was observed that the velum was in a lower position for vowels close to nasal consonants than for vowels in a non-nasal context (Dickson 1961; Moll 1962). This basic finding was further confirmed by other investigators using a combined cine-radiography–electromyography (EMG) technique (Lubker 1968) or through endoscopy (Ushijima and Sawashima 1972). Furthermore, it was found that nasality may also affect non-adjacent consonants (Moll and Daniloff 1971; Kent, Carney and Severeid 1974).

Concerning the influence of vowel environment on nasal consonants, the occurrence of a rounded /n/ allophone in the sequence 'since true' was found by Daniloff and Moll (1968). In agreement with earlier X-ray data collected by Harrington (1944), it was observed through cineradiography (Moll and Shriner 1967) and endoscopy (Bell-Berti *et al.* 1979) that the velum was higher for nasal consonants in a close-vowel context than in an open-vowel context.

Taken together, these results suggest that there is a strong interaction between oral and nasal sounds. Bladon and Nolan (1977) rank nasals among sounds with the lowest degree of coarticulatory resistance.

Acoustic evidence

Compared to the extensive amount of available physiological data, there is a relative lack of acoustic data on nasal sounds. There are several possible explanations. The acoustic study of the influence of vowels on consonants has been achieved using such different analysis techniques as spectrography, analysis-by-synthesis and sweep-tone measurements. Noticeable frequency shifts of nasal resonances and anti-resonances in consonant spectra were found in several languages, e.g. American English (Fujimura 1962), French (Delattre 1954), Russian (Fant 1960) and Swedish (Fant 1973). Moreover, Su, Li and Fu (1974) showed that the consonant /m/ was more sensitive to the vocalic environment than /n/ because of the greater freedom of the tongue to antici-pate the vowel position.

The contextual influence of nasal consonants on vowel formant frequen-cies was even more difficult to assess. Stevens and House (1963) did not include nasal consonants in their study because of the difficulty of measuring the acoustic modifications due to the changes of the consonantal place of articulation and to the intrinsic oral/nasal coupling of the various vowels. Instead, investigators have focused on the vowel onset/offset frequencies as cues for detecting nasal consonants in the applied domain of automatic speech recognition (Mermelstein 1977; Gubrynowicz 1983).

Lastly, still more problematic was the analysis of nasal vowels in languages where the oral/nasal opposition is distinctive. As most of the investigations were based on the use of spectrography (e.g. Delattre 1954, for French and de Lacerda and Head 1963, for Portuguese), conflicting data often resulted from these descriptive studies. Later, more reliable information on the spectral char-acteristics of nasal vowels was collected in French by means of a multiple anal-ysis procedure (Lonchamp 1978) and through the simulation of the pole-zero pairs (Maeda 1984; Feng 1986). However, most of this work concerns isolated vowels or vowels occurring in a single consonantal context. No acoustic study concerning the contextual influence of nasal vowels has been conducted so far.

Perceptual evidence

Most of the research on the perception of nasal coarticulatory effects has focused on the influence of the vocalic environment on nasal consonants. Concerning /m, n, ŋ/, it was generally agreed that two cues, i.e. formant tran-sitions and nasal murmurs, were mainly responsible for the identification of these sounds. In seeking to determine the vowel contextual influence, several investigators have used either synthetic speech (Liberman *et al.* 1954) or natural speech (Kuehn and Moll 1972; Repp 1986a) to demonstrate that formant transitions are perceptually more salient in a low-vowel context than in a high-vowel context. According to Sharf and Ohde (1981) this trend can be ascribed to the fact that low vowels have a greater intrinsic intensity. The importance of the nature of the adjacent vowel on the consonant's perception was confirmed by Zee (1981). In an experiment on the effect of vowel quality, he used natural speech signals with different signal-to-noise ratios to demon-strate that, whereas /m/ and /n/ are often misidentified after the front vowels

/i/ and /e/, the same consonants are correctly perceived after the vowel /a/ even in the noisiest conditions. However, it should be pointed out that, in addition to the intensity factor, the spacing of formant transitions, may play an important part as well. Sussman, McCaffrey and Matthews (1991) and Sussman, Hoemeke and McCaffrey (1992) have shown a high correlation between the locus equation coefficients and consonant place of articulation. Among other things, it was demonstrated that, whereas the place-dependent transitions for any manner of consonant (nasal or stop) are very much alike near /i/ (this being also true for labials and velars near /u/), formant transitions are clearly separated close to /a/.

Carlson, Grandstrom and Pauli (1972) reported an inverse relationship in terms of vowel contextual influence. In a perceptual experiment based on synthetic stimuli, they found that the perceptual relevance of the nasal murmur Fn2 was greater in a high-vowel context for the nasal consonants /m, n/ in Swedish. Further evidence of this interactive influence was provided by Abramson *et al.* (1981) who demonstrated through articulatory synthesis that, in American English, the perceptual boundary along an acoustic continuum /d–n/ shifted as a function of the adjacent vowel height.

At this point, attention should be drawn to the fact that results obtained from speech synthesis experiments do not necessarily extrapolate to real speech. To explain some of the phenomena which may give rise to distinctive nasality, Kawasaki (1986) used natural utterances to test the perceptual hypothesis of Hyman (1975), according to which the phenomenon of denasalization leads to the reinforcement of the perceived contrast between oral and nasal vowels. For this purpose, the amplitude level of the initial and final nasal consonants of the syllables /mɪm, mam, mum/ was reduced gradually in relation to the vowel nucleus. Results show that the stimuli with the vowel /i/ are perceived as less nasal than those with the vowels /a/ and /u/. Moreover, in accordance with the predicted theory, the degree of perceived nasality of a vowel is enhanced by the reduction of the adjacent nasal consonant's amplitude. Conversely, the presence of a nasal consonant does favour the perceived nasality of the neighbouring vowel. This finding validates not only Hyman's hypothesis, but also gives credit to Trager's earlier remark that 'nasal vowels are most nasalized when they are not adjacent to a nasal consonant' (Trager 1971: 31). This experiment contributes to establishing a strict dichotomy between physiological nasalization and perceptual nasalization.

The effect of the consonantal environment on vowel perception was investigated further by Krakow *et al.* (1988) who examined the influence of a consonantal nasal and non-nasal context on perceived vowel height. The experiment showed that the perception of the height dimension of nasalized vowels was dependent not only on their spectral characteristics but also on the adjacent consonantal context. In a related study, Krakow and Beddor (1991) tested the effects of different oral, nasal and null contexts on the perception of vowel nasality. The results showed that listeners were less accurate at judging a vowel as nasal in an appropriate N–N context than in an inappropriate C–C (where C = a non-nasal consonant) or #–# context. Thus, in agreement with the results obtained by Kawasaki (1986), it is suggested that the presence of a contiguous nasal consonant did not necessarily favour the perception of vowel nasality.

Viewed as a whole, the results obtained in these experiments suggest that perceptual effects of formant transitions, nasal murmurs and vowel height are strongly context dependent and that there exists a complex interaction between oral and nasal sounds at the perceptual level (for a comprehensive review of perceived vowel nasality in various phonetic contexts, see Beddor 1993).

Direction and extent of nasal coarticulation

Once it had been established that nasal sounds were strongly coarticulated with adjacent segments, the question was raised as to the direction in which nasality produced its greatest effects. In other words, which type of coarticulation, anticipatory or carryover, prevailed in the spreading of nasality to neighbouring units? An issue which is closely related to this question and which is crucial for the evaluation of coarticulation models concerns the extent of nasal coarticulation. This issue may be broken down into several specific questions.

Are the coarticulatory effects of nasality limited to adjacent sounds? Does this influence extend to other units across syllable and word boundaries or higher order syntactic boundaries? Are nasal coarticulatory effects time-locked or do they vary as a function of the number of phonetic units? Lastly, are nasal coarticulation effects perceptually salient?

Physiological evidence
Anticipatory coarticulation
Concerning the spreading of nasality, noticeable anticipatory effects were found through direct observation of velum movements by X-ray cineradiography (Moll and Daniloff 1971), oral endoscopy (Benguerel *et al.* 1977a; Bell-Berti 1980), measurement of the EMG activity of the levator palatini muscle (Ushijima and Hirose 1974; Benguerel *et al.* 1977b) and measurement of the level of nasal sound pressure (Clarke and Mackiewicz-Krassowska 1977).

Concerning the extent of coarticulation, it was found that anticipatory coarticulation was not limited to a single adjacent sound but could affect several preceding segments. Moll and Daniloff (1971) showed that in a CVVn sequence, the opening of the velopharyngeal port may be initiated as early as the first consonant. This observation, valid for the English language, was also found to apply to French (Benguerel *et al.* 1977a).

As to the effect of juncture boundaries on the extent of coarticulation, it was found that nasal coarticulation was not hindered by syllabic or word boundaries in several languages, including American English (Moll and Daniloff 1971; McClean 1973), French (Benguerel *et al.* 1977a) or Hindi (Dixit and MacNeilage 1972). In contrast it was reported that in Japanese, the presence of a syllabic boundary may prevent the spreading of nasality to preceding segments (Ushijima and Sawashima 1972). However, conflicting data have often been obtained for the effects of syllabic junctures and marked/unmarked word boundaries. Much of this controversy probably stems from the fact that different languages, speakers, instrumental procedures and utterances have been used. Obviously, additional information is needed in this domain.

Carryover coarticulation

It has been demonstrated by means of various instrumental techniques, that nasal carryover coarticulation can have a noticeable effect in various languages. In spite of difficulty assessing its temporal extent through electromyographic measurement, Lubker (1968) showed in a combined EMG-X-ray study of American English that an /a/ followed by an /m/ was characterized by a lower activity of the levator palatini (correlated with a lower velar height) than an /a/ uttered in isolation.

Such a progressive nasal effect was also found in Japanese by Ushijima and Hirose (1974) and in French by Benguerel *et al.* (1977b) who reported a minimal effect of this type. This effect was also found by Bonnot *et al.* (1980) who showed that the latency of the levator palatini varied as a function of the duration of the consonantal segment, i.e. simple versus geminate.

Through aerometry and the examination of airflow traces, a nasal lag was found on the fricative segment in nasal–fricative clusters (Ali, Daniloff and Hammarberg 1979). By means of dynamic electropalatography, Recasens (1984) showed that in Catalan, the alveolo-palatal consonant /ɲ/ was subject to greater carryover effects from V_1 than anticipatory effects from V_2. Lastly, using the latter technique simultaneously with aerometry, Farnetani (1986b) found that in Italian, the nasality from the consonant /n/ extended more into the following vowel than into the preceding one.

To conclude, most investigators agree that nasal carryover coarticulation is essentially due to the mechano-inertial properties of the velopharyngeal system, thus confirming the earlier speculations of Daniloff and Hammarberg (1973).

Acoustic evidence

Detecting the onset/offset of nasality through the examination of spectral changes has always been a major problem in acoustic research (Fant 1960). Consequently, few studies have been undertaken to compare the effects of anticipatory versus carryover coarticulation.

Concerning the spectral characteristics of the consonant /m/ in various vowel environments, Su, Daniloff and Hammarberg (1975) showed that there is a close relationship between higher level boundaries and the concomitant reduction of anticipatory effects.

In spectral studies, Stevens and House (1963) and Öhman (1966) showed that in CVC syllables, the initial consonant had a greater effect on the medial vowel than the final consonant, suggesting a stronger carryover coarticulatory influence. This finding was confirmed by Schouten and Pols (1979b) who examined the effect in Dutch of variable vowel environment(s) on the initial and final second-formant frequencies in an /n/ context. In accordance with the results obtained in earlier experiments, they found a greater consonantal effect on the vowel in CV units than in VC units.

Using an acoustic method aimed at measuring 'nasalance', i.e. the ratio of the sound intensity radiated at the lips to that radiated at the nose, Flege (1988) determined the duration of vowel nasalization before and after the /n/ sound. His study showed that, contrary to some expectations based on prior physiological evidence (Moll and Daniloff 1971), the extent of nasal carryover coarticulation is greater than that of anticipatory coarticulation at both normal and fast speech rates.

Using the Kay Elemetrics Nasometer, Rochet and Rochet (1991) compared assimilation patterns in French and English as a function of vowel height. In both languages, high vowels exhibited more assimilating nasality than low vowels. A comparison of the proportional carryover and anticipatory coarticulation effects revealed important differences across languages. Whereas anticipatory effects prevailed in English, greater carryover effects were found in French but these applied to high vowels only and not to low ones. In general, French showed less assimilating nasality than English, which was attributed to the fact that English does not have phonemic nasal vowels and thus can tolerate higher levels of assimilating nasality.

Perceptual evidence

Most perceptual studies have concentrated on determining the effects of nasal anticipatory coarticulation as an additional cue to the perception of contiguous segments. In various studies on natural speech, it was demonstrated that anticipatory coarticulatory effects were used by the listener for the perception of both nasal/nasalized vowels and nasal consonants.

Using a tape-splicing procedure, Malécot (1960) found that in American English, a vowel was still perceived as nasalized even when the following nasal consonant was completely cut out. Such perceptual effects were also observed in French by Benguerel and Lafargue (1981) who showed that the degree of perceived nasalization increased with the opening of the velopharyngeal port, and that the perception of nasal quality was the result of some temporal integration.

Concerning the identification of nasal consonants, it was shown that spliced nasals in final position could be predicted from the information encoded in the preceding vowel (Ali *et al.* 1971). Further evidence about the greater magnitude of anticipatory versus carryover effects was provided by Ostreicher and Sharf (1976). In a study on the influence of consonants on vowel perception and vice versa, /m, n/ were presented in various syllabic utterances and deleted using a tape-erasing procedure. The results revealed higher identification scores from the preceding sounds than from the following ones, especially in a high-vowel context; this supported prior evidence obtained through vocal analogue simulation (House and Stevens 1956).

As to the extent of perceptible coarticulated nasality, the anticipatory influence was shown to extend over more than one sound beyond a word or syllabic boundary. Kuehn and Moll (1972) demonstrated that initial /m, n/ sounds could be predicted above chance level with various silent intervals between the consonant and the final segment of a carrier phrase. In a related study, Sharf and Ostreicher (1973) showed that, while coarticulated nasality may extend perceptually across syllable boundaries, its influence can be hindered by one or two intervening sounds.

However these findings, which attest to the reality of perceptual anticipatory effects in natural speech conditions, have not been corroborated in experiments on synthesized speech. In a pioneering study on formant transitions as perceptual cues (Liberman *et al.* 1954) and later in a study on categorical perception (Larkey, Wald and Strange 1978), synthetic stimuli were used in an identification task of /m, n, ŋ/ in final position. By reversing the tape, syllable-final consonants were heard as syllable-initial consonants. In general, no significant differences in the identification scores were found between the original stimuli and their backward versions, which implies that for these authors neither directional influence prevails. Yet Kuwahara and Sakai (1972) have found evidence of the importance of both directional effects on the identification of nasal consonants in different syllabic units in Japanese. Lastly, in connection with previously collected acoustic data, Maturi (1991) has examined the perceptual relevance of nasality in Italian. Results of various experiments based on the inversion of the final vowel in natural sequences lead to the following conclusions:

- the perception of the nasality–non-nasality feature in the consonantal opposition /n/–/d/ and /m/–/b/ is affected by the presence/absence of the same feature in the following vowel;
- the nasality feature has not the same perceptual weight for vowels and consonants as it appears to be more important for the former speech sounds than the latter, at least in this language.

Future directions

Certain aspects of nasal coarticulation research have received more attention than others. In the following section, we shall attempt to point out some of the most apparent weaknesses in past research. We shall emphasize the gaps which in our opinion need to be filled and make some suggestions for future research.

Acoustics

It is evident that there is a definite imbalance between the considerable amount of physiological data gathered by means of various instrumental techniques and the relative scarcity of presently available acoustic data. This imbalance is probably due to the fact that for many years it was easier to interpret articulatory data than acoustic data. With the improvement of acoustic methods for detecting nasality, fast progress should be made in this domain as there is a need for reliable data in applications such as text-to-speech synthesis, automatic speech recognition and speaker identification. Inconsistent findings about nasal coarticulatory effects are often due to differences in measurement techniques and more particularly to the use of physiologically invasive techniques as opposed to acoustic non-invasive techniques. Whenever it is possible, data from studies using different measurement techniques should be brought together to assess the relevance of the results obtained.

Spontaneous speech

Investigators have generally used nonsense utterances embedded in a carrier phrase or sometimes minimally contrastive contexts to study the effects of nasal coarticulation. Although such carefully controlled conditions are necessary to investigate the separate effects of a given contextual environment, it nevertheless remains true that results originating in such studies are only valid for so-called laboratory speech and not for everyday speech. Following the recommendations of several authors (Kohler 1990; Keating 1991; Nolan 1992), there has been a renewed interest in the study of connected speech in the past few years. From the analysis of stimuli excised from a two-hour conversation in French, Duez (1995) has reported that the oral voiced stop /d/ was perceived as the nasal homorganic consonant /n/ due to the presence of one or more adjacent nasal vowel(s) or a close nasal consonant. In a preliminary study of connected speech in Hindi, Ohala (1996) has noticed the presence of epenthetic nasals at the junction between a word-final vowel and a following word-initial voiced stop, thus confirming previous findings (Ohala and Ohala 1991). Moreover, she reported that the velar nasal /ŋ/ may be frequently produced as a glide with an incomplete oral closure.

Although acoustic data remain scarce in the present state of phonetic research, there is no doubt that the study of the acoustic structure of nasal sounds in more natural speech conditions will be a noteworthy asset in the understanding of the diachronic process of sound changes.

Suprasegmentals

Most investigators have focused on the importance of segmental factors as it has been shown that the nasal feature may extend its influence to other phonemic units through anticipatory or carryover coarticulation. Comparatively speaking, the effects of suprasegmental factors such as stress or speech rate have received little attention, yet evidence has been provided from the analysis of CVn utterances that velum height and velocity, as well as the timing of velum gestures, may differ in stressed or unstressed environments (Vaissière 1988). Moreover, significant differences in nasalization duration have been reported as a function of normal versus fast speaking rate (Flege 1988). These findings are important, for they imply that velum movement patterns, and hence the extent of nasalization, may be enhanced or reduced in accordance with suprasegmental factors.

Similarly, it has been reported for several languages that velum height may vary as a function of word position, being in fact at its highest in word-initial rather than in word-final position (Ohala 1975; Fujimura 1977). This finding was more recently confirmed by Krakow (1986). It might be that such positional target values would not be found across syllable or word boundaries, if speech rate and stress conditions varied, and that the extent of nasal coarticulation would be different across languages, as demonstrated by Solé and Ohala (1991).

Although valuable information has been gathered recently in this domain, the influence of suprasegmental factors on the spreading of nasalization represents a large field of investigation which remains largely unexplored in many languages. This issue will no doubt arouse the interest of researchers in the years to come.

Languages

As early as the mid-sixties, Öhman (1966) noticed that coarticulation might be different across languages, since minimal V-to-V coarticulatory effects were found in Russian. Later, it was found that this observation also applied to nasal coarticulation, as Clumeck (1976) observed early velum lowering in American English and Brazilian Portuguese, whereas lowering was initiated later in French, Chinese, Swedish and Hindi. Concerning this latter language, Clumeck's opinion conflicts with Ohala's view. She reports an early lowering of the velum in the process of nasalization of vowels in Hindi (Ohala 1974). From the examination of nasographic tracings, she showed that velic opening is about the same for 'distinctive nasalization' and 'nondistinctive nasalization'; nasalization may extend across several segmental units, thus confirming the previous findings of Dixit and MacNeilage (1972); word boundaries may have a different delaying effect on the anticipatory velic opening across languages, e.g. noticeable differences were observed with English (Ohala 1971); nasalization is predominantly anticipatory in Hindi, a fact which supports the claim that in general a preceding nasal consonant is less influential in affecting the nasalization of the vowel than a following nasal.

This varying degree of nasal anticipatory coarticulation has been explained in terms of perceptual distinctiveness. The amount of coarticulation in a language is constrained by the need to maintain a distinction between vowels and thus varies inversely with the number of vowels in the language. Although cross-linguistic studies on nasal coarticulatory effects are of great interest in the field of applied linguistics (Delattre 1951) and in the search for perceptual correlates in the non-nasal/nasal distinction of vowels as in the comparative study of American English and Gujarati by Hawkins and Stevens (1985), few contrastive studies are found in the literature.

Lately, there has been a renewal of interest in this type of study for several languages, i.e. American English versus Hindi (Henderson 1984), American English versus French, (Rochet and Rochet 1991), American English versus Spanish (Solé 1992). Nevertheless, the fact remains that additional comparative research about nasal coarticulatory patterns is still needed in several other languages and especially those in which nasality has a distinctive function, as in French and Portuguese.

4

Lingual coarticulation

DANIEL RECASENS

Introduction

The review of lingual coarticulation presented here is organized with reference to different vowel and consonant gestures. A rationale for this methodological approach is that a specific lingual region may exhibit different coarticulatory behaviours depending on its involvement in gestural production. Thus, for example, the tongue blade should be more resistant to coarticulatory effects during the production of dentoalveolar consonants than of velar consonants since it participates actively in the formation of a dentoalveolar closure or constriction. Coarticulatory sensitivity for a given lingual region will be shown to depend not only on place and manner of articulation requirements but also on mechanical restrictions such as flexibility and coupling with other lingual regions.

A goal of this study is to approach the problem of articulatory control in speech production. Our hypothesis is that the degree of coarticulatory variability exhibited by a given tongue region is in many respects indicative of the degree of control exerted upon it by the speaker: thus, an increase in articulatory control should cause a decrease in coarticulatory sensitivity. It seems that in some cases we must neutralize the influence of possible mechanical constraints in order to draw significant inferences about articulatory control; thus, a given tongue region may be resistant to coarticulatory effects just because it happens to be coupled with a primary articulator (e.g. the tongue predorsum during the production of laminal stops). The data reviewed here have been collected using different techniques for articulatory analysis (electropalatography, cineradiography, electromyography), and occasionally using acoustic analysis as well. Our terminology for the articulatory zones and for the lingual regions is consistent with that proposed by Catford

(1977); a close correspondence obtains between the two, namely, tip and blade and alveolar zone, predorsum and prepalate, mediodorsum and medio-palate, postdorsum and postpalate, and tongue root and pharynx.

This chapter takes a view of coarticulation as temporal coproduction of gestures. This view works quite successfully for independent articulatory structures (i.e. lips, tongue and velum) but less so for specific tongue regions; in fact, while the tongue tip, the tongue blade and the tongue dorsum clearly behave as different articulators (and thus one can refer to apical, laminal and dorsal gestures), it is not clear whether the tongue dorsum ought to be treated as a single articulator or as a multiarticulatory structure involving separate predorsal and mediodorsal activation. Moreover, a distinction should probably be made between coarticulation proper and gestural overlap: inspection of articulatory data reveals, for example, that the gesture for a vowel may coarticulate slightly with that for a following consonant before the well-defined onset of the consonantal gesture actually occurs. Unfortunately much of the data reported in the literature have been taken at individual points in time along particular utterances and thus, do not allow disentangling these two notions.

Spatial variability

A lingual gesture can undergo articulatory changes as a function of other lingual gestures for adjacent phonetic segments. This section reviews context-dependent effects in lingual activity during the production of lingual gestures for vowels and consonants.

Vowels

Front vowels

The vowel [i] allows little tongue dorsum variability (Hoole, Gfroerer and Tillmann 1990), presumably since the tongue body becomes highly constrained when fronted and raised simultaneously. This vowel is more resistant to consonant-dependent coarticulation in F2 frequency than most vowels in several languages (Catalan: Recasens 1985; Dutch: Pols 1977; American English: Stevens and House 1963).

A variability minimum occurs at regions which are directly involved in the formation of the vowel constriction, either at the mediodorsum (American English: Perkell and Nelson 1985; Catalan: Recasens 1991a) or at the blade (Japanese: Kiritani *et al.* 1977). These literature sources report the existence of more variability at regions located behind the constriction, which is in agreement with [i] undergoing raising and fronting of the back of the tongue dorsum surface under the influence of an adjacent velar (MacNeilage and DeClerk 1969; Kiritani *et al.* 1977; Alfonso and Horiguchi 1987). A decrease in palatal contact for the vowel is caused by some consonants, presumably because of manner requirements associated with their production: apicoalveolar lateral [l] (Ohala and Kawasaki 1979; Farnetani and Recasens 1993), especially if velarized (Catalan: Recasens 1991a); apicoalveolar trill [r] (Recasens 1991b); alveolar fricatives (Farnetani and Recasens 1993), even though [i] may not show a deep tongue dorsum grooving in this consonantal environment (Stone *et al.* 1992). Articulatory and acoustic data (F1 raising and F2 lowering effects) indicate that [i] undergoes tongue dorsum lowering and retraction when adjacent to velarized consonants (Russian: Kuznetsov and Ott 1987) and pharyngealized consonants (Arabic: Al-Ani 1970; Ghazeli 1977; Yeou 1995).

Coarticulatory effects at the palatal zone appear to increase with a decrease in dorsopalatal constriction width for front vowels of different height in the progression [i]>[e]>[ɛ] (see Recasens 1991a for some palatographic evidence).

Back vowels

The tongue body shows considerable context-dependent variability for back vowels (Perkell and Cohen 1989; Hoole, Gfroerer and Tillmann 1990). Concerning [a], dentoalveolar and alveolopalatal consonants cause some raising and stretching of the tongue dorsum and blade (Gay 1974, 1977; Recasens 1991a) while velars cause considerable tongue postdorsum raising (MacNeilage and DeClerk 1969; Kiritani *et al.* 1977). High vocalic F2 frequencies suggest that palatal and palatalized dentoalveolars exert tongue dorsum raising effects on [a] (Recasens 1985; Kuznetsov and Ott 1987).

Dental, alveolar, alveolopalatal and palatal consonants cause some tongue dorsum stretching and some raising of the tongue tip and blade during the production of the labial vowels [u] and [o] (Butcher and Weiher 1976; Kiritani *et al.* 1977; Alfonso and Horiguchi 1987; Recasens 1991a). A high F2 frequency for those vowels with adjacent palatalized dentoalveolars (Kuznetsov and Ott 1987) suggests that a similar lingual coarticulatory mechanism is at work in this case. Tongue fronting during the production of labial vowels in the vicinity of dentoalveolars may take place in order to facilitate the lip protrusion gesture.

Recent ultrasound data reveal groove formation along the tongue dorsum surface for low and mid back vowels as a function of adjacent lingual fricatives and [l] (Stone *et al.* 1992).

Schwa and lax vowels

The absence of obvious articulatory requirements upon the formation of a lingual constriction for [ə] explains why the tongue body is highly variable during the production of this vowel. Electropalatographic data on C-to-V coarticulation for [ə] show lingual contact at the centre and/or sides of the palate surface extending until the alveolar zone in the vicinity of dental and alveolar consonants, until the prepalatal zone with adjacent alveolopalatals and palatals, and along the mediopalatal zone with adjacent velarized [ɫ], velars and labials.

F2 data reported by Stevens and House (1963) indicate that lax vowels (e.g. English [ɪ], [ʌ]) are more sensitive than tense vowels to consonant-dependent coarticulatory effects which may be said to conform to durational and articulatory differences between the two sets of sounds (i.e. in comparison to their tense correlates, lax vowels are shorter and are produced with more neutral articulatory configurations, Perkell 1969).

Discussion

Data reported in this section provide good evidence for large coarticulatory effects at tongue regions not intervening directly in the formation of a vowel constriction. It would be, however, premature to interpret this finding in support of the hypothesis stating that articulatory control for vowels is exerted upon specific constriction locations (such as palatal, velar, upper pharyngeal and lower pharyngeal, Wood 1979) rather than upon entire tongue body configurations (high front, high back, mid back and low back, Perkell 1969). One problem is that we do not know how much variability in lingual activity is allowed at the assumed constriction locations and thus, for example, whether low vowels allow larger or smaller coarticulatory effects in tongue root fronting than in tongue dorsum raising. Some scant data (for [a] in Perkell and Nelson 1985; for [u] in Hoole, Gfroerer and Tillmann 1990) suggest that lingual variability around the constriction locations is less than at other tongue regions and are thus in support of the constriction-dependent hypothesis of articulatory control for vowels.

Unconstricted tongue regions may exhibit different degrees of articulatory variability because they are subject to mechanico-inertial requirements of unequal strength; thus, larger coarticulatory effects at the tongue front for back vowels than at the tongue back for front vowels may be related to the former lingual region being less constrained than the latter in this case. Articulatory compatibility plays a role as well; the fact that the tongue dorsum must achieve a certain height in order to allow for the formation of a front lingual constriction may explain why consonants such as [s] exert larger coarticulatory effects on [a] than on [i].

Another issue which deserves further investigation is the coarticulatory outcome of conflicting lingual gestures; it has been shown in this respect that

[i] is sensitive to consonant-dependent effects in tongue predorsum lowering and tongue body retraction. Another research topic is whether vowels articulated with two lingual regions are resistant to coarticulatory effects because of being subject to high control requirements (e.g. pharyngealized vowels in Caucasian languages and vowels produced with tongue root activation in West African languages, Ladefoged and Maddieson 1990).

Consonants

The production of consonants requires the formation of a closure or one or two constrictions (Perkell 1969). Alveolopalatal and palatal consonants are treated here as non-complex segments involving a lamino-predorsal gesture (as opposed to two gestures, i.e. laminal and dorsal). Coarticulatory effects on the activity of the primary articulator may depend on the following factors.

Articulatory flexibility

Differences in coarticulatory sensitivity among primary lingual articulators may be associated with their being more or less flexible when performing articulatory movements.

Concerning dentoalveolar consonants, laminal fricatives ([s], [z], [ʃ] and [ʒ]) appear to be more resistant than apicals ([t], [d], [n] and [l]): while laminals do not usually allow tongue tip raising effects from adjacent apical consonants, apicals tend to become laminal when adjacent to laminals (British English, Bladon and Nolan 1977). These English data have been corroborated by reports on vowel-dependent variability at the tongue front for consonants in other languages: the degree of variability usually decreases in the progression [n] > [l] > [d] > [t] > [s] (German: Hoole, Gfroerer and Tillmann 1990; Kühnert *et al.* 1991). Catalan electropalatographic data in figure 4.1 reveal indeed lesser vowel coarticulation at the place of articulation for lingual fricatives than for [n] and [ɬ]. The apicoalveolar tap [ɾ] is also highly sensitive to coarticulatory effects at the place of articulation (Japanese: Sudo, Kiritani and Yoshioka 1982; Catalan: Recasens 1991b). Articulatory flexibility is probably related to manner requirements: while laterality and rothacism favour apical activation, laminal activation facilitates the intraoral pressure build up for oral stops and the formation of a lingual constriction for the passage of airflow for fricatives. Specific coarticulatory effects in apicolaminal activity for dentoalveolars are characterized later.

Laminodorsal and dorsal consonants are more resistant than apical and laminal consonants to vowel-dependent effects at the place of articulation, namely, at the alveolo-prepalatal zone for the former (usually [ɲ] and [ʎ]) and at the palatal zone for the latter (often [j]) (Catalan: Recasens 1984b; American English: Kent and Moll 1972a). This trend is shown for [ɲ] in figures 4.1 and 4.2. The American English dorsopalatal approximant [r] undergoes fronting and backing effects at the tongue dorsum sides (as a function of front versus back vowels) but is quite resistant to coarticulation in constriction width (Miyawaki 1972; Zawadzki and Kuehn 1980; Dagenais, Lorendo and McCutcheon 1994). Considerable coarticulatory resistance for laminodorsal and dorsal consonants should be partly attributed to their involving a large closure or constriction with a sluggish tongue dorsum articulator.

Interarticulatory coordination, coupling and antagonism
Coarticulatory trends at the place of dentoalveolar articulation are often conditioned by tongue dorsum positioning. Closure location for English alveolar [t] may be fairly front when the tongue dorsum is lowered with adjacent [a] and more laminal and retracted when the tongue dorsum is raised with adjacent [i]; on the other hand, Italian apicodental [t] is highly resistant to such vowel-dependent coarticulatory effects, presumably because it is articulated further away from the tongue dorsum (Farnetani, Hardcastle and Marchal 1989). As shown in figures 4.1 and 4.2, Catalan [n] shows a fronted laminoalveolar closure when the tongue dorsum is raised (for [ini]) and a retracted apicoalveolar closure when the tongue dorsum is either lowered and/or retracted (for [ana] and/or [unu]) (Recasens, Fontdevila and Pallarès 1992). Apical consonants [r] (Sudo, Kiritani and Yoshioka 1982; Recasens 1991b) and non-velarized [l] (German: Recasens, Fontdevila and Pallarès 1995b) also become more laminal and show more alveolar contact with adjacent [i] versus [a], [u].

Figures 4.1 and 4.2 also confirm the fact that front fricatives [s], [z], [ʃ] and [ʒ] may exhibit a narrower constriction at the place of articulation when the tongue dorsum is raised in the vicinity of [i] versus [a] and [u] (Australian English: Clark, Palethorpe and Hardcastle 1982; Italian: Faber 1989; Swedish: Engstrand 1989). Their constriction location is usually quite stable across contextual conditions.

In some instances the tongue front articulator is required to adopt a certain configuration in order not to interfere with the activity of the tongue dorsum. The Hindi retroflex stop [ʈ] is produced at the alveolar zone in the context of back vowels and at the dentoalveolar zone in the context of [i], presumably because the curling back of the tongue front for the execution of the consonant is hard to reconcile with the simultaneous raising of the tongue dorsum (Dixit 1990; Dixit and Flege 1991). Examples of articulatory repositioning due to gestural antagonism in consonant clusters are given later.

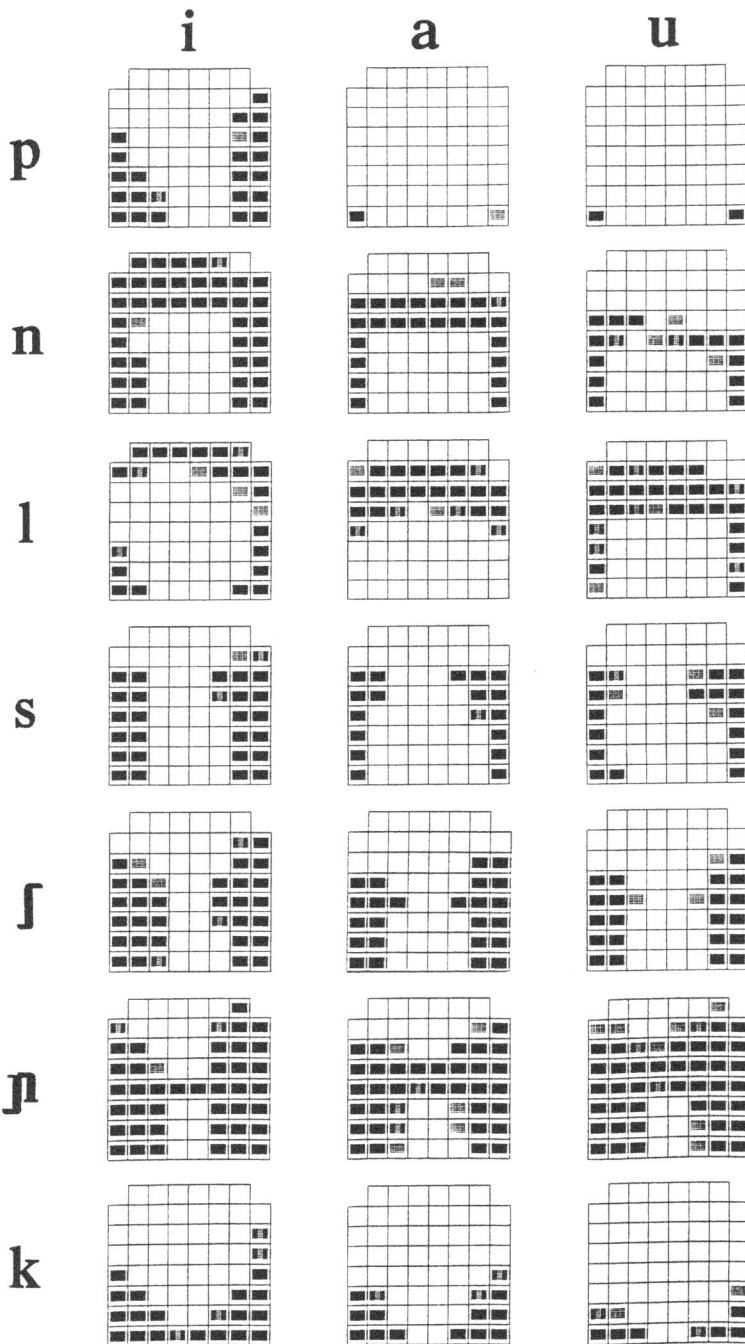

An interaction between lingual activity and labial activity may occur when both articulatory structures intervene simultaneously in the production of a given phonetic segment. Thus, tongue fronting at the constriction location for [s] in the sequence [usu] may be associated with vowel-related effects in lip protrusion (Italian: Faber 1989; American English: Carney and Moll 1971).

Blending
Two adjacent segments produced at neighbouring tongue regions may be realized by means of a single gesture at an intermediate articulatory location (Browman and Goldstein 1989). In Catalan, the sequence composed of dental [t] and following alveolar [n] may be realized at the juncture between the teeth and the alveolar ridge ([dn]), and the cluster composed of [ʃ] and following [s] is realized as a palatalized laminoalveolar fricative ([ʃʲʃʲ], [ʃʲ]). Progressive temporal overlap between the front constriction for word final [s] and the back constriction for following word initial [j] results in intermediate centroid values falling over the course of the fricative (Zsiga 1995); a similar finding has been reported by Nolan, Holst and Kühnert (1996) for the sequence [sʃ] in British English.

Velar consonants are realized at the medio-postpalatal zone before [i] and other front vowels (American English: Kent and Moll 1972a; MacNeilage and DeClerk 1969; Swedish: Öhman 1966); EPG data for the Catalan speakers in figures 4.1 and 4.2 reveal indeed that the dorsal closure for [k] is more fronted when the consonant is adjacent to [i] than to [a] and [u]. According to data on Japanese VCV sequences (Wada *et al.* 1970), velars present as many places of articulation as constriction locations for the adjacent vowel. Recent EMMA (electromagnetic midsagittal articulography) data for German VCV sequences (Mooshammer and Hoole 1993) reveal tongue dorsum movement towards the medio-postpalatal zone during the velar stop closure period even when [i] is absent.

Blending between two successive consonants produced at adjacent places

Figure 4.1 Linguopalatal configurations at the period of maximal closure or constriction for different Catalan consonants in symmetrical VCV sequences with the vowels [i], [a] and [u] (speaker JP). Consonants can be characterized as follows: bilabial stop [p]; alveolar nasal [n]; velarized alveolar lateral [ɫ]; alveolar fricative [s]; postalveolar or prepalatal fricative [ʃ]; alveolopalatal nasal [ɲ]; velar stop [k]. Data have been recorded with the Reading EPG system and averaged across five repetitions. Percentages of electrode activation: (black) 80–100%; (striped) 60–80%; (dotted) 40–60%; (white) less than 40%. The four front rows of electrodes on each graph correspond to the alveolar zone; the four back ones belong to the palatal zone.

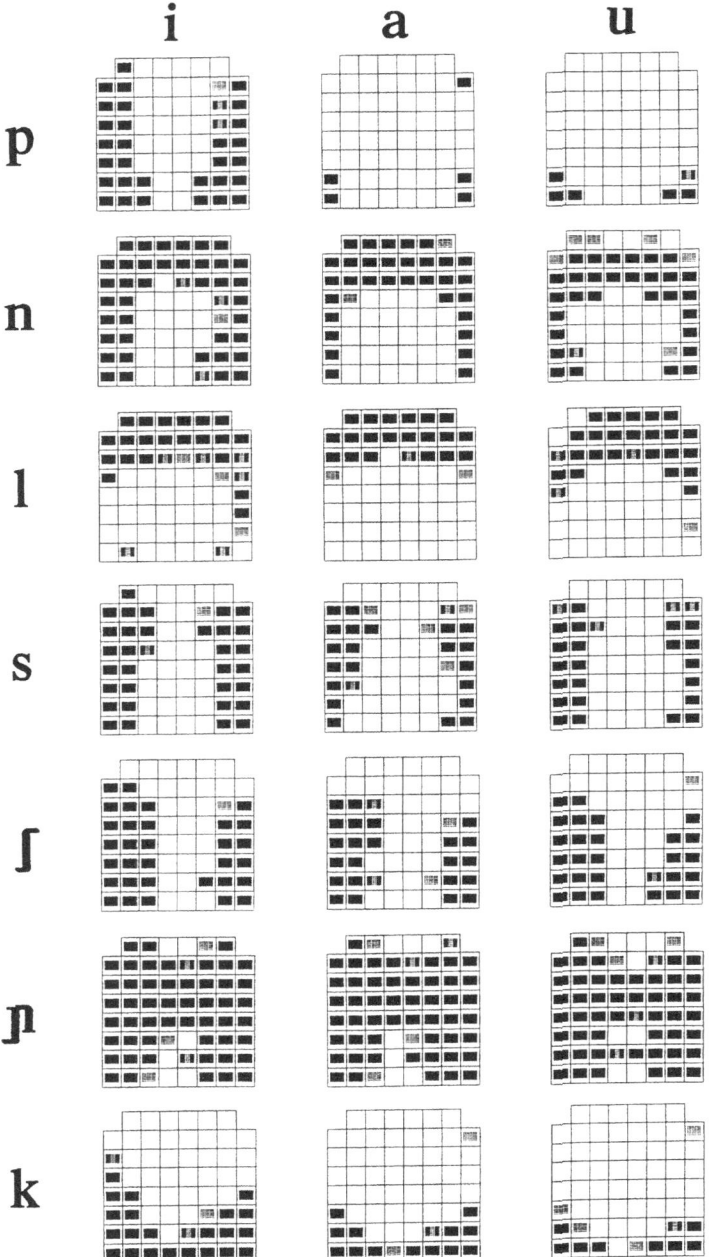

Figure 4.2   EPG contact displays for another Catalan speaker (speaker DR). See details on figure 4.1 captions

of articulation may not occur if one of them involves higher requirements than the other or if the lingual articulator moves fast enough to produce the two consonants at different places. EMMA data for the Catalan clusters [zð] and [ʒð] (Recasens 1995) reveal tongue front movement from C_1 to C_2 with alveolar C_1 keeping the same constriction place as that found in intervocalic position and dental C_2 undergoing significant retraction. On the other hand, alveolar C_1 and dental C_2 achieve their normal place of articulation during the production of the sequence [ɾð].

Unconstricted lingual regions

The degree of coarticulatory sensitivity at tongue regions which are not directly involved in the formation of a closure or constriction is conditioned by whether they are more or less coupled with the primary lingual articulator.

- Labials
  Vowel-dependent coarticulatory effects in tongue body activity are larger for labial stops and for labiodental fricatives than for lingual consonants, since this articulatory structure does not intervene in the production of the former consonantal category (Carney and Moll 1971; Hoole, Gfroerer and Tillmann 1990; Farnetani 1991). Dorsopalatal contact during the [p] closure period in figures 4.1 and 4.2 is indeed somewhat larger when the bilabial stop is adjacent to [i] than to [a] and [u]. Effects from [t] and [k] on adjacent [p] at the tongue front and dorsum are also documented (Recasens, Fontdevila and Pallarès 1993).

- Dentoalveolars
  Coupling between the tongue front and the tongue dorsum for dentoalveolar consonants is not strong enough to prevent tongue dorsum coarticulation from taking place. As discussed above, coarticulatory variability is less considerable for these consonants than for labials and labiodentals. During dentoalveolar consonant production, tongue dorsum height (and dorsopalatal contact size) usually changes as a function of the adjacent vowel in the progression [i]>[u]>[a]. This has been found to be the case for the following consonants: stop [t] (Farnetani, Vagges and Magno-Caldognetto 1985), stop [d] (Öhman 1966), stop [n] (Recasens 1984b; Engstrand 1989), fricatives [s] and [z] (Carney and Moll 1971; Kiritani and Sawashima 1987), non-velarized lateral [l] (Italian: Recasens and Farnetani 1990; Swedish: Engstrand 1989)

and tap [ɾ] (Sudo, Kiritani and Yoshioka 1982; Recasens 1991b). Vowel-dependent differences in dorsopalatal contact for [n] and [s] in figures 4.1 and 4.2 conform to the coarticulatory trends summarized here.

Anticipatory effects in tongue dorsum raising are also exerted by dorsal consonants on dentoalveolars in clusters [tk] (Marchal 1985), [dg] (Byrd 1996) and [sk] (Kent and Moll 1975). Moreover, the degree of coarticulatory sensitivity at the tongue dorsum for dentoalveolars is probably conditioned by differences in tongue body backing, which is more pronounced for apicals than for laminals (Stevens, Keyser and Kawasaki 1986; Dart 1991).

- Postalveolars, alveolopalatals and palatals
  In comparison with dentoalveolars, laminodorsal and dorsal consonants are less sensitive to coarticulatory effects at the tongue dorsum region behind the place of articulation in line with strong coupling effects with the primary articulator. This is the case for postalveolar [ʃ] and [ʒ] (Engstrand 1989; Recasens 1989; Hoole, Gfroerer and Tillmann 1990), alveolopalatals [ʎ] and [ɲ], and palatal [j] (Italian and Catalan: Recasens 1984a; Farnetani 1990; Recasens *et al.* 1993). Analogously to dentoalveolars, [ʎ] allows effects in vowel height and in vowel fronting; consonants involving more dorsopalatal contact ([j] and [ɲ]) show effects in vowel height only. Data in figures 4.1 and 4.2 show similar amounts of dorsopalatal contact for [ɲ] in all vowel contexts; the fricative [ʃ] allows some more palatal coarticulation.

- Velars and pharyngeals
  Velars show lamino-predorsal fronting and raising as a function of adjacent front versus back vowels (MacNeilage and DeClerk 1969); analogous effects are exerted by [t] on [k] in the cluster [kt] (Recasens, Fontdevila and Pallarès 1993). Overall, velars exhibit more coarticulatory variability at the tongue front than dentoalveolars and less so than labials (Hoole, Gfroerer and Tillmann 1990), which is consistent with this tongue region not being involved in the formation of a closure or constriction.

  As expected, the tongue dorsum surface is quite free to adapt to all vowels ([i], [a], [u]) during the production of Arabic pharyngeal approximants [ħ] and [ʕ] (Al-Ani 1970).

- Clusters
  Vowel-dependent coarticulatory effects in lingual activity during stop consonant clusters vary inversely to the degree of linguopalatal contact for the consonantal sequence, in the progression [kp], [pk]> [tp], [pt]> [tk], [kt] (Recasens, Fontdevila and Pallarès 1993). Coarticulation during C_1 and C_2 occurs mostly at unconstrained lingual regions, namely, at the tongue front for [k], at the tongue back for [t] and at both regions for [p].

Overall tongue body configuration

Some requirements on consonantal production (e.g. on manner of articulation, on the formation of a double lingual constriction, etc.) affect the configuration of the entire tongue body rather than that of specific lingual regions. Lingual coarticulatory effects are strongly dependent on such production constraints.

- Voicing
  The tongue body is more sensitive to contextual effects for voiced than for voiceless labial and dentoalveolar stops (Engstrand 1989; Farnetani 1990; Hoole, Gfroerer and Tillmann 1990). This contrast is associated presumably with differences in intraoral pressure level between the two voicing groups and accords with the existence of a larger oral cavity and less linguopalatal contact for the voiced correlate than for the voiceless one (Shibata 1968; Perkell 1969; Farnetani 1989).

- Frication
  Fricatives [s], [z], [ʃ] and [ʒ] allow significant vowel-dependent coarticulatory effects in constriction width but not so (or less so) in constriction location and length (Clark, Palethorpe and Hardcastle 1982; Engstrand 1989). A wider alveolar channel has also been found for [s] before [t] than before other consonants (Hasegawa *et al.* 1979).

  Fricatives often allow less tongue dorsum coarticulation than stops (and laterals) of the same or a close place of articulation and voicing class. This is so for labiodental fricatives versus bilabial stops and for alveolar fricatives versus dentoalveolar stops (Bladon and Nolan 1977; Hoole, Gfroerer and Tillmann 1990; Farnetani 1991). It appears that tongue dorsum grooving for the passage of airflow prevents too much tongue dorsum raising from occurring as a function of high vowels [i] and [u] (Farnetani 1991; Scully,

Grabe-Georges and Badin 1991); in spite of this constraint, [s] shows some more tongue dorsum contact when adjacent to [i] versus lower vowels (Stone *et al.* 1992).

Vowel-dependent coarticulation for [s] may be less obvious at the alveolar place of articulation than at the palatal zone: the tongue dorsum can adapt to the vowel environment while the constriction remains quite fixed (Recasens, Fontdevila and Pallarès 1992).

- Trill production
  Apicoalveolar trills involve precise requirements on tongue body positioning, i.e. some predorsum lowering and some postdorsum backing in order to allow for the production of two or more successive apicoalveolar closures. This lingual configuration is highly resistant to changes in closure location, and in tongue dorsum raising and fronting associated with adjacent [i] (Recasens 1991b).

- Laterality and velarization
  Non-velarized ('clear') [l] in French, Italian and Spanish is particularly sensitive to coarticulatory effects from adjacent vowels, both at the tongue tip and the tongue dorsum: high front [i] causes some tongue dorsum raising and some laminal involvement at the closure location; the consonant is produced with less dorsopalatal contact and an apical closure when adjacent to [a] (Farnetani 1991). The tongue dorsum is more constrained for German non-velarized [l] and thus less sensitive to coarticulatory effects from [i] versus [a] (Recasens, Fontdevila and Pallarès 1995a).

  Velarized ('dark') [ɫ] in Russian, Catalan and American English can be characterized as a complex segment produced with a primary front lingual gesture and a secondary dorsal gesture, and highly resistant to coarticulatory effects in overall tongue body configuration. Small tongue dorsum raising and fronting effects associated with adjacent [i] occur in these circumstances (Giles and Moll 1975; Bladon and Al-Bamerni 1976; Recasens and Farnetani 1990; see later). Moreover the primary tongue front articulator remains quite fixed independently of variations in tongue dorsum position: the need to lower the predorsum for the production of velarized [ɫ] may explain why vowel-dependent effects in tongue dorsum raising in the sequence [iɫi] are not large enough to cause much laminal involvement at the alveolar zone (Recasens, Fontdevila and Pallarès 1995b).

In languages such as Russian and Irish Gaelic, velarized labials and dentoalveolars are produced with a tongue dorsum backing and lowering gesture (the latter are often apicodental); on the other hand, velarized velars show a dorsovelar place of articulation in both front and back vowel contexts, and some tongue predorsum lowering. Vowel-dependent effects in lingual activity for all these consonants are absent or quite small (e.g. some tongue predorsum raising effects have been observed for non palatalized velars; Ní Chasaide and Fealey 1991), which suggests that the tongue dorsum is highly constrained during their production. Other double articulations such as pharyngealized consonants in Arabic have been reported to be highly resistant to vowel coarticulation as well (formant data can be found in Yeou 1995).

- Palatalization
  Palatalized labials and dentoalveolars in languages such as Russian and Irish Gaelic involve active tongue dorsum raising and fronting; coupling effects between the tongue front and the tongue dorsum cause palatalized apicoalveolars to become laminoalveolar. Palatalized velars show a medio-postpalatal place of articulation in all vowel contexts.

  The tongue dorsum is highly constrained and quite resistant to coarticulatory effects during the production of all these consonants. Some effects in tongue dorsum raising from [i] versus [a] have been found for palatalized alveolars (behind the place of articulation) and for velars (in front of the place of articulation) (Irish: Ní Chasaide and Fealey 1991; Estonian: Eek 1973; Russian: Derkach, Fant and Serpa-Leitaō 1970).

Discussion
Differences in coarticulatory sensitivity at the place of closure or constriction (for apicals > laminals > dorsals) depend on factors such as flexibility for the primary articulator and on the particular relationship between the primary articulator and other lingual or non-lingual regions. They also vary with manner of articulation requirements (for fricatives or stops versus other consonants). Coarticulatory sensitivity at unconstricted lingual regions is conditioned by coupling effects and increases as the place of articulation for the consonant occurs at more extreme locations within the vocal tract, for dentoalveolars (at the tongue back) and velars (at the tongue front) versus palatals; non-lingual consonants, i.e. labials, allow more tongue body

coarticulation than lingual consonants. Alveolopalatal and palatal consonants are produced with a high degree of tongue body constraint thus preventing coarticulatory effects from taking place at all lingual regions.

More research is needed on coarticulatory effects between adjacent phonetic segments specified for highly constrained antagonistic lingual gestures (e.g. tongue dorsum raising and fronting for [i], and tongue dorsum lowering and backing for velarized consonants or [r]). Preliminary data reveal a trend for the vowel to show more tongue body repositioning than the consonant in this case, thus indicating the existence of stronger C-to-V than V-to-C effects. This outcome suggests the need for an articulatory model of lingual coarticulation instead of models predicting the amount of undershoot from the acoustic distance between adjacent phonetic segments. Such models cannot explain why, given a fixed acoustic distance between two succesive segments (e.g. velarized [ɫ] and high front [i]), one phonetic segment will undergo more undershoot than the adjacent one. Articulatory models are also needed to account for differences in coarticulatory sensitivity between velarized and palatalized consonants.

Temporal aspects

Spatial coarticulatory effects in lingual displacement associated with a given phoneme may begin and end at adjacent or more distant phonetic segments. This section investigates the temporal effects in articulatory activity for different lingual gestures in different contextual conditions.

Consonant-dependent effects

Several factors may affect the onset time of lingual activity for a target consonantal gesture. Anticipatory effects take place if the phonetic segment preceding the target segment (e.g. a vowel) allows coarticulation to occur; thus, a low vowel usually allows for larger coarticulatory effects in tongue dorsum activity than a high vowel (see earlier). Those effects also depend on the articulatory distance between the two adjacent phonetic segments, as shown by the onset of apical activity for [t] occurring earlier during a preceding low versus a high vowel (Gay 1977). Moreover, the onset time of anticipatory activity is directly related to the size of the C-to-V effects and thus to the involvement of the lingual articulator in the formation of the consonantal closure or constriction; thus, the onset of tongue dorsum movement varies in the progression [k]>[t] (during preceding [ə]; Perkell 1969) and [ʃ]>[z]>[d]> non velarized [l] (during preceding [a]; Farnetani and Recasens 1993). Data on English VCCV sequences also reveal a stronger anticipatory influence from $C_2 = $ [k] versus [t] on the F2 and F3 transitions extending from

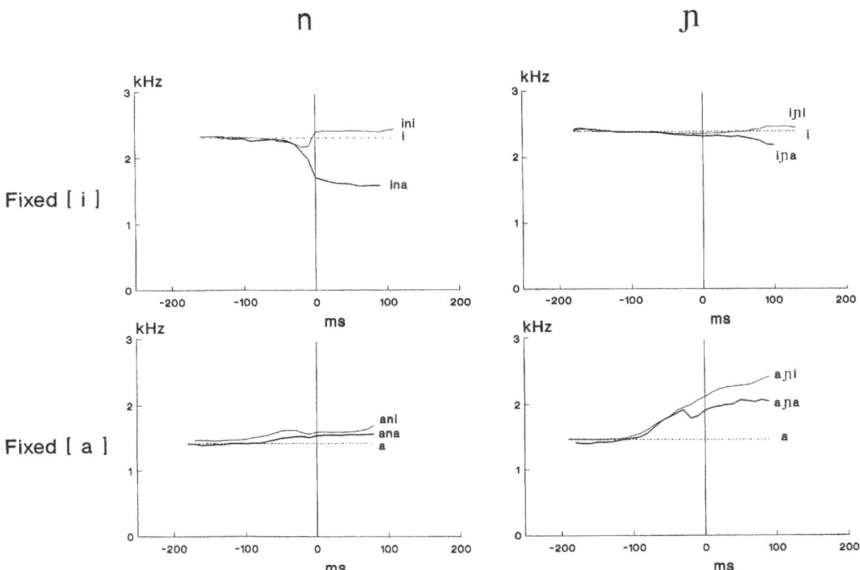

Figure 4.3   Average F2 data representing C-to-V and V-to-V anticipatory effects in VCV sequences with alveolar [n] and alveolopalatal [ɲ] (Catalan speaker JP). C-to-V anticipatory effects take place along the consonantal period to the right of the 0 line or closure onset (positive values). They correspond to F2 differences between a given [iCi] trajectory and the dotted line for steady state [i] (top) and between a given [aCa] trajectory and the dotted line for steady state [a] (bottom). Steady state vowel values were established at half of the V_1 duration. V-to-V anticipatory effects occur to the left of the 0 line (negative values) when an F2 difference between V_2 of [iCi] and [iCa] (top) and V_2 of [aCi] and [aCa] (bottom) extends into V_1.

V_1 to C_1 (Zsiga 1992). Alveolopalatal [ɲ] and velarized [ɫ] require large antic-ipatory effects because they are produced with very salient lingual gestures. F2 data in figures 4.3 and 4.4 reveal indeed an earlier onset of consonant-related activity for [ɲ] than for [n] in the fixed [a] condition; this timing difference is in accordance with differences in the size of the C-to-V anticipatory effects. Consonantal anticipation is less salient when the fixed vowel is [i].

An interesting research topic is the relative salience of the anticipatory versus carryover coarticulatory effects. Variations in mediodorsum activity for vowels ([i], [e], [a], [o] and [u]) as a function of adjacent consonants (bila-bial, dentoalveolar and velar) in Japanese CVC sequences are two times larger at the carryover level (C_1-to-V) than at the anticipatory level (C_2-to-V) (Kiritani *et al.* 1977). A similar trend has been reported for F2 coarticulation on [a] as a function of consonants differing in place of articulation (Catalan:

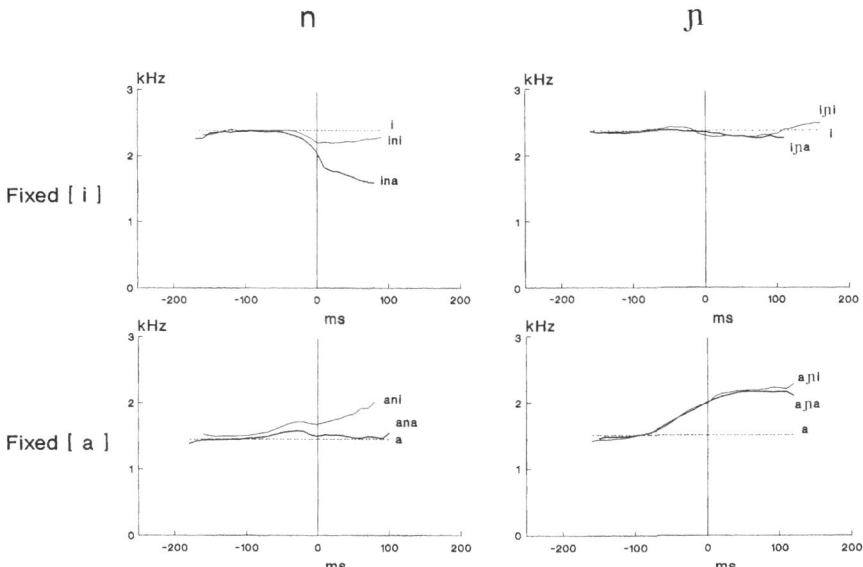

Figure 4.4   F2 coarticulatory effects for the Catalan speaker DR. See details on figure 4.3 caption.

Recasens 1986). As discussed below, the dominance of carryover over anticipatory coarticulation in such cases may be associated with the inertial properties of the sluggish tongue dorsum. The opposite trend, i.e. larger C-to-V anticipation versus carryover, may occur from an alveolar trill [r] or a velarized lateral [ɫ] on the vowel [i], and is related to the high lingual demands for the consonant (Recasens and Farnetani 1992); a similar rationale may account for the presence of large C_2-to-C_1 anticipatory effects at the tongue front in the cluster [kl] (Catalan velarized [ɫ]: Gibbon, Hardcastle and Nikolaidis 1993).

An experiment was designed in order to investigate the temporal differences between anticipatory and carryover C-to-V coarticulation (Recasens 1989). Effects in dorsopalatal contact and F2 frequency associated with [ʃ] versus [t] were measured along preceding [VC$_1$ə] and along following [əC$_2$V] where C_1 and C_2 were [ʃ] or [t]. Results show that the onset of dorsopalatal contact is constrained to occur during the preceding schwa in the two C_1 conditions (somewhat earlier or later depending on the spatial extent of the consonantal gesture; Farnetani and Recasens 1993). The offset of the consonant-dependent carryover effects is more variable than the onset of the anticipatory effects, and may last until the following schwa (when $C_2 = $ [ʃ]) or until C_2

(when $C_2 = $ [t]). This finding suggests that the articulatory anticipation is pre-programmed and that the extent of the carryover effects is determined by the production requirements of the contextual phonetic segments.

Vowel-dependent effects

The magnitude and extent of the vowel-dependent effects in VCV sequences is related to the tongue body demands for the production of the adjacent and distant phonetic segments.

Adjacent consonant

V-to-V effects in tongue dorsum activity have been reported across non-dorsal consonants, i.e. [b] and [d] (Öhman 1966), non-velarized [l] and [ɾ] (Recasens 1987), [t] (Butcher and Weiher 1976; Farnetani, Vagges and Magno-Caldognetto 1985; Butcher 1989). Dorsal consonants allow less transconsonantal coarticulation, as for [k] (Butcher and Weiher 1976; Butcher 1989) and for [ʎ], [ɲ] and [j] (Recasens 1984b). Vowel-dependent effects associated with [i] versus [a] in figures 4.3 and 4.4 also last longer across [n] versus [ɲ], clearly so when the fixed transconsonantal vowel is [a]. V-to-V effects are also very small or absent across palatalized, velarized and pharyngealized consonants (Öhman 1966; Derkach, Fant and Serpa-Leitaõ 1970; Purcell 1979; Recasens 1987; Hussein 1990; Ní Chasaide and Fealey 1991). In summary, the onset of vowel-dependent coarticulation appears to vary inversely with the degree of tongue dorsum constraint for the immediately preceding consonant. Researchers invoking a C-to-V mode of coarticulation (see next paragraph) have reported a longer delay in onset of vowel-related tongue dorsum activity with the degree of tongue dorsum involvement for the preceding consonant (for [k] > [t] > [p]).

Some researchers advocate the view that tongue body displacement for V_2 in VCV sequences starts during the closure period (for example, tongue dorsum lowering for [a] during preceding [k], [t] and [p] in English; Gay 1977). This finding suggests that there is a tongue body target for those consonants and/or that the consonantal release and the articulatory movement towards the vowel are linked in a basic gesture. A delay in the onset of lingual activity for V_2 in Swedish [VpV] sequences has also been attributed to some active tongue body relaxation during the closure period which could be related to the presence of aspiration in the stop (Engstrand 1988).

Opposite vowel

V-to-V coarticulatory effects in tongue blade and tongue dorsum activity and in F2 frequency, usually extend into adjacent [ə], [a] or [u] but much less so or not at all into adjacent [i] (Italian: Farnetani, Vagges and Magno-Caldognetto 1985; Spanish and Catalan: Recasens 1987; Japanese: Magen 1984b). This situation applies to the F2 data for fixed [i] and [a] in figures 4.3 and 4.4. Differences in onset time of anticipatory coarticulation may be due to differences in degree of tongue dorsum constraint for the vowel ([i]>[a]) or in articulatory distance between the vocalic and consonantal targets ([a]>[i]).

Another issue is whether vowel-dependent effects in lingual activity in VCV sequences may reach the steady-state of the opposite vowel or affect the vowel transitions only. While some studies reveal the rarity of long-range temporal effects (Carney and Moll 1971), other literature sources suggest that long-range effects extending beyond the VCV domain occur more frequently than previously thought. As indicated in the next section, Recasens (1989) reported long-range carryover effects in F2 frequency. Magen (1989) found early F2 anticipatory effects from $V_2 = $ [i] versus [a] during V_1 in [$bV_1bəbV_2b$] sequences; however, Fowler and Saltzman (1993) have suggested that the temporal extent of these effects is in fact quite restricted (about 200–250 ms) and conforms to the predictions of a time-locked model of coarticulation.

Coarticulatory directionality

A relevant issue in coarticulation theory is the relative salience of the anticipatory effects versus carryover effects. The view of coarticulatory directionality presented in this section is in accordance with predictions from the DAC ('degree of articulatory constraint') model of coarticulation (Recasens, Pallarès and Fontdevila 1997).

- Consonantal class
  Vowel-dependent carryover effects have been reported to exceed vowel-dependent anticipatory effects at and across dorsal consonants of different place of articulation; this trend has been documented for dorso(alveolo)palatals (Recasens 1984b; Farnetani 1990), palatalized dentoalveolars (Ní Chasaide and Fealey 1991) and dorsovelars (Bell-Berti and Harris 1976; Gay 1977). The reason why vocalic carryover exceeds vocalic anticipation in VCV sequences with dorsal consonants follows from the considerable strength of the C-to-V carryover effects; indeed, prominent carryover effects associated with the biomechanical constraints for the consonantal dorsal gesture prevent much vowel-related anticipation from occurring.

When VCV sequences include more unconstrained intervocalic consonants there may be a predominance of either the vowel-related anticipatory or carryover component, depending on factors such as degree of tongue dorsum raising, stress condition and speech rate (see Huffman 1986). Predominance of vowel-dependent carryover effects at and across such consonants have been reported for bilabials (Bell-Berti and Harris 1976; Magen 1984b; Manuel and Krakow 1984; Recasens 1987), dentoalveolar stops (Bell-Berti and Harris 1976; Farnetani, Vagges and Magno-Caldognetto 1985; Farnetani 1990), alveolar taps and flaps and non velarized [l] (Shibata 1968; Recasens 1987, 1991b; Farnetani 1990). Other accounts indicate however that the vowel-dependent anticipatory component may prevail upon the vowel-dependent carryover component. Consistently with this view, Hoole, Gfroerer and Tillmann (1990) have shown that anticipatory effects may be larger than carryover effects at a more flexible articulator such as the tongue front; moreover, a decrease in tongue dorsum involvement may cause an increase in vowel-dependent anticipatory coarticulation (for labials > dentoalveolars > velars), and larger anticipatory than carryover effects (labials in German: Hoole, Gfoerer and Tillmann 1990; labials and dentoalveolars in English: Butcher 1989; Magen 1997). In agreement with this trend, [ʃ] favours carryover over anticipatory effects from adjacent vowels to a larger extent than [s] (Hoole, Nguyen-Trong and Hardcastle 1993).

Recent linguopalatal contact and F2 data on coarticulation in VCV sequences with non-dorsal consonants (Recasens, Pallarès and Fontdevila 1997) show that vocalic anticipation is blocked when [i] contributes to the raising of the tongue dorsum during non-dorsal consonants such as [n] which causes an increase in the degree of tongue dorsum constraint for the consonant. Consequently, in comparison to C-to-V anticipatory effects, C-to-V carryover effects become more prominent for [ini] than for [ana]; on the other hand, V-to-C and V-to-V effects from [i] versus [a] in VCV sequences with [n] favour the carryover over the anticipatory direction to a larger extent when the transconsonantal vowel is [i] than when it is [a].

A third consonantal group is made up of consonants requiring a much stronger anticipatory versus carryover component (velarized [ł], trill [r], lingual fricatives). Data on V-to-V coarticulation across velarized [ł] and an alveolar trill often reveal larger anticipatory versus carryover vowel-dependent coarticulation (or, at least, a significant reduction of the latter). Predominance of vocalic anticipation over vocalic carryover in this case occurs since vowel anticipation is not much affected by the carryover effects associated with the consonant because these, as pointed out above, are less salient than the consonantal anticipatory effects. Lingual fricatives however appear to favour the opposite trend, i.e. larger vowel-dependent carryover versus anticipatory effects (Hoole, Nguyen-Trong and Hardcastle 1993); this accords with data on VCV coarticulation reported by Farnetani and Faber (1991) showing that the tongue dorsum activity for [s] and [ʃ] blocks V-to-V anticipatory effects associated with [i] versus [a] but not V-to-V carryover effects associated with those same vowels.

- Other conditioning factors
  Differences in gestural compatibility between adjacent segments may determine the relative strength of the anticipatory versus carryover effects. While tongue dorsum raising for [k] may occur quite early during the closure period of [t] in the cluster [tk], anticipatory activity for [t] in the cluster [kt] requires tongue body repositioning (Hardcastle and Roach 1979). For similar reasons, C_2 anticipation is more feasible in the clusters [fl] and [pl] versus [kl] (Giles and Moll 1975) and in the cluster [sʃ] versus [ʃs] (Perkell, Boyce and Stevens 1979).

  Vowel-dependent effects may also differ in the temporal extent and in the variability of onset and offset times. In the same experiment reported earlier (Recasens 1989), coarticulatory effects in dorsopalatal contact and in F2 frequency associated with [i] versus [a] were measured along preceding $[C_1 \ni C_2 V]$ and along following $[VC_1 \ni C_2]$ where C_1 and C_2 were [ʃ] or [t]. Anticipatory effects show two outcomes: they are blocked by a conflicting consonant (i.e. when $C_2 = [ʃ]$); they begin during the opposite vowel schwa if articulatory conflict is not involved (i.e. when $C_2 = [t]$). The offset of the carryover component is more variable and depends to a larger extent on the articulatory requirements for the contextual segments. It may occur during the schwa in the highly constrained sequence [VʃəʃV] or during C_2 in the more unconstrained string [VtətV]; moreover, longer V_1-dependent effects in the sequence [VʃəʃV] than in the sequence [VʃətV] are associated with the need to keep a large linguopalatal contact size along a [iʃəʃV] string.

Occasionally anticipatory effects occur to emphasize the production of a given phonetic segment in a similar contextual environment, e.g. [j] before [i] in the sequence [Vji] as opposed to [Vja] and [Vju]. On the other hand, the presence of carryover V-to-V effects in dorsopalatal contact for [ija] versus [aja] may reflect the synergetic contribution of V_1 and C and thus can be interpreted as a case of articulatory overshoot (Recasens 1984b).

Discussion

An increase in gestural conflict and in articulatory distance between two adjacent phonemes causes an earlier onset time of C-to-V coarticulation (e.g. an earlier tongue dorsum activity for velarized [ɫ] after [i] versus [a]) and a later onset time of vowel-dependent coarticulation (e.g. a later onset of tongue dorsum activity for [a] during a preceding palatal versus dentoalveolar consonant).

If there is gestural compatibility between two adjacent phonetic segments, the onset of anticipatory effects in lingual activity is quite fixed and predictable: vocalic effects often begin during the first vowel in VCV sequences (e.g. tongue dorsum raising anticipation from [i] in the sequence [əti]), and consonantal effects do not usually extend into the preceding consonant in CVC sequences (e.g. tongue dorsum raising anticipation from [ʃ] in the sequence [təʃ]). Moreover the larger the articulatory displacement for the target segment, the earlier the onset of anticipatory coarticulation (e.g. effects in tongue dorsum raising for [ɲ] versus [t] during preceding [a]). Anticipatory effects are most noticeable at lingual regions which are flexible or not directly involved in the making of a closure or constriction.

Our model of coarticulatory directionality predicts that the weight of the vowel-dependent anticipatory component varies inversely with the prominence of the consonant-dependent carryover component. This explains why V-to-V effects in VCV sequences are mostly carryover across dorsopalatal consonants, mostly anticipatory across velarized [ɫ] and [r], and may favour both coarticulatory directions across consonants produced with a quite unconstrained tongue dorsum configuration depending on contextual and prosodic factors (labials, non-fricative dentoalveolars). The model needs to be partly refined in order to account for some directionality effects in VCV sequences with lingual fricatives.

Data on the temporal extent of lingual coarticulation (mostly in tongue dorsum activity) reported here confirm the view that the onset of the anticipation effects is more precise than the offset of the carryover effects. This view follows from the former reflecting gestural formation events and the latter being particularly sensitive to mechanico-inertial contextual factors. In agreement with this observation, tongue dorsum carryover effects may be cumulative with the tongue dorsum activity for the following segment (for example, tongue dorsum raising for [ʃ] is enhanced by a preceding [i]).

Prosodic factors

Syllable position

Coarticulatory sensitivity for a given phoneme may vary as a function of contextual position within the syllable, word, foot or sentence. In general, consonants are more sensitive to coarticulatory effects in syllable-final versus syllable-initial position which accords with differences in articulatory and acoustic salience between the two allophonic types (Ohala and Kawasaki 1984). Thus, for example, data on American English reported by Kiritani and Sawashima (1987) show larger vowel-dependent effects in tongue dorsum displacement on syllable-final versus syllable-initial [p] and [s]. On the other hand, syllable-final [l] is more velarized and more resistant to coarticulatory effects than syllable-initial [l] in languages such as English and Catalan, which is in accordance with the former versus the latter consonantal allophone exhibiting a more prominent dorsal component (Giles and Moll 1975; Bladon and Al-Bamerni 1976; Recasens and Farnetani 1990; Sproat and Fujimura 1993). The finding that there are larger vowel-dependent effects for the American English flap (Zawadzki and Kuehn 1980) in syllable-final versus syllable-initial position is in agreement with the syllable-final allophone being produced with a more vowel-like articulatory configuration involving more tongue dorsum bunching and more tongue front retraction.

Stress

The articulatory characteristics of consonants and vowels vary as a function of stress. In comparison to their unstressed correlates, stressed consonants are often articulated with more linguopalatal contact (stops: Farnetani 1990; Dixit and Flege 1991) and possibly greater lingual displacement and higher peak velocity. Stressed vowels are less centralized, thus involving more extreme articulatory configurations (Kent and Netsell 1971).

Assuming that articulatory salience is positively correlated with articulatory constraint, coarticulatory sensitivity ought to be less for stressed than for unstressed phonetic segments. Indeed smaller V-to-C effects in linguopalatal contact have been found for dental stops in stressed versus unstressed syllables (Farnetani 1990); moreover, acoustic data reveal that stressed vowels are less sensitive to context-dependent effects than unstressed vowels (Nord 1974;

Fowler 1981b). In agreement with these findings, vowel-related tongue movements and /p/ closure overlap to a larger extent in unstressed versus stressed VCV utterances (Engstrand 1988).

Speech rate

An increase in speech rate causes segmental shortening as well as articulatory and acoustic undershoot for vowels (Lindblom 1963b; Gay *et al.* 1974) and consonants (Kent and Moll 1972a; Zawadzki and Kuehn 1980; Farnetani 1990). There is more overlap in lingual activity between adjacent phonetic segments in fast versus slow speech; this has been shown to be the case for V-to-C effects (Giles and Moll 1975; Zawadzki and Kuehn 1980; Gay 1981; Engstrand 1989; Farnetani 1990), for C-to-C effects (cluster [kl]; Hardcastle 1985) and for C-to-V effects (Farnetani and Recasens 1993). A similar outcome results from the embedding of speech sounds in continuous speech as opposed to isolated utterances (Farnetani and Recasens 1993). A topic which deserves further investigation is the extent to which changes in speech rate affect the relative salience of the anticipatory versus carryover effects.

An increase in gestural overlap resulting from an increase in speech rate may give rise to an assimilatory process. Recent evidence for English (Barry 1985) and German (Künhert 1993) indicates that segmental assimilations are often incomplete with the assimilated segment preserving a residue of the originary lingual gesture (e.g. $C_1 = /t/$ shows some lateral alveolar contact in the English sequence 'late calls').

Segmental duration

V-to-C effects at closure mid-point are slightly smaller for long versus short /t/ and /d/ (but roughly the same for long versus short /n/ and /l/) in Italian (Farnetani 1986b, 1990). Coarticulatory sensitivity appears to be negatively correlated with linguopalatal contact size in this case given the fact that geminates may involve more linguopalatal contact than non-geminates (Italian /t/ and /d/ in Farnetani 1990; see also F2 data in Bladon and Carbonaro 1978).

Larger vowel-dependent effects in linguopalatal contact (in the progression [i]>[u]>[a]) upon the fricative component of palatal affricates than upon isolated fricatives are associated presumably with the shorter duration of the former versus the latter (American English: Dagenais, Lorendo and McCutcheon 1994).

Acoustic data reported by Zsiga (1992) show a significant correlation between the V_1/C_1C_2 duration ratio and the degree of C_2-to-V_1 coarticulation (measured at the V_1 formant transitions) in English /VdkV/ sequences: the shorter the cluster duration with respect to the V_1 duration, the more prominent the coarticulatory effects.

Syntactic and phonological boundaries

Coarticulatory effects in lingual activity may vary inversely to the strength of a linguistic boundary between two adjacent phonetic segments. Thus, it has been shown that C_1 and C_2 in the cluster [kl] overlap to a lesser extent across a sentence or a clause boundary than across a word or a syllable boundary (Hardcastle 1985); smaller vowel-dependent coarticulatory effects on a bilabial nasal stop have also been found in the former versus latter boundary condition (Su, Daniloff and Hammarberg 1975). Other sources confirm the presence of coarticulatory effects in tongue body activity between vowel gestures across a word boundary (Kent and Moll 1972b).

Conclusion

Data on coarticulation are useful in order to infer mechanisms of articulatory control in speech production. For that purpose we need to increase our knowledge about the degrees of variability allowed by different lingual regions during the production of different speech sounds as well as about the size and temporal extent of the coarticulatory effects among adjacent consonants and vowels in speech sequences. A crucial research aspect is to disentangle context-free mechanisms from those which are more dependent on contextual changes and on articulatory mechanico-inertial constraints in general. Modifications in contextual composition can be carried out so as to induce differences in variability of the onset and offset times of coarticulation or in the predominance of a given coarticulatory direction.

5

Laryngeal coarticulation

Section A: PHILIP HOOLE

Section B: CHRISTER GOBL and AILBHE NÍ CHASAIDE

Introduction

At one level, voicing coarticulation has frequently been studied as a temporal phenomenon, i.e. as the extension of $\pm$ periodicity from one segment to another adjacent one (differently specified phonologically). To take a simple example, consider the devoicing of /l/ in English words such as 'plead'. There is universal agreement that this can be explained by the influence of the adjacent voiceless /p/. In other words, minimal pairs such as 'plead' and 'bleed' have not been used to suggest that English has a phonemic contrast between voiced and voiceless laterals. Such combinations of voiceless obstruent + sonorant sequences are probably the consonant clusters that have been most extensively investigated (see below and especially Docherty 1992, for further references), at least in terms of acoustic measurements of the timing of voicing – and they represent one of the two main topics covered in the section on coarticulatory investigations of the devoicing gesture. Of course, there are many other potential sequences of consonants in which the individual members of the sequence differ with respect to voicing specification, and can accordingly influence one another (Westbury 1979; Docherty 1992).

Yet, consideration of even apparently simple coarticulatory phenomena such as the /pl/ case leads inevitably to a widening of the perspective to include questions of interarticulator coordination, in other words the formation and the release of oral constriction for /p/ and /l/, and their temporal relationship to the devoicing gesture. In this respect, coarticulation with respect to the laryngeal system requires an approach somewhat different from that traditionally followed, for example, for labial and velar coarticulation. In the latter cases it is legitimate to examine issues such as relative extent of carryover and anticipatory effects, explanatory adequacy of feature-spreading versus time-locking models etc. (for example for lip rounding), without explicit consideration of details of *inter*articulator coordination (implicitly, all the above concepts of course require a further articulatory system as reference for the analysis of the coarticulatory behaviour of the targeted articulatory sub-system). The situation can be summarized by observing that while simple alternating CV sequences have provided a point of departure for coarticulatory studies in almost every other articulatory system, for an understanding of oral–laryngeal coordination one would need to look at more complex environments.

The phonatory system differs from other sub-systems used in speech production (such as the lips, velum and tongue) in that the acoustic output is less directly or transparently determined by the articulatory (laryngeal) gestures. Simply knowing the precise configuration of the glottis at one instant in time does not in itself permit us to specify whether the acoustic signal at that point is voiced or voiceless. The initiation, maintenance or cessation of phonation depend on the interplay of a number of factors: muscularly controlled adjustments of the vocal folds which determine whether and to what degree they are abducted or adducted as well as the precise configuration of the glottis when adducted; aerodynamic conditions at the glottis, and in particular, the transglottal pressure, which is sensitive not only to respiratory factors, but also to the degree and duration of any supraglottal occlusion; the intrinsic elasticity of the vocal folds and the muscularly controlled tension in the folds. During phonation, variation in any of these factors will also affect their mode of vibration, and hence the auditory quality of the voice produced.

Some recent investigations have suggested that the mode of phonation of a vowel may indeed be affected in rather subtle ways by adjacent consonants (specifically voiceless consonants). To the extent that these effects appear, the simple measure of the timing of voice onset or offset ($\pm$ periodicity in the acoustic signal) underestimates the coarticulatory influence of consonants on vowels (and presumably on adjacent voiced segments generally). They further provide insights into the control mechanisms that may be involved in the regulation of voiceless consonants.

The two sections of this chapter deal with very different aspects of laryngeal coarticulation. In the first section Philip Hoole deals with the spatial and temporal organisation of the laryngeal devoicing gesture, dealing in particular with interarticulator coordination in single voiceless consonants as well as in clusters (the relevant instrumental techniques are presented in chapter 15 section A). In the second section Christer Gobl and Ailbhe Ní Chasaide deal with the variations which may be found in the vowel's mode of phonation in the vicinity of certain consonants. In this section a number of illustrations are presented, based on a rather fine-grained analysis of the voice source (this methodology is described in chapter 15 section B). The implications of these data for our understanding of laryngeal control mechanisms are discussed.

Section A: Coarticulatory investigations of the devoicing gesture: Philip Hoole

Introduction

As just discussed in the general introduction to this chapter, investigation of coarticulation with respect to the devoicing gesture almost inevitably requires consideration of the interarticulatory organization of consonantal sequences, rather than of simple alternating sequences of single consonants and vowels. The first main topic to be discussed under this heading – as already mentioned – will be the organization of sequences of voiceless obstruent plus sonorant. The second main topic follows on from observations made by Yoshioka, Löfqvist and Hirose (1981), who point out in a paper examining consonant clusters in American English that in terms of coarticulation at the laryngeal level it can be revealing to examine sequences of purely *voiceless* consonants, since this can provide insight into the organizational principles according to which individual gestures blend and mutually influence one another (coarticulation as coproduction). This topic will accordingly provide the second main area to be addressed below. Again, as with the first topic, we will be arguing that it is difficult to divorce the question of laryngeal coarticulation and coproduction from the question of laryngeal–oral interarticulator coordination. Having brought the question of interarticulator coordination into play we must now also make clear what aspects of this all-embracing topic we will *not* be considering here: in fact, we will be ignoring what has probably been the major topic in laryngeal–oral coordination over the last thirty years, namely the role of laryngeal timing in voicing contrasts in stop consonants, developed under the influence of the work of Lisker and Abramson (e.g. 1964) and with its important implications for the status of time and timing in phonological representations (cf. Löfqvist 1980). There is now a very substantial literature on the physiological and kinematic aspects of the mechanisms of stop consonant voicing control employed in many different languages (e.g. for laryngeal–oral timing patterns ranging from preaspiration, via unaspirated and postaspirated to voiced aspirated). Nonetheless, we will preface the discussion of the two main topics in this part of the chapter with consideration of some of the basic kinematic properties of laryngeal articulation in single voiceless plosives and fricatives to form a background for the central discussion of longer consonantal sequences. As we will see, some interesting questions already emerge here, that can then be picked up again with respect to these longer sequences. A useful group of illustrations showing some of the interarticulatory relationships discussed below for single consonants and clusters in terms of transillumination and EMG (electromyography) signals is to be found in Löfqvist (1990), figures 5 to 7.

Properties of single voiceless consonants

We will organize this section around a series of comparisons: in the first part with respect to manner of articulation (i.e. plosives versus fricatives) and in the second part with respect to place of articulation. Within each sub-section we will compare various aspects of the amplitude and timing of the devoicing gesture. (Refer to figure 15.1, for an illustration of the time-course of laryngeal abduction and adduction in an utterance containing several voice-less sounds.)

Manner of articulation

It has frequently been reported in the literature that the amplitude of the devoicing gesture is larger for fricatives than plosives (Munhall and Ostry 1985; Löfqvist and McGarr 1987; McGarr and Löfqvist 1988). (Admittedly, the ultrasound measurements in the former yielded a mere 0.25 mm difference in the amplitude of vocal fold abduction for plosives and fricatives, though this was still significant.) A group of papers in which clusters rather than single voiceless sounds were examined points clearly in the same direction (Löfqvist and Yoshioka 1980a, 1980b; Yoshioka, Löfqvist and Hirose 1980, 1981). Summarizing these latter studies, Yoshioka, Löfqvist and Hirose (1980a: 306) go as far as to say regarding the more vigorous abduction in fric-atives that 'this finding for fricatives is also consistent with our recent studies using American English, Icelandic and Swedish although the phonologies differ, among other things, in the significance of stop aspiration. Therefore, we are inclined to conclude that at least the difference in the peak value between a voiceless fricative and a voiceless stop is universal.'

In fact, this may slightly overstate the situation: the amount of aspiration required for stops in specific languages may occasionally override this ten-dency. In an extensive study of Danish (with the unusually large number of five subjects in the kinematic part of her study) Hutters (1984) found slightly but significantly larger peak glottal opening in aspirated stops than in frica-tives.[1] She notes that aspiration is more extensive in Danish than, for example, Swedish. She also notes the possibility, in view of the subtlety of the differences, that differences in larynx height for the different sounds compared may interfere with the interpretation of the amplitude of the transillumina-tion signal.

With regard to the timing of the devoicing gesture, one robust difference between fricatives and (aspirated) plosives that emerges clearly from the literature is that the onset of glottal abduction is earlier for fricatives, relative to the formation of the oral closure (e.g. Butcher 1977; Hoole, Pompino-Marschall and Dames 1984; Hutters 1984; Löfqvist and McGarr 1987; for further comparative information on glottal timing in fricatives and aspirated stops see Löfqvist and Yoshioka 1984). The reason is probably to be found in the aerodynamic requirements of fricative production. Löfqvist and McGarr (1987) discuss reasons for the larger glottal gesture in fricatives, but their remarks could equally well apply to the early onset of abduction in fricatives: 'the larger gesture for a voiceless fricative is most likely due to the aerodynamics of fricative production, in that a large glottal opening not only prevents voicing but also reduces laryngeal resistance to air flow and assists in the build-up of oral pressure necessary for driving the noise source' (399). The aerodynamically crucial phase of a fricative is probably its onset, whereas for an aspirated plosive the crucial phase is the offset (in addition, Löfqvist and McGarr suggest that early onset of glottal abduction is avoided in English stops as inappropriate preaspiration might otherwise occur). Related to this is a tendency for fricatives to show higher velocities and tighter timing control in the abduction phase compared with the adduction phase on the one hand, and compared with plosives on the other hand. However, the picture to be found in the literature is not completely consistent (cf. Löfqvist and McGarr 1987).

Another way of looking at the early onset of glottal abduction in fricatives is with respect to the onset of the preceding vowel. It is well known that vowels tend to be longer before fricatives. Hoole, Pompino-Marschall and Dames (1984) suggested (on the basis of not ideally suited material) that the timing of glottal abduction could be identical for plosives and fricatives when viewed from the onset of the previous vowel. However, the more balanced material of Hutters (1984) failed to confirm this, since although the expected differences in vowel length were found, they were not large enough to completely compensate for the difference in time of glottal abduction relative to fricative constriction and stop closure; significant timing differences between stops and fricatives remained. Nonetheless, the theme of the relative amount of reorganization of laryngeal and oral articulations is one to which we will be returning.

Place of articulation

There are surprisingly few studies that compare the laryngeal devoicing gesture with respect to place of articulation. Regarding the amplitude of the gesture Hutters (1984) found in Danish that peak glottal opening was

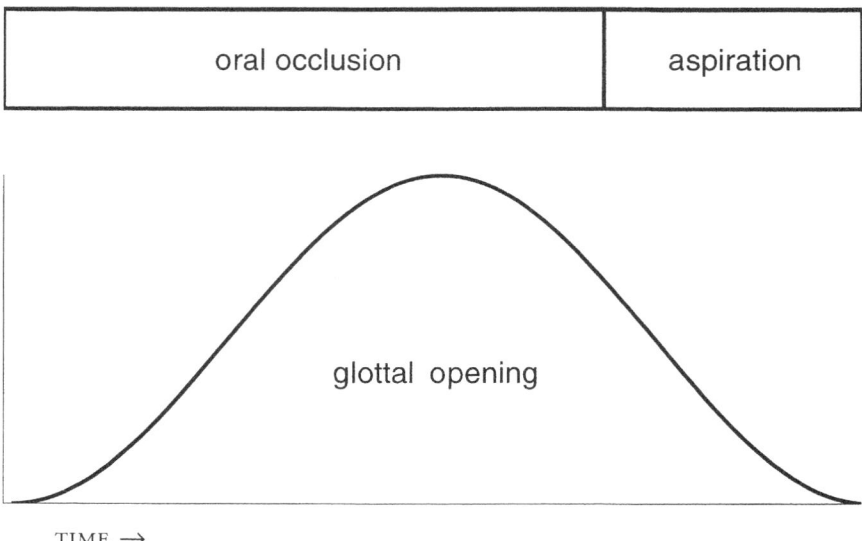

TIME →

Figure 5.1   Typical pattern of laryngeal–oral coordination in aspirated stops

greater for /s/ than for /f/, and for /t/ than for /p/ (although the latter comparison did not reach statistical significance, perhaps being complicated by the fact that /t/ is affricated in Danish). Cooper (1991) compared the stops /p, t, k/ in two speakers of American English and found a significant place of articulation effect for peak glottal opening, but the pattern of results was not straightforward since the different stops were differently affected by the experimental variation of stress and position of the stop in the word.

Probably the more interesting issue is whether the timing of the devoicing gesture is influenced by place of articulation, particularly in aspirated stops. Refer to figure 5.1 for a schematic illustration of the relation between the time-course of a typical devoicing gesture and the oral occlusion and aspiration phases in such sounds.

The interest derives from the widespread observation that place of articulation has a significant effect on VOT (voice onset time). The most robust finding is that /p/ has shorter VOT than /t/ or /k/. Whether there is a general relationship of the form p<t<k (i.e. longer VOT for more retracted consonants) is more open to debate (see e.g. Docherty 1992 for discussion). Disregarding possible additional aerodynamic effects for the moment, this suggests that peak glottal opening is timed earlier with respect to release for /p/ than for the other plosives (see e.g. Jessen 1995). On the other hand, /p/ also generally has a longer occlusion duration than the other stops. Taken

together this raises the possibility that the devoicing gesture has essentially the same duration for all stops, and that the differences in VOT are a simple passive effect of different oral occlusion durations superimposed on a constant laryngeal gesture. A suggestion along these lines has been put forward by Weismer (1980) and by Suomi (1980; cited in Docherty 1992: 137) on the basis of durational analysis of acoustic data. Hutters (1985) also presents some evidence for a similar effect operating across languages rather than across place of articulation: i.e. languages with short occlusion phases have long aspiration phases, and vice versa. Docherty notes that Suomi's conclusion was based on consideration of mean duration (occlusion, VOT, total devoicing) for each stop category and himself applies what he regards as a more stringent test of the hypothesis: in addition to examining mean duration values (which confirmed the existence of a reciprocity between occlusion and VOT duration) he also tested for a negative correlation between the two variables, since under the hypothesis of an invariant gesture a strong negative correlation should occur. The evidence for this was, however, rather weak. In comparison with the rather weak negative correlations for occlusion versus VOT, Docherty found fairly strong positive correlations between total abduction duration and VOT, which can be seen as a test that there *are* laryngeal differences, and these are responsible for VOT.[2]

Of the few relevant transillumination studies, Hoole, Pompino-Marschall and Dames (1984) found over the German stops /p/ and /t/ a reciprocal relationship between occlusion duration and the duration of the interval from peak glottal opening to release, but did not test the constancy of the devoicing gesture directly. Hutters' (1984) Danish data (leaving /t/ out of consideration in view of its affrication) showed that occlusion release comes earlier relative to peak glottal opening for /k/ than for /p/ but there were no differences in either occlusion duration or vowel-plus-occlusion duration for these stops; the interval from vowel onset to peak glottal opening did in fact turn out to be shorter for /p/ than for /k/, so there do appear to be some active laryngeal differences between the two stops. The most direct test of this question is to be found in Cooper (1991), where /p/, /t/ and /k/ were compared. He found the expected reciprocal relationship between duration of oral occlusion and VOT, /p/ contrasting with /t, k/ (VOT was shorter in /p/), but neither his acoustic data nor the associated transillumination data allowed a strict interpretation in terms of an invariant laryngeal gesture over place of articulation. The duration of the devoicing gesture was longer for /t/ than for /k/. But it is not clear what the motivation for this difference could be since it was not, for example, related to duration of VOT. VOT *was* directly related to the timing of peak glottal opening relative to release, and this probably reflects an active process of interarticulator timing, rather than emerging passively from variation of occlusion duration. But it is still not clear *why* this form of organization should occur.

The idea of an invariant glottal gesture for all stops thus does not appear completely justified by the data. Weismer (1980) even went so far as to suggest an invariant gesture for stops and fricatives – which as we have seen is also probably not justified. Nevertheless it is interesting at this juncture to pick up Weismer's conjectures as to why voiceless fricatives have a constriction duration that is clearly longer than the occlusion duration of voiceless plosives. Assuming that it is inappropriate for fricatives to be aspirated (at least for English) then it may be easier 'to "fit" the supraglottal constriction to the time-course of the devoicing gesture' (436) than vice versa. This concept may still have some merit (cf. the similar discussion of clusters below) even if the invariance of the devoicing gesture is not correct in a hard and fast sense (see also Shipp's 1982 suggestion that the highly preprogrammed nature of the abductory–adductory cycle may make the larynx 'one of the basic metronomes of the speech production process', 111).

Devoicing organization in consonant sequences
Coarticulatory devoicing in stop-sonorant and fricative-sonorant sequences

As outlined in the introduction we will move here from consideration of the coarticulatory effects themselves to discussion of the implications of the available data for more general issues of interarticulator coordination. The most accessible source of systematic data is Docherty's (1992) acoustic investigation, and this will accordingly form the basis for much of the discussion.

Two simple regularities can at once be stated for sequences of stop or fricative plus sonorant:[3] (a) VOT (i.e. the period of voicelessness following release of the stop or fricative) is longer in these sequences than in simple CV sequences; (b) it is well documented that stops and fricatives generally have a shorter occlusion duration when they occur in clusters (e.g. Haggard 1973; Klatt 1973; Hawkins 1979). Docherty notes that there have been virtually no attempts to explain the longer VOTs in stop–sonorant clusters. One exception discussed further by him is a speculative suggestion by Hoole (1987)[4] that the above two findings can be simply related in a manner entirely analogous to the attempt (discussed above) to explain place of articulation differences in VOT in terms of the superimposition of different occlusion durations on an invariant devoicing gesture. In other words, pairs such as English 'keen' and 'clean' may have the same glottal gesture, but a shortened occlusion duration of /k/ in 'clean', resulting in an essentially voiceless /l/. In terms of the schematic illustration given in figure 5.1 one can think of the devoiced sonorant replacing the phase labelled 'aspiration', this phase being proportionally longer and the preceding phase labelled 'oral occlusion' proportionally shorter in the consonant clusters under discussion here than in the simple aspirated plosives.

As with the place of articulation data above, Docherty's acoustic data did not, however, provide much support for this hypothesis: in the stop–sonorant–vowel case the total duration of devoicing was *longer* than in the simple stop–vowel case; in other words there was a greater increase in VOT than could be accounted for by the reduction in stop occlusion duration alone. We find this result most intriguing, perhaps more so than Docherty himself seems to do, since it is difficult to think of a speech production model that could predict this finding. In rather overstated terms, it appears that the effect of adjoining a voiced consonant to a voiceless aspirated plosive is to *increase* the magnitude of the devoicing gesture, which is most definitely not how coarticulatory effects are generally considered to work. Before indulging in further speculation we must hasten to point out that there may well be one simple passive explanation for the unexpected fact that the stop–continuant cluster has a longer period of devoicing than the simple stop, namely that the aerodynamic conditions in the continuant are not conducive to initiation of phonation (due to the fact that the oral tract is still partially occluded). Thus the acoustically measured period of voicelessness may not be an accurate reflection of the duration of the laryngeal gesture itself. Further articulatory data may thus still save the invariant laryngeal gesture hypothesis, although Docherty seems to be of the opinion that the magnitude of the effects makes this rather unlikely.

Even if it remains an open issue whether devoicing duration is genuinely longer in stop–sonorant clusters, it does seem to be clear that devoicing duration is not *shorter*. This is in itself a significant finding since given the shorter occlusion duration a shorter devoicing could well be expected under the plausible assumption that the component gestures of an aspirated plosive become modified in parallel. For example, working within the framework of the Task-Dynamics model, Saltzman and Munhall (1989) point to evidence from perturbation experiments that the laryngeal gesture is modified when the bilabial closure for /p/ is interfered with experimentally. They cite this as evidence for a level of intergestural cohesion that undoubtedly must exist (cf. VOT). These workers further introduce a concept of gestural 'dominance' (Saltzman and Munhall 1989: 349): in other words, different segments have a different degree of dominance over the timing of the glottal peak. This concept is used to explain the ways in which glottal gestures merge in voiceless clusters (see below). The problem in the present context is that in /kl/ clusters, for example, no other segment should be competing with /k/ for dominance of the larynx, yet it may be necessary to assume that the position of peak glottal opening relative to /k/ release is shifted from the non-cluster case. Kingston's (1990) concept of binding (of laryngeal to oral articulations) would seem to run into similar problems.[5]

One way around this problem, which would certainly be in the spirit of the task-dynamics approach, is that in clusters the acoustic manifestation of occlusion duration in plosives or constriction duration in fricatives is no longer very directly related to the underlying gestural activation. For example, in /#sm/ it is conceivable that the acoustic manifestation of /s/ is partly 'hidden' and thus shortened by an overlapping bilabial gesture (cf. Borden and Gay 1979), and that in /#sl/ the manifestation of /s/ is truncated by the /l/ competing for the tongue tip articulator. In both cases the underlying lingual input for /s/ may have remained constant, together with the glottal timing with respect to this input.

Is it possible to come up with an explanation as to why the devoicing gesture conceivably lengthens? In an analysis of voiceless clusters (to which we return below) Browman and Goldstein (1986) come to the conclusion that it can be stated as a regularity of English that a word (syllable) can only begin with one devoicing gesture.[6] This idea could be extended, certainly with a good deal of violence to the authors' original intentions, to suggest that in some sense the devoicing gesture is a property of the whole syllable onset. The devoicing gesture may then lengthen as the syllable onset becomes longer. With regard to their two rules, there is, however, the possibility that they might not be strictly correct, because of the change of the temporal relationship between peak glottal opening and oral occlusion in clusters (but note the distinction just made between surface manifestation and underlying input).

An alternative, more output oriented style of explanation might be that it is perceptually important to have a substantial amount of devoicing on the second element in a cluster (e.g. to separate 'played', 'blade', 'prayed', 'braid'). A further alternative is that given the aerodynamic conditions in the vocal tract, early adduction might not lead to reliable re-initiation of voicing anyway, so speakers find it easier to use a somewhat longer gesture (note, according to Docherty 1992: 147, the VOT of English phonologically voiced stops is also slightly longer in stop–sonorant sequences, such as /bl/, than in the singleton case).

Docherty's results for fricative–sonorant sequences are essentially comparable to those for stop–sonorant sequences. For /s/ plus nasal sequences the constriction duration for /s/ was reduced in comparison with single /s/, but total devoicing duration increased, so again it seems that the amount of nasal devoicing does not simply result from the reduction in /s/–duration. The other fricative–sonorant combinations mostly indicated the same pattern. One interesting exception was that /f/–sonorant clusters did not show a significant increase in total devoicing duration, leading Docherty to speculate that this may be related to the potential for coproduction of the oral components of the cluster (which is presumably higher in the labiodental fricative case; in fact the labial stop in Docherty's data also shows a relatively weak increase in devoicing duration in clusters). Thus, in the /sl/ case, with little coproduction possible he suggests that 'one might hypothesize the existence of a temporal constraint delaying voicing onset until the lateral gesture is complete' (Docherty 1992: 154). This seems to be close to the suggestion made above that the devoicing gesture may be influenced by the length of the whole syllable onset – independently to some extent of the intrinsic voicing characteristics of the segments making up that onset. If rules of this kind should prove necessary they would have interesting implications for the patterns of intergestural coordination that a production model would have to account for.

In conclusion here, it can safely be said that some fairly straightforward transillumination or fibrescopic data on clusters with mixed voicing characteristics (in plentiful supply in languages such as English and German) could swiftly resolve some of the speculative discussion above and already prove illuminating for our understanding of laryngeal–oral coordination. The more demanding task will be to link the laryngeal findings to improved understanding of the organization of supraglottal gestures in clusters.

Devoicing patterns in voiceless clusters

As outlined in the introductory section, clusters of voiceless consonants provide one of the most suitable fields for examining processes of coarticulation or coproduction at the laryngeal level by studying how the simple, ballistic-looking pattern of abduction and adduction found in single consonants is modified when sequences of voiceless consonants occur. The most convenient source of information on this topic is a series of articles published some ten years ago by Löfqvist and colleagues, in which sequences of voiceless sounds in American English, Swedish, Icelandic, Dutch and Japanese were studied (Löfqvist and Yoshioka 1980a, 1980b, Yoshioka, Löfqvist and Hirose 1980, 1981; Yoshioka, Löfqvist and Collier 1982). These papers have the advantage of sharing a common methodology, namely transillumination or fibreoptics together with EMG (the latter not for Icelandic). The corpora are also quite comparable, consisting for the four Germanic languages mainly of combinations of /s/ and a stop to left and right of a word boundary – giving sequences of up to five voiceless consonants. For Japanese, which does not have clusters of this kind, long voiceless sequences were obtained by exploiting the phenomenon of vowel devoicing, preceded and followed by voiceless stop or fricative.

One emphasis in these papers is in arriving at a qualitative understanding of the time-course of laryngeal abduction and adduction as a function of the structure of the consonant sequence, i.e. in predicting where one, two or more peaks in the transillumination signal will occur (in addition these articles also provided the consistent result of larger, faster abduction in fricatives versus stops, as dicussed above).

In a later paper (Munhall and Löfqvist 1992) the question of the relationship between the number of peaks in the transillumination signal and the number of underlying laryngeal gestures is examined – specifically whether a single peak in the surface behaviour can plausibly be regarded (in appropriate contexts) as a blending of two (or more) underlying gestures. In Saltzman and Munhall (1989) some of the additional assumptions likely to be required to predict the details of the blending process are discussed. Each of these developments will be discussed briefly in turn.

With regard, then, to the observable kinematics of laryngeal behaviour in voiceless consonant sequences the results have been summarized by Löfqvist (1990: 296) that 'sounds requiring a high rate of airflow, such as fricatives and aspirated stops, are produced with a separate gesture'. Perhaps the clearest example of this behaviour is to be found in fricative–plosive clusters. For the three Germanic languages English, Swedish and Icelandic, when these clusters occur word-initially or finally (e.g. /#sp/ or /sp#/) the plosive is unaspirated, and only one abduction peak occurs. When the cluster spans a word boundary the stop is aspirated in all languages, and two peaks are found. As the number of voiceless segments in the cluster increases, then more peaks can occur, e.g. /sks#k/ (or equivalent thereof) showed three peaks in all three languages. On the other hand, there are a number of cases when fewer peaks are observed than the above summary might lead one to expect. For example, the long voiceless sequence /ks#sp/ showed only one peak in all three languages. This may well be related to the homorganicity of the fricatives: simple /s#s/ sequences also showed only one peak in English, Icelandic and Dutch (the corresponding Swedish data was not shown). /k#k/ in English showed only one peak, whereas the non-homorganic sequence /k#p/ in Swedish had two.[7] Compared with the Germanic languages Japanese appears to show in general a weaker tendency to multiple peaks. A sequence such as stop–devoiced-vowel–geminate stop shows only one; even the very long voiceless sequence fricative–devoiced-vowel–geminate–fricative showed only comparatively weak evidence of more than one peak. Possibly this situation is related to the fact that aspiration is not a prominent feature of Japanese stops, so the air-flow requirements in sequences involving stops may not be particularly stringent.

Following these qualitative remarks, we immediately reach the stage, of course, at which it becomes important to distinguish between the observable kinematic behaviour and the putative underlying gestural input. Clearly a homorganic cluster could be realized with a particularly large degree of overlap of discrete underlying oral and laryngeal gestures (though note also that haplology is a productive phonological process). However, here we reach the limits of the interpretability of this group of papers since no figures are given allowing, for example, fricative-constriction duration to be compared in the singleton versus the homorganic cluster case. Nonetheless, the authors did note in the Icelandic paper that where different repetitions of a given cluster were spoken with widely varying durations then the number of observable peaks might be less at the shorter duration, e.g. for /t#k/ two peaks clearly corresponding to each stop at the long duration, only one peak at short durations. It is then tempting to assume that underlyingly two peaks are present at the shorter duration, too; they have simply become merged together. This is illustrated schematically in figure 5.2.

Munhall and Löfqvist (1992) then examined the plausibility of this assumption more systematically by running an experiment in which only one cluster was examined (/s#t/ from 'kiss Ted') but where a wide range of speech rates was elicited (and stress was also varied) in order to obtain something approaching a continuum of cluster durations. The result showed by and large a gradual merging from two separated gestures at the slowest rates via a more complexly shaped movement at intermediate rates to a simple single-peaked movement at the fastest rates. Single-peaked patterns for this kind of cluster may thus be seen as simply one end of a continuum, rather than a completely different mode of organization compared with the multi-peaked tokens. For the cross-word clusters examined here, and for example the /s#s/ homorganic clusters mentioned above, the approach is undoubtedly rather persuasive. Whether word-initial clusters (e.g. /#sp/) can by the same line of reasoning (cf. Saltzman and Munhall 1989; Löfqvist 1990; also Pétursson 1977) be regarded as underlyingly two gestures is more contentious (see below); they never, as far as we know, show two gestures on the surface. Munhall and Löfqvist are also quick to admit that alternative explanations are not completely ruled out:

> One problem in the area of coarticulation and in the present study is that it is difficult, in practice, to distinguish between alternative explanations. At the fastest speaking rates in the present data, a single movement is observed. By examining the kinematics of these movements in isolation it

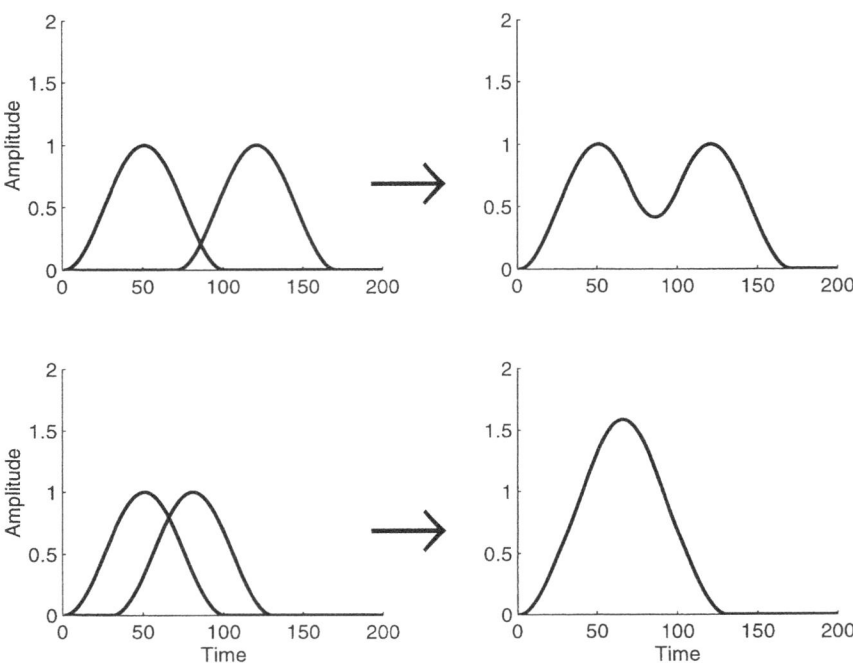

Figure 5.2   Simplified illustration of relationship between hypothesized underlying gestural input (left panels) and observable behaviour (right panels) at different degrees of gestural overlap (top versus bottom). Amplitude of the basic laryngeal gesture has been arbitrarily set to 1, and duration to 100. See Munhall and Löfqvist (1992, figure 5) for a wider range of more realistic simulations.

is impossible to determine the nature of the underlying control signal. For two reasons, we have favored the overlap account for the present data. While any individual movement could be accounted for by many approaches, it is more parsimonious to attribute all the data to a single pattern of serial ordering. It would appear, particularly from the intermediate rate observations, that two separate gestures are blended. This style of coordination can produce the full range of observed data and thus seems a likely candidate even for the fastest speaking rates. A second factor that supports this approach is evidence from other motor activities. . . . (1992: 122)

This remains a significant experiment for coarticulatory studies as a whole (one might even say that it was long overdue, following the pioneering studies discussed at the beginning of this section): the great simplicity of the devoicing gesture (in spatial terms) in comparison, for example, to tongue movements makes it probably the speech sub-system where the existence of blending processes can be most convincingly demonstrated.

Some suggestions for principles underlying the details of the blending process are to be found in Saltzman and Munhall (1989). As mentioned above, they make use of the concept of dominance:

> The dominance for a voiceless consonant's oral constriction over its glottal timing appears to be influenced by (at least) two factors. The first is the *manner* class of the segment: Frication intervals (at least for /s/) dominate glottal behavior more strongly than stop closure intervals. . . . The second factor is the presence of a word-initial boundary: Word-initial consonants dominate glottal behavior more strongly than the same nonword-initial consonants. (p. 369)

Motivation for the idea of fricative dominance is developed especially in Goldstein (1990). In particular this determines the order of the two rules given in footnote 6.

Saltzman and Munhall illustrate the process first with some unpublished data on word-final clusters. English /s#/, /ks#/, /sk#/ all have only one glottal peak, which for single /s/ is smaller than in the other two cases (observable in Yoshioka, Löfqvist and Hirose 1981), suggesting that in the cluster case blending of two gestures is involved. The specific location of the peak glottal opening in the clusters could be interpreted as indicating that /s/ is the 'dominant' partner, but with the location of the peak being perturbed slightly away from mid-frication by the adjacent stop (mid-frication being the normal location of peak glottal opening in isolated fricatives). It will be recalled that one motivation for this kind of approach is that a more parsimonious analysis results if the single glottal peak can be assumed to be the result of two underlying gestures. The only problem in the above example is that word-final voiceless plosives in English are often glottalized (see e.g. Yoshioka, Löfqvist and Hirose 1981). Thus some additional rule is in any case required to state when the laryngeal gesture for a word-final voiceless plosive can be reorganized from devoicing (abduction) to glottalization (adduction) (on the problem of glottalization see Browman and Goldstein 1992, and Kingston and Cohen's 1992 comment).

In a further example Saltzman and Munhall compare such word-final clusters with corresponding word-initial clusters. We have already noted that in /#st/ only a single peak occurs. We have also mentioned that for Munhall and Löfqvist the 'kiss Ted' results make it reasonable to assume that these single-peaked word-initial clusters consist underlyingly of two blended gestures. On the other hand, we have further noted that for Browman and Goldstein (1986) it is a significant generalization of the (articulatory) phonology of English that a word can begin with no more than one glottal gesture.[8] There is thus an interesting divergence of views even among quite closely related approaches (cf. Saltzman and Munhall 1989: 365).

Saltzman and Munhall state that for these word-initial clusters in English peak glottal opening occurs at mid-frication in both single /s/ and in /st/ and thus that, in contrast to the word-final case, location of peak glottal opening has not been perturbed by the adjacent plosive. In terms of the dominance concept, this would be due to the intrinsically high dominance of /s/, reinforced by its word-initial position. In fact, however, as far as we can tell, the relevant literature does not state that peak glottal opening in /st/ is at mid-frication, only that it is during the frication phase (Pétursson 1977 not cited by Saltzman & Munhall, in fact notes that in Icelandic it occurs in the first half of the frication phase; Goldstein 1990 on the other hand notes that it may be delayed somewhat, i.e. later than mid-frication). This reflects a paucity in the literature of precise information on constriction and occlusion duration in those clusters for which we have information on the laryngeal kinematics. There is also some ambivalence in the literature as to what constitutes a clearly more extensive devoicing gesture. The blending hypothesis would lead us to expect a larger gesture on /st/ than on /s/. Almost the only accessible source of numeric data showing this to be the case is for one American speaker in McGarr and Löfqvist (1988). For Swedish, Löfqvist and Yoshioka (1980b) say /#sp/ is similar to /s/, as do Yoshioka, Löfqvist and Collier (1982) for Dutch. Goldstein (1990: 447), following on from the articulatory phonology analysis, also seems to view the gestures as about the same size. Finally, in order to link up with the discussion of mixed-voicing clusters above, it should be noted that even if the laryngeal gesture for /st/ does indeed turn out to be reliably larger than for /s/ then this may not be sufficient grounds for suspecting the presence of two underlying gestures if, in turn, it emerges that such sequences as /pl/ and /sl/ also have a larger devoicing gesture than the singleton case.

Concluding this topic, the aim of this review is not so much to arrive at a conclusion as to what is the more persuasive analysis of fricative–stop clusters, on which there is a substantial further literature of both phonological and phonetic orientation (see references in Pétursson 1977; Ewen 1982; Browman and Goldstein 1986), but rather to highlight the still existing gaps in our knowledge about the relevant articulatory interrelationships.

Let us return briefly to the second factor suggested by Saltzman and Munhall (1989) to determine dominance strength, namely position of the consonant in the word. This is a very reasonable principle since it is quite clear that the devoicing gesture for a word-final fricative is smaller than for a word-initial one (see Yoshioka, Löfqvist and Hirose 1981), while for stops Cooper (1991) has also shown clear effects of stress and position in the word (see also discussion of reduction of devoicing gestural magnitude in Browman and Goldstein 1992). However, some aspects of cross-word boundary clusters do not seem to quite accord with expectations. American English, Swedish and Icelandic all have data for sequences with a structure like /st#st/ (American English has /sk#sk/), i.e. the same kind of cluster before and after the word boundary. In all these cases two peaks are observable, but the first one (presumably corresponding to the word-*final* position) generally appears to be higher. Similarly, for American English and Dutch, in /s#s/ only one peak occurs, but it is skewed to the left (not, however, in Icelandic, where /s#s/ also occurs), suggesting more vigorous devoicing early in the sequence. On the other hand American English /k#k/ peaks late in the sequence (skewed to the right). These examples suggest that the amplitude of the devoicing gesture may also be modulated on-line depending on the aerodynamic conditions in the vocal tract: as already mentioned above, the critical laryngeal phase of a fricative is the onset, since voicing must be terminated and air-pressure built up to drive the frication source. However, once these demands have been met the requirements for the following devoicing gesture (i.e. for the second /sk/ in /sk#sk/, or the second /s/ in /s#s/) are probably not so stringent, and the amplitude may then be smaller. For plosives the reverse applies: the more stringent demands are at offset rather than onset. In short, the procedures by which dominance is determined in any particular case may have to make more explicit reference to the airflow demands of the sequence of sounds being produced.

At the conclusion of this section it should be said the great advantage of the rather specific proposals for blending and dominance put forward in Saltzman and Munhall (1989) resides in the fact that they provide a very efficient framework for pinpointing the current state of our knowledge.

Conclusion to section A

This review of laryngeal coarticulation has shown that we have quite a good understanding of the organization of the laryngeal devoicing gesture both in simple and more complex sequences of sounds. However, some gaps remain. Some should be easy to fill, for example with respect to the amplitude and duration of laryngeal activity in voiceless–voiced consonant sequences. Others, particularly those relating to the details of laryngeal–oral coordination will be more difficult; in fact what is required is not so much better knowledge of laryngeal behaviour *per se*, but rather improved insight into the organization of labial and lingual gestures in consonant sequences. In view of the considerably greater complexity of supraglottal articulations compared to laryngeal articulations this will be no mean task.

Section B: Voice source variation in the vowel as a function of consonantal context: Christer Gobl and Ailbhe Ní Chasaide

Introduction

Traditionally, acoustic studies of coarticulation were based on temporal measurements: in the example mentioned in the general introduction above, coarticulatory devoicing of the /l/ of the English word 'plead' is measured as the duration of the voiceless interval from stop release to the onset of voice in the lateral. In some languages, such as Irish, extensive devoicing may also be found in laterals before voiceless stops. In these cases, coarticulation is measured as the interval from voice offset in the lateral to stop occlusion.

Recent work has shown that the coarticulatory influences of voiceless consonants may extend well beyond the instant of voice onset (or offset). Fine-grained analyses of the voice source have shown that during a voiced segment the mode of phonation may vary as a function of the nature of an adjacent consonant, and this forms the central topic of the remainder of this chapter. The types of effects which (particularly voiceless) stops and fricatives may have on the mode of phonation of the adjacent voiced segment, here a vowel, are illustrated later. For reasons that have to do with the limitations of the current methodology, the data are far from exhaustive, but they do suggest that these influences on the vowel's mode of phonation depend both on the manner of articulation of the consonant (e.g. stop versus fricative) and on the language or dialect. The data yield a number of insights into the underlying control strategies that may be involved in the regulation of these consonants, and these are discussed later.

The data on which the following illustrations are based are for the most part drawn from Ní Chasaide and Gobl (1993) and Gobl and Ní Chasaide (1988) and concern detailed analyses of the vowel in the stressed syllable followed or preceded by the phonologically voiceless and voiced consonants /p(ː), b(ː), v(ː), f(ː)/ in five languages: French, Italian, Swedish, German and English (further details below). Although each of these languages has a two-way phonological voicing contrast, we should note that the phonetic realization of the stops is not the same in all these languages. In French and Italian, the opposition is between a strongly voiced [b] and the voiceless unaspirated [p]. In English, Swedish and German the opposition is between [b] and the aspirated [pʰ], and the precise realizations are more variable in different contexts: the voiced stop may tend toward devoicing in certain environments, and for [pʰ], the duration of aspiration varies according to a number of factors, being for example much longer in the initial prestressed environment than in the medial poststressed one.

As it is pertinent to later discussions, we will briefly review here the received wisdom concerning the laryngeal gestures associated with the three phonetic categories of stops that we are dealing with – voiced, voiceless unaspirated and voiceless aspirated (i.e. postaspirated). For the voiced category, the glottis is adducted and vibrating. Voicing is often seen to weaken or even disappear towards the end of stop closure; when this happens, it is generally thought to be due to passive aerodynamic forces rather than to active laryngeal adjustments. The voiceless categories involve active abduction and, of course, subsequent adduction of the vocal folds. (We are here not concerned with glottalized stops such as occur in specific environments for certain dialects of English and which involve a rather different mechanism of devoicing.) It is a widely held view that the difference between the unaspirated and the postaspirated stop depends essentially on a difference in the timing of the laryngeal gesture relative to the oral closure, particularly of glottal adduction relative to stop release (see for example Löfqvist 1980; Goldstein and Browman 1986). For both types of stop, glottal abduction is thought to begin at approximately the moment when oral closure is formed. In the unaspirated stop, peak glottal opening is reached at about the middle of the interval of closure duration for the stop. The relatively early onset of adduction ensures that the vocal folds are in an appropriately adducted state for the initiation of voicing at or around the time of oral release. For the aspirated stop, glottal abduction continues throughout the stop closure. Peak glottal opening occurs at approximately the time of oral release, and is of a considerably greater amplitude than for the unaspirated stop (see for example Kim 1965). According to what we might term the 'timing' model of glottal control, this amplitude difference is explained as a consequence of the relatively later timing of glottal adduction. Furthermore, aspiration is taken to be effectively the interval during which the folds adduct to the point where voicing resumes. According to this view, the presence, absence or indeed the duration of aspiration can be explained in terms of a difference in the timing of an otherwise similar glottal gesture: slightly longer or shorter aspiration reflects a slightly later or earlier onset of the adduction gesture. Preaspiration can similarly be accounted for by this 'timing' model: whereas in unaspirated and postaspirated stops the abduction gesture is assumed to be synchronized with the oral closure for the stop, preaspiration occurs when the abduction is timed to begin before oral occlusion.

Data and analytic methods

The data analysed involved the stressed first vowel of $C_1V_1C_2V_2$ nonsense utterances in five languages, French, Italian, Swedish, German and English, where $V_1 = $ /a/, $C_2 = $ /p(:), b(:), v(:), f(:)/; $C_1 = $ /p, b/. Recordings were made of four informants (including male and female) of each language.

Note that in a language where vowels have contrastive length, the short vowel was used. Consequently, in Italian and Swedish, the postvocalic consonant is a geminate, this being the only possibility following a short vowel. High quality digital recordings as well as separate oral airflow recordings were made, and full details concerning the recording conditions are included in chapter 15B.

The analytic methods are also outlined in detail in chapter 15 section B. To recap briefly here, the main acoustic analysis tool is inverse filtering, whereby the effects of the vocal tract filter are eliminated to yield the glottal flow derivative. A model of the source flow (the LF model) is matched to the output of the inverse filter as a way of measuring salient aspects of the source data. Both of these procedures involve manual interactive editing of individual glottal pulses. As this is a time-consuming and difficult procedure, the quantity of data subjected to detailed source analysis was limited to the following. First of all, one full set of data for all combinations of pre- and postvocalic stops was analysed for each speaker of each language (eighty utterances). Subsequently, for a comparison of postvocalic stops and fricatives, more numerous repetitions of utterances where C_2 = each of the stops and the fricatives, and C_1 = /b/ were analysed for one speaker of French (five repetitions), Italian (five repetitions) and Swedish (three repetitions), yielding an additional fifty-two utterances.

The source data were supplemented by more extensive oral airflow data, which can be very illuminating in particular cases and which help us to establish the likely generality of our voice source data for each speaker. For a further discussion of this point, see Gobl and Ní Chasaide (1988). In addition, spectral measurements of the speech output, in particular a comparison of the levels of F1 and F0 are included as useful indicators of source behaviour.

The source data in the following section are presented in terms of glottal flow parameters and the reader is again referred to chapter 15 section B where these are fully explained. Here we will simply gloss some that appear in the illustrations below. EE, the excitation strength, is a good overall indication of the amplitude of the source signal; RA, the dynamic leakage, is a good indicator of breathiness in the glottal pulse and high RA value is associated with a loss of energy in the higher harmonics in the speech output; FA is a measure of the frequency above which energy is lost in accordance with the RA value for a particular f_0; RK is a measure of the symmetry or skew of the glottal pulse: a high RK shows a symmetrical glottal pulse.

Illustrations of anticipatory and carryover effects

The main effect observed concerned voiceless consonants. Where such effects are found, one finds an appreciable difference in the voice source characteristics for the vowel in the voiced and voiceless context. Among the stops there appeared to be some striking cross-language differences, both in terms of the directionality as well as the degree of the effect observed. Insofar as we could ascertain, fricatives appeared to be more consistent across languages.

We illustrate the data below in some detail, dealing separately with anticipatory and carryover effects, before proceeding to a discussion of the possible control strategies that may be involved in the regulation of these voiceless consonants. We would stress from the outset that the data analysed are quite limited, in terms of the quantity of data analysed, the numbers of subjects and of the phonetic environments investigated. While the data may usefully point to likely tendencies, further investigations will be needed to establish a definitive account in any particular language.

Anticipatory effects: stops

Among the stops striking cross-languages differences were observed, with Swedish and French at opposite ends of a continuum. The differences between them are illustrated in figure 5.3, where EE and RA values are superimposed for the /p–p(ː)/ and /p–b(ː)/ contexts in German, French, Swedish and Italian. The traces shown are for single utterances and for averages and fuller illustrations, see Ní Chasaide and Gobl (1993). The traces for the two contexts have been aligned to the oral closure of the intervocalic consonant (C_2 of the nonsense utterance). In the Swedish utterance, before the voiceless stop, the source pulse exhibits an increasingly weak excitation (EE), increasing dynamic leakage (RA) and becomes increasingly symmetrical (increasing RK values, not shown here). This is consistent with an increasingly breathy mode of phonation, corresponding to a weakening acoustic signal with particular loss of energy in the higher frequencies. As these effects are absent when the following stop is voiced, there is effectively considerable information even during the vowel on the nature of the upcoming consonant.

In contrast, the French data exhibit virtually none of the effects associated with the voiceless stops in Swedish. The vowel has a constant quality regardless of the upcoming stop. Very tiny differences do show up but they are confined to the last glottal pulse or two. Note also that the duration of the vowel is fairly similar for both contexts, unlike the large differences that can be seen for the Swedish data.

Vowel offsets in German are rather similar to the French: the voiced/voiceless nature of the postvocalic stop appears to have little differential effect on the vowel's mode of phonation. Note the falling excitation strength and rise in dynamic leakage before both consonants. This may indicate some adduction or slackening of the vocal folds but, as it is associated with both contexts,

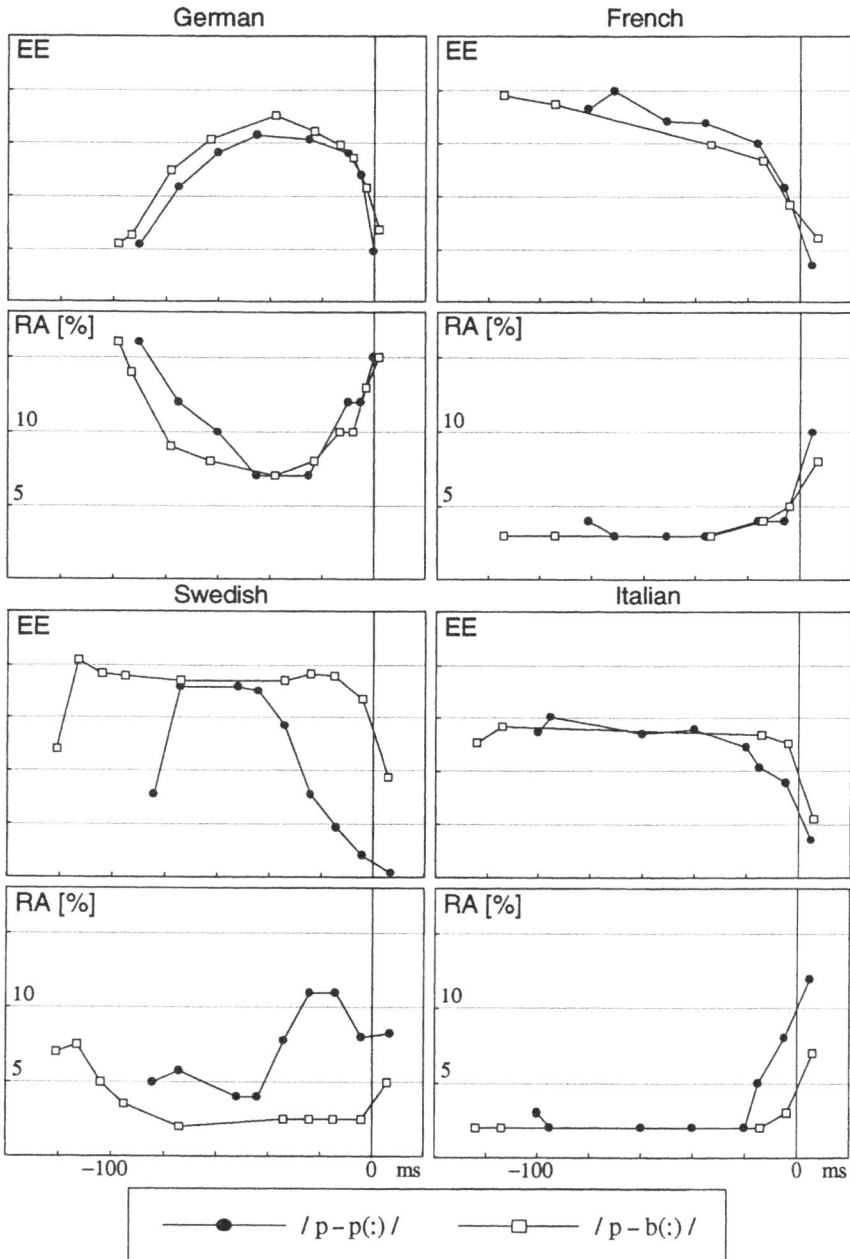

Figure 5.3   EE and RA values superimposed for the /p–p(:)/ and /p–b(:)/ contexts in German, French, Swedish and Italian. Traces are aligned to oral closure (= 0 ms).

it does not serve to differentiate between them. The Italian data showed some of the effects observed in Swedish before the voiceless stop. The extent of the effect is however much smaller. Furthermore, the duration of the Italian vowel in this context was considerably longer, and therefore, the breathy offset occupies proportionally much less of the vowel's duration.

A visual inspection of the oral airflow signal in these languages (figures 5.4a and 5.4b) completes the picture. Note in figure 5.4a for Swedish, the sharp rise in airflow in the vowel before /–p:/. From the point where the oral airflow rises, one can also see a gradual decay in the amplitude of voicing in the vowel. This contrasts sharply with the same vowel in the /–b(:)/ environment. The rise in airflow associated with the voiceless stop of Swedish almost certainly reflects a very early abduction of the vocal folds. This study did not include any direct record of glottal behaviour, but the illustration of the glottal gesture in the Icelandic word /la^{h}pa/ should serve to illustrate the point (figure 5.5). Note that the intervocalic stop in this instance is a preaspirated stop. The reader should observe how the glottal opening gesture for the preaspirated stop (point A in this figure) coincides closely with the rise in oral airflow. Note also that as the vocal folds open they continue to vibrate: the amplitude of voicing decays gradually up to a point (somewhere around B in this figure) where it gives way to voiceless aspiration. We would suggest that oral airflow can be a very good indicator of glottal abduction, provided it occurs before the oral occlusion.

As one would expect, the voiced/voiceless nature of the intervocalic stop in French has little effect on the airflow signal of the preceding vowel, which also shows strong voicing right up to oral closure. The same is true of the German data, whereas for Italian, we find evidence of early glottal abduction in the airflow peak associated with the /–p:/ context. This accords well with the source data. The spectral data in figure 5.6 also serve to illustrate some of these cross-language differences. In this figure the levels of F1 are shown relative to the levels of F0 (i.e. L1–L0) for the vowel in the /–p(:)/ and /–b(:)/ contexts for French, German, Swedish and Italian. Note in particular the weakening in F1 before the voiceless consonant of Swedish and the similar though less extensive effect in Italian.

The comparison of L1 and L0 is a useful measure: by normalizing to L0 we can compare spectral level data for different speakers/languages. Using L0 for normalization across a whole utterance is justified insofar as L0 tends to remain rather stable. This is illustrated in figure 5.7, which shows for the Swedish vowel in the /b–b:/ and /b–p:/ environments respectively: the speech waveform, Osc., the differentiated glottal flow, Ug'(t), the true glottal flow, Ug(t), the excitation strength, EE (shown here in dB), the amplitude of the first harmonic, L0, and the peak flow of the glottal pulse, U$_p$. Note during the breathy

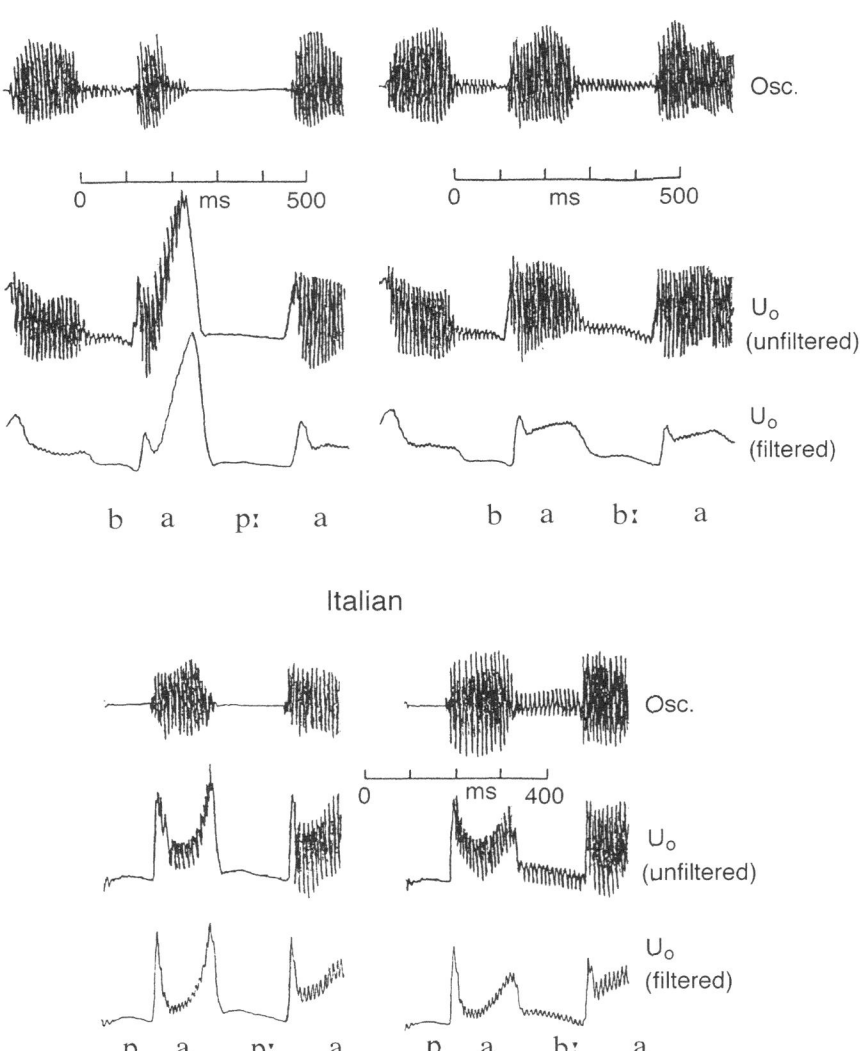

Figure 5.4a   Oral airflow and speech waveform illustrating contrasting intervocalic bilabial stops in Swedish and Italian.

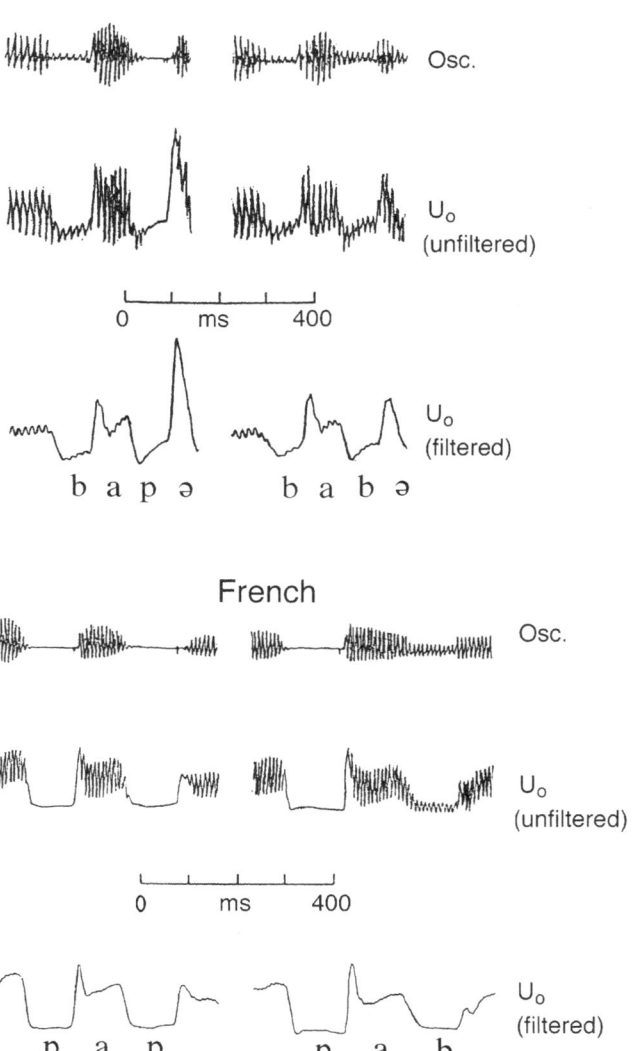

Figure 5.4b   Oral airflow and speech waveform illustrating contrasting intervocalic bilabial stops in German and French.

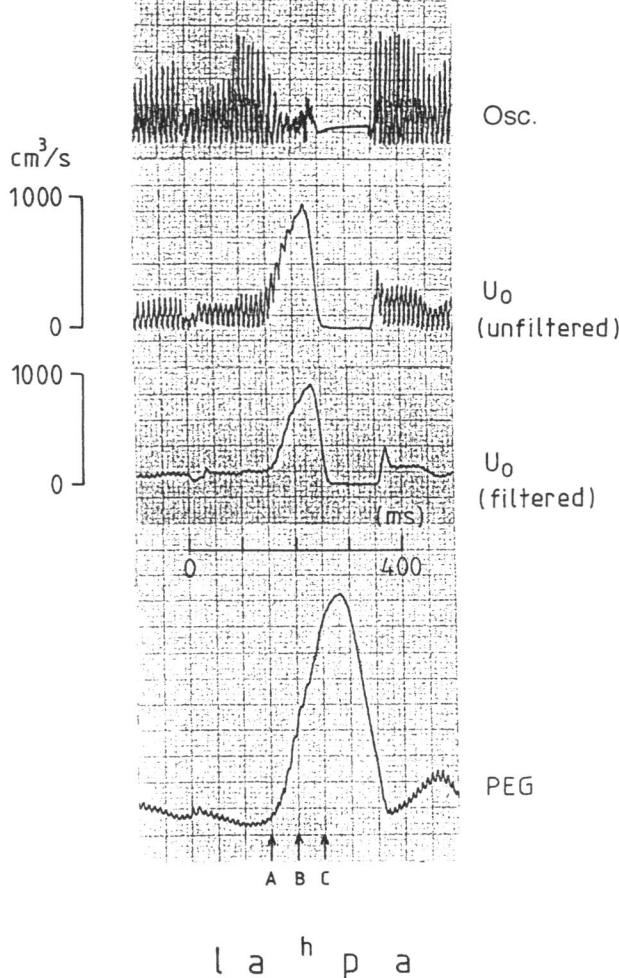

Figure 5.5   Multi-channel recording of the Icelandic word /laʰpa/. Time points A, B, and C refer respectively to the beginning of vocal fold abduction, termination of vocal fold vibration, and oral closure. Osc. = speech waveform, U_0 = oral airflow and PEG = photo-electric glottograph signal.

voiced offset of the vowel in the /–p:/ context, while EE drops in amplitude, L0 remains rather constant up until the last glottal pulse. Note also the relative constancy of U_p and of the total volume of the glottal flow pulse for the same interval. It has been pointed out by Fant (1980) and Bickley and Stevens (1986) that the level of the low frequency spectrum is basically proportional to

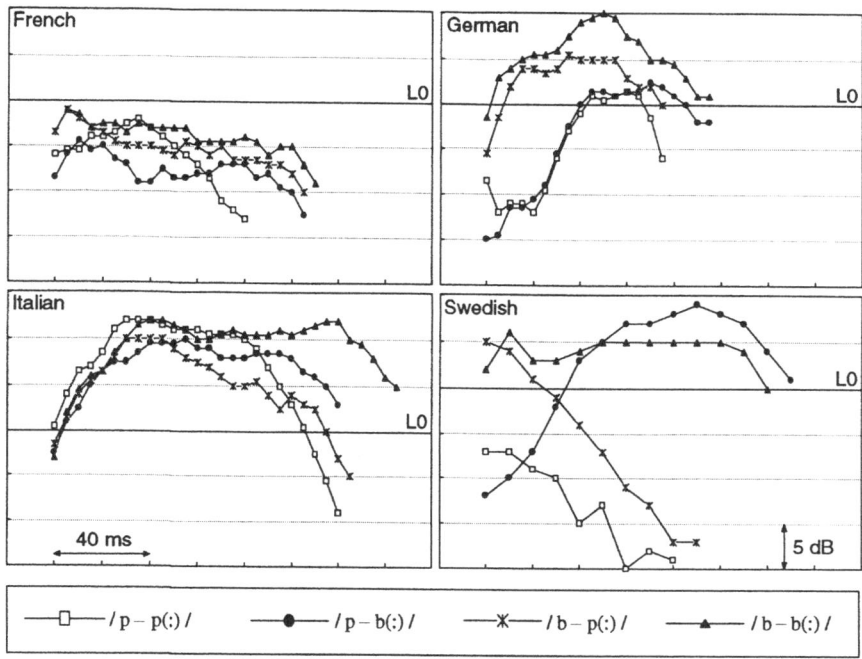

Figure 5.6   L1 relative to L0 for the contexts /p–b(ː)/, /b–p(ː)/, /p–b(ː)/ and /b–b(ː)/ in French, German, Italian and Swedish. Traces are aligned to vowel onset.

the total volume of the glottal pulse, and this explains the close correspondence between the glottal flow signal and L0. This rather constant L0 was observed for most of the data examined. An exception was the voice onset in the German data following /p/, and this is discussed where relevant below.

The English data (not shown here) were subjected to a similar analysis and were rather curious in that two distinct trends were observed. Two of the speakers exhibited large source differences for the two contexts: the data here were quite similar to the Swedish case. The other two showed only slight effects and were more like the French data or somewhere between the French data and the Italian. These data are illustrated and discussed more fully in Ní Chasaide and Gobl (1993).

Anticipatory effects: fricatives

A visual inspection of our airflow recordings suggest that the vowel before voiceless fricatives exhibits the type of gradual breathy voiced offset described above for the stops of Swedish. Voice source data showing the EE, RA and RK parameters are shown in figure 5.8 for the vowel before fricatives

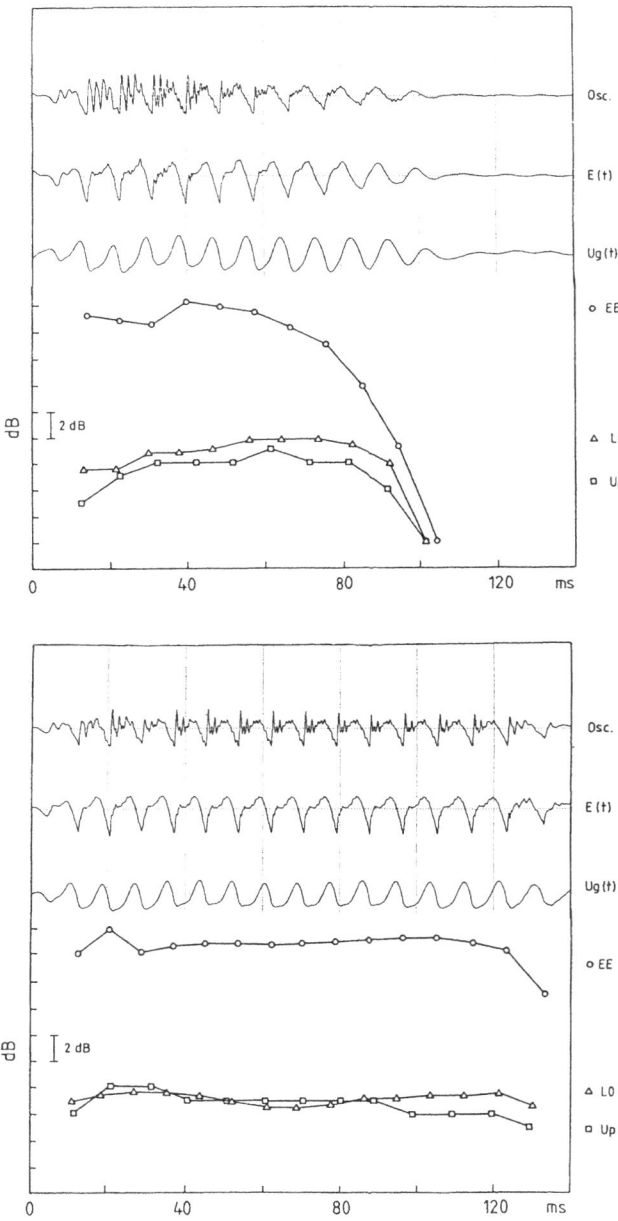

Figure 5.7   For the first vowel of the Swedish words /bab:a/ and /bap:a/ are shown:
Osc. = speech waveform, E(t) = differentiated glottal flow, Ug(t) = true glottal flow,
EE = excitation strength (here in dB, for comparability with L0), Up = peak flow of
the glottal pulse and L0 = the amplitude level of F0.

as compared to stops for a speaker of Swedish, Italian and French. The three languages were chosen for the fricative analysis, as they represent the full range of variation found for the stops. Values in this instance are averaged over a number of repetitions (see earlier). Insofar as was possible, the traces have been aligned to the closure of the stops and to the onset of frication in the fricative. Fairly typical oral airflow signals are also shown in figure 5.9 for these same languages.

The similarity of the vowel source characteristics prior to the voiceless fricative is rather striking for the three languages. Note the gradually falling excitation strength, EE, along with the rising dynamic leakage, RA, and the increasingly symmetrical shape of the glottal pulse, RK, in the vowel. Note also the sharp rise in the oral airflow before it drops in a way that reflects that the oral stricture is accomplished. All the indicators are that the glottal abduction gesture is initiated substantially before the oral stricture, and that devoicing has been accomplished before the onset of frication.

The most striking point is perhaps the cross-language similarity for the voiceless fricatives, bearing in mind that these three languages exhibit rather different patterns in their voiceless stops. And although the sample is small to serve as a basis for generalization, these data do corroborate the articulatory data reviewed in section A of this chapter. On the basis of both types of evidence, we would hypothesize that early glottal abduction (relative to oral stricture) and a gradual, breathy voiced decay to the vowel may be a general, universal feature of fricatives (more on this below). But whereas the articulatory data presented in section A led to the suggestion that glottal abduction in fricatives is earlier than in stops, we would argue on the basis of the present data that there is no general rule. Glottal abduction in stops may be earlier or later depending on the language or dialect looked at. Thus in Swedish, the timing of glottal abduction is very similar in stops and fricatives, and is very early for both. In French, early abduction pertains only to the fricative and so the timing rules differ for the two manners of articulation.

Carryover effects: stops

Carryover effects were also examined for initial prevocalic stops. Compared to the anticipatory effects, there was on the whole less evidence of a left to right influence on the vowel's mode of phonation from a preceding voiceless consonant. The source parameters EE and RA are shown for Italian, French and German in figure 5.10 for comparable pairs of utterances where the initial consonant differed. In Italian the /p–p:/ and /b–p:/ contexts are contrasted, in French the /p–p/ and /b–p/ contexts and in German the /p–b/ and /b–b/ contexts. The traces were aligned to vowel onset. We should note

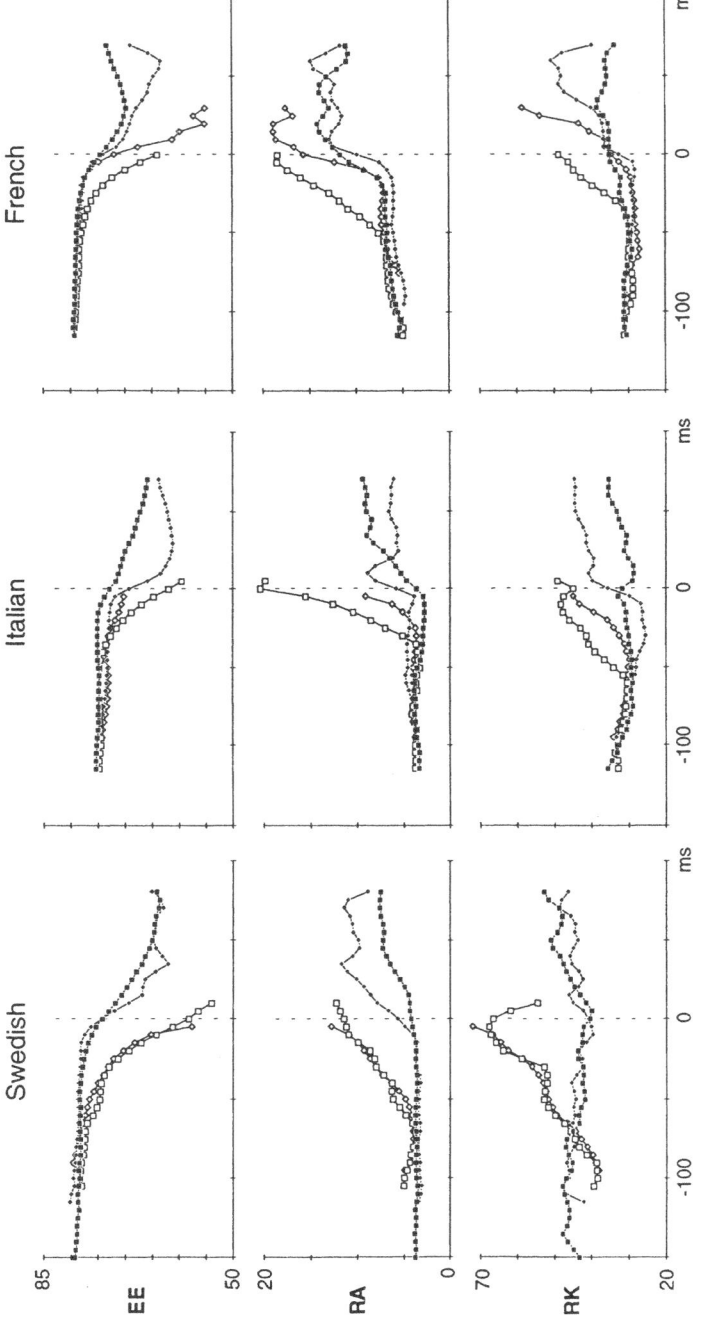

Figure 5.8   Averaged EE, RA and RK values superimposed for the contexts /p–/, /b–/, /f–/ and /v–/ in Swedish, Italian and French. Traces are aligned to vowel onset (= 0 ms).

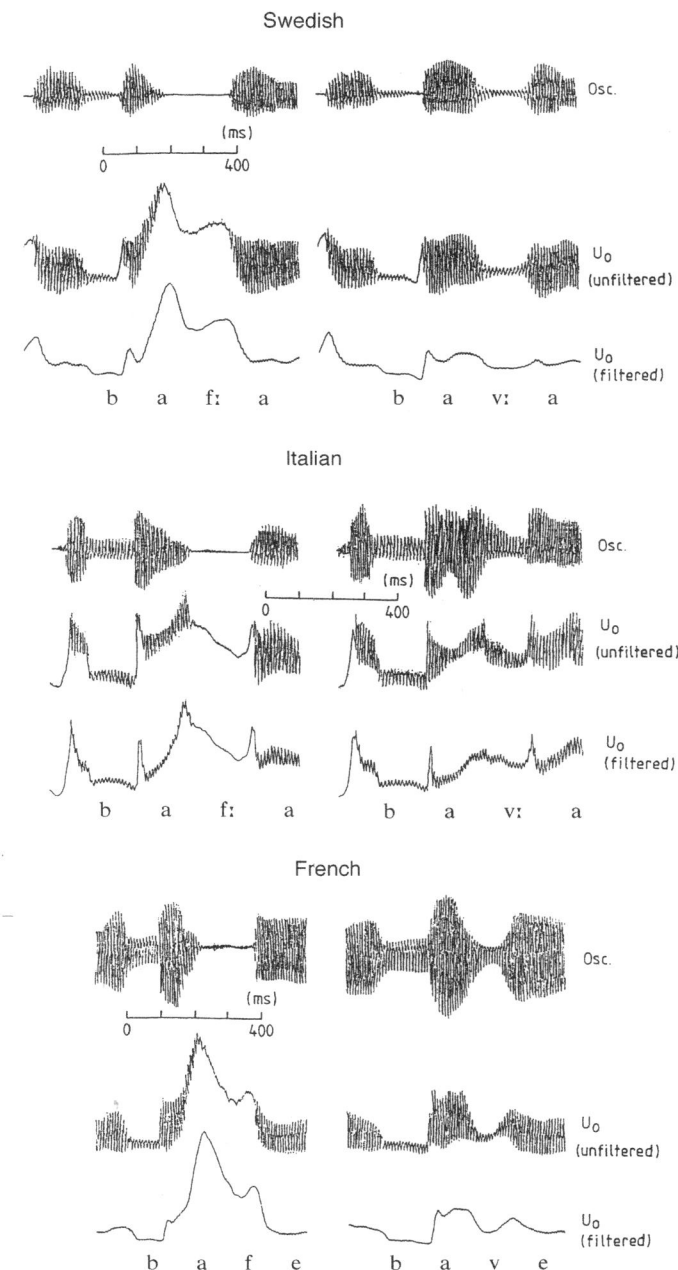

Figure 5.9   Oral airflow and speech waveform illustrating contrasting intervocalic labiodental fricatives in Swedish, Italian and French.

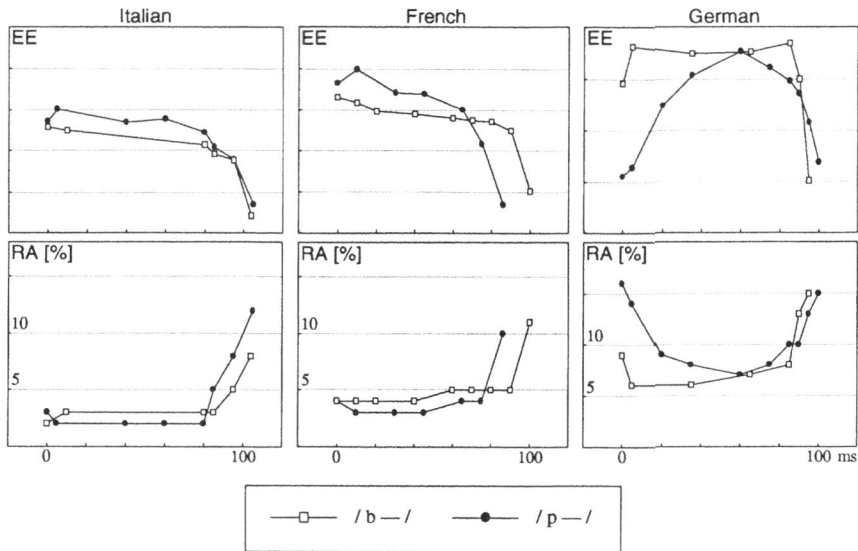

Figure 5.10   EE and RA values superimposed for the /p–/ and /b–/ contexts in Italian, French and German. Traces are aligned to vowel onset (= 0 ms).

that in Italian and French the contrast is realized as a voiced [b] versus voiceless unaspirated [p]. In English, German and Swedish /p/ is realized as a post-aspirated stop [pʰ], whereas /b/ was typically voiced [b]. (Note that as the utterances were read in a frame, the initial consonant is intervocalic. It therefore does not generally exhibit the devoicing typical for the initial variant, though some such instances were observed in English and German.)

In Italian and French there was effectively no carryover coarticulation from the preceding consonant. The vowel achieved high excitation strength more or less immediately and there was little evidence of dynamic leakage. Efficient voicing is therefore achieved right from the onset of the vowel. In German, there were major source differences in the vowel onset for the two contexts. At the onset of the vowel following /p–/, the excitation, EE, is very weak, dynamic leakage, RA, is very high and the shape of the glottal pulse is very symmetrical (high RK, not shown in figure). This contrasts sharply with the efficient voicing for vowel onset following /b–/. This breathy mode of vibration of the former changes gradually so that values for the two contexts become more similar in the later part of the vowel: yet it is clear that much of the vowel is affected. We would conclude that for these German data, the post-aspirated stop [pʰ] has a major effect on the quality of voicing of the following (stressed) vowel.

One might have expected to find similar effects in Swedish and English, where the same categories of stops are contrasted. A few instances of a similarly gradual onset were observed, particularly in the English data. However, the most typical onset pattern following postaspirated stops in our Swedish and English data was rather of efficient voicing at the vowel onset. Note in figure 5.11 below, where two instances of the vowel onset following [pʰ] are shown for Swedish, the rather instantaneous rise in EE values. The RA values, though fairly low, were nevertheless somewhat higher at vowel onset than were generally found following the voiced stop. For these instances it would appear that although voicing is strong at onset, there may nevertheless be incomplete glottal adduction (see more on this below).

The spectral measure of L1 relative to L0 can be seen in figure 5.6 for the four contexts /p–p(ː)/, /b–p(ː)/, /p–b(ː)/ and /b–b(ː)/ in French, German, Italian and Swedish. Traces in all cases are aligned to the onset of the vowel and this facilitates comparison of the effects of the initial consonant. In French and Italian the vowel onset looks similar regardless of the initial vowel. In Italian it can be seen that L1 (relative to L0) increases sharply over the first 25 ms or so, suggesting damping in the first few glottal pulses. More importantly however, this effect is found following both the voiced and voiceless consonants so the effect can not be attributed to the voicing characteristics of the consonants as such. The spectral differences observed for the two contexts at vowel onset for Swedish are rather more surprising, as the source values for the voiceless consonants in these instances showed a strong excitation, with a slightly raised RA value. L1 following [pʰ] is low, attaining full strength after about 40 ms. This clear damping of F1 does indeed suggest incomplete glottal adduction at voice onset following [pʰ] and yet we should note that even with partial abduction, the source excitation EE is strong. Source and spectral data for these same contexts for Swedish are shown together in figure 5.11. FA values indicate the cutoff frequency for the increased spectral tilt which results from RA values (FA is derived from RA and f_0, see formula in chapter 15 section B). As FA values are from 400–600 Hz, which is lower than the F1 frequency of /a/ (here approximately 600 Hz), we would estimate that the F1 amplitude would be attenuated by approximately 3–5 dB. This is considerably less than the attenuation observed in our spectral measures and so much of the attenuation must be attributable to a wider B1, due to higher coupling to the subglottal system.

In German L1 is initially weak following [pʰ] and rises gradually through most of the vowel. The difference here between the voiced and the voiceless context is striking and although generally consistent with the source data of figure 5.10, is in fact here underestimated. As was explained above in relation

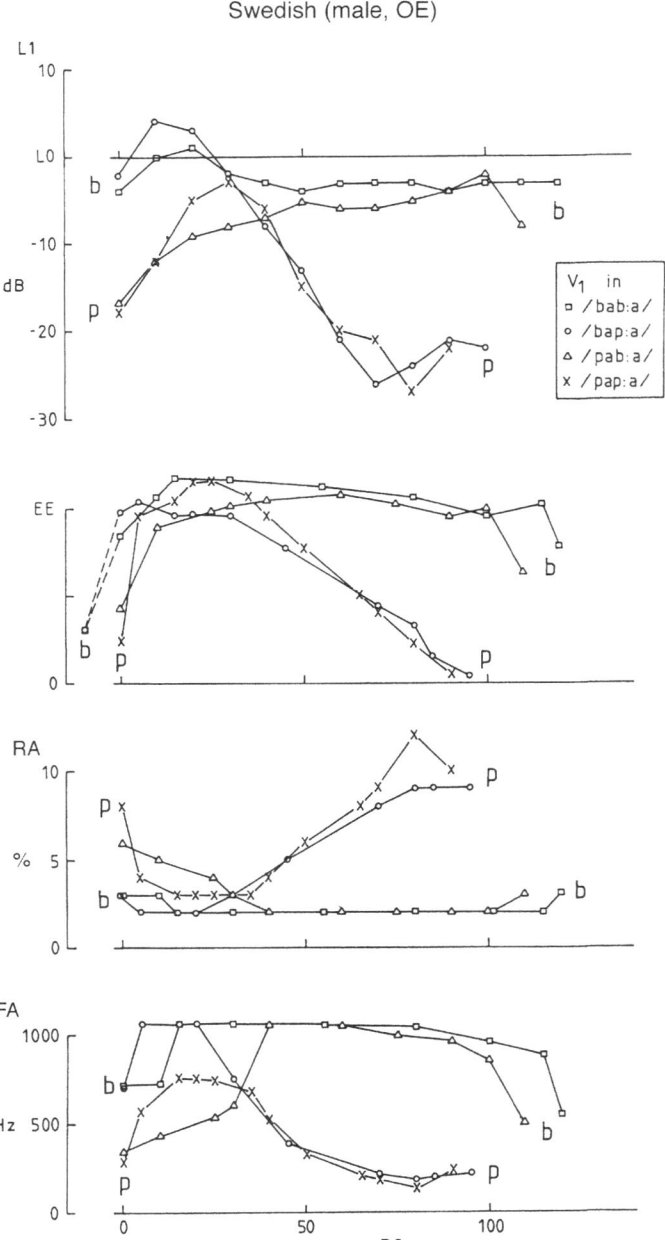

Figure 5.11   Spectral (L1 relative to L0) data and source parameters EE, RA and FA for the Swedish /a/ in the contexts /b–b:/, /b–p:/, /p–b:/ and /p–p:/

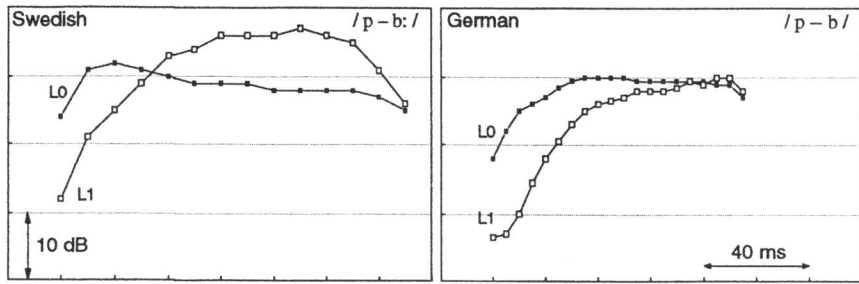

Figure 5.12   Levels of F0 (L0) and F1 (L1) in the vowel following the post-aspirated stop in Swedish and German

to figures 5.6 and 5.7, the L1–L0 measure is a useful basis for comparison provided L0 remains fairly constant as it usually does. An exception to this generally observed tendency concerned voice onset in German, where L0 rose gradually, attaining fairly constant values only after 30 ms or so. The spectral comparisons are somewhat misleading for Swedish and German. Figure 5.12 presents absolute L1 and L0 values for the two languages in a /p–b(:)/ context. Note that L1 damping is more extensive in the German case than would be inferred if shown only relative to L0. We should further note in figure 5.6 that for German but not Swedish, L1 values following /p/ simply never attain similar amplitudes to the levels following /b/.

Inferences on glottal control mechanisms

The anticipatory effects observed reflect, we suggest, differences in the timing of the glottal abduction gesture, and are thus compatible with what we have termed the 'timing' model of glottal control. In other words, the breathy voiced interval need not be directly controlled as such and may simply be the consequence of the fact that the vocal folds abduct while the vocal tract is unoccluded. The elastic nature of the folds and the fact that they are already vibrating ensures that voicing (of an increasingly breathy quality) persists for some time. This same phenomenon has been discussed for the preaspirated stops of Icelandic and Scottish Gaelic (Ní Chasaide 1985; on Scottish Gaelic see also Shuken 1980) and was illustrated in figure 5.5. In passing it may be worth noting that perceptual tests on Icelandic indicate that this breathy voiced interval can alone be sufficient to cue preaspiration (Ní Chasaide 1985, 1986).

When the laryngeal abduction is more tightly synchronized to the oral closing gesture, as was the case for French, the cessation of voice is achieved more rapidly. This is due to the fact that with the build up in oral pressure, the transglottal pressure drop is rapidly neutralized. It is perhaps worth noting that some pulses of intrusive voicing were observed for French, but that voice offset is nevertheless rapidly achieved.

To sum up we would suggest that the differences observed in the vowel before /–p/ in, say, the Swedish, Italian and French data can be accounted for in terms of differences in the timing of the glottal abduction relative to oral occlusion. We cannot exclude the possibility of there being other differences, e.g. in laryngeal tension settings. However, there does not seem to be any necessity to invoke such parameters to account for the data.

In the case of the fricatives, it would appear that the relative timing of laryngeal and oral gestures is more similar across languages. The voice source measures and the airflow data presented here complement the articulatory findings reviewed by Hoole in section A of this chapter and add further substance to the suggestion that laryngeal abduction in voiceless fricatives always substantially precedes the oral gesture so that devoicing is essentially achieved before the onset of oral frication. Further phonological evidence of a breathy offset of vowels before voiceless fricatives is provided in Ohala (1993a). In Ohala and Busá (1995) such an effect is also invoked to explain a widespread sound pattern where nasals are deleted especially before voiceless fricatives. We would therefore hypothesize that the way in which the glottal gesture is controlled in fricatives may be a universal, unlike the case of stops, where there is clearly a good deal of variability. An explanation for the apparently more universal tendencies for fricatives is most likely to be found in the production constraints pertaining to this class of consonants. Two potentially complementary explanations suggest themselves and have been mentioned earlier in section A. First of all, the requirement of generating high airflow at the point of oral constriction may be facilitated by early glottal abduction and might be rendered more difficult to achieve in time if glottal abduction were relatively later and synchronized with the oral gesture. Another explanation concerns the need to achieve voicelessness and to prevent intrusive voicing during the interval of frication. The fact that the vocal tract is only partially occluded means that it contributes less to the suppression of voicing in fricatives as compared to stops. In an articulatory modelling experiment, Castelli (1993) has shown that a later glottal abduction for the voiceless fricative results in intrusive voicing, not a desirable situation if one wants to retain a robust contrast of the voiced and voiceless pairs.

Unlike these anticipatory effects it does not seem likely that the carryover effects observed for German can be explained in terms of the timing of the laryngeal gesture alone. At first glance, the breathy voiced onset of the vowel found in German following [pʰ] looks rather like the breathy voiced offset observed in the Swedish data before [pʰ]. In principle, the German onset phenomenon could be a mirror image of the Swedish, insofar as the glottal adduction gesture and the initiation of voice occurs when the vocal tract is unoccluded (after stop release). However, we would suggest that the underlying mechanisms that produced these effects may be rather different. As is clear from the majority of the Swedish and English tokens, the initiation of voice following [pʰ] can be quite abrupt, with a strong excitation, and does not necessarily involve the weak, very gradual onset typical of our German data. This we feel indicates that the initiation and cessation of voice when the vocal tract is unoccluded are not identical. A brief glance at source parameter values for Swedish in /p–/ and /–p/ in figure 5.11 should serve to illustrate this point. Whereas voice initiation is accomplished with a rapid introduction of efficient voice source excitation, voice cessation yields a very gradual decay.

We would therefore suggest that the differences observed between the voice onset in German following [pʰ] and the typical Swedish onset in this environment may reflect differences in some other control parameter, such as vocal fold tension. It might be worth noting that in a language such as Hindi where a breathy voiced versus a full voice onset is exploited for phonological purposes (in the contrast of breathy voiced stops with other categories of stops such as voiced, voiceless-unaspirated and voiceless-aspirated) less activity of the cricothyroid muscle has been reported for the former case, reflecting a relatively slacker setting of the vocal folds (Dixit 1989). Clearly, direct investigations will be called for here. We would simply speculatively suggest that a 'timing model' alone does not appear to explain the data and that the involvement of some additional control parameter such as glottal tension may be implicated.

Conclusions

Detailed source analysis showed up some striking coarticulatory effects. The phonatory quality of the voiced vowel was to vary both as a function of the consonant's manner of articulation (stop versus fricative) and as a function of the language or dialect. The cross-language differences appeared only for stops. Languages or dialects differed both in the extent in which they exhibited coarticulatory effects and also in the directionality of these effects.

These data yield insights into laryngeal behaviour and permit us to formulate tentative hypotheses concerning the control strategies that might be involved in regulating voiceless consonants. We can list these hypotheses as follows:

(1)　In voiceless fricatives early vocal fold abduction relative to the oral constriction may be a strategy whose function might be to aid the production of these fricatives, ensuring that devoicing has been achieved before the onset of frication and that sufficiently high pressure is built up behind the oral constriction.

(2) For voiceless stops there is considerable latitude in when exactly abduction begins. The differences seemed to reveal language/dialect specific tendencies. Insofar as these limited data can be generalized, we would suggest that they reveal high level differences in the timing control for glottal abduction, part of the rule-governed behaviour of a language or a dialect.

(3) The initiation of voicing and its cessation when the vocal tract is unoccluded yield acoustic phenomena which are not entirely identical. The cessation of voicing appears to involve a very gradual transition through a breathy voiced mode of phonation with a gradually weakening excitation. This we would suggest occurs generally in voiceless fricatives, in preaspirated stops and sometimes in other voiceless stops (traditionally described as postaspirated or unaspirated) where the glottal abduction occurs prior to the oral closure. The initiation of voicing under similar conditions (unoccluded vocal tract) can be either very gradual or rather abrupt. The differences here may depend on different tension settings of the vocal folds, and not purely on differences in the timing of the glottal abduction gesture.

Acknowledgments

The authors would like to acknowledge that much of the work discussed in this chapter was carried out within the framework of the EC-funded ESPRIT-ACCOR I and II project. Our special thanks to Peter Monahan for assistance with the figures.

Notes

1 There is also a report by Butcher (1977) for one (probably) English speaker showing greater peak glottal opening on plosives than fricatives; but very few experimental details are given, so the significance of this result is difficult to assess.
2 It should be noted, however, that the interpretation of these latter correlations is somewhat problematic, as they are part–whole correlations (cf. Benoit 1986).
3 We will restrict consideration here to word-initial clusters. See e.g. Docherty (1992) and Dent (1984) for investigations of coarticulatory devoicing in such clusters across word-boundaries.
4 We call the suggestion speculative since it was not based on any data for English, but resulted from the attempt to place some findings on devoicing in Icelandic in a coarticulatory perspective. Specifically, Icelandic shows essentially a mirror-image

of the phenomenon being discussed here: for example, sequences of voiceless nasal or lateral plus stop. These can be regarded as (voiced) sonorants coarticulated with a following pre-aspirated stop. The temporal relationships were such that a very similar devoicing gesture occurred for simple pre-aspirated stops and for the continuant–stop sequences, while the occlusion duration of the stop shortened in the latter case.

5 It is also unclear whether current formulations of the dominance and the binding concepts can handle the different timing of peak glottal opening relative to release for different places of articulation.

6 The relevant laryngeal–oral coordination patterns are captured in two rules (Browman and Goldstein 1986: 228): (a) if a fricative gesture is present, coordinate the peak glottal opening with the mid-point of the fricative, (b) otherwise, coordinate the peak glottal opening with the release of the stop gesture.

7 This may also be related to a greater tendency of Swedish to aspirate and a lesser tendency to glottalize word-final plosives than English.

8 Pétursson (1977) points out that this may be a generalization that is specific to the Germanic languages. Some Indian languages contrast unaspirated stop with aspirated stop following /s/ (within the same word). In the latter case it can probably be assumed that two peaks in the glottal abduction will be observed.

6

Labial coarticulation

EDDA FARNETANI

Introduction

The labial system plays an important role in speech production: the lips act as primary or secondary articulators in the production of a number of segments. With respect to all other speech structures, the lips have the advantage of being readily observable, and the facial muscles responsible for lip movements that of being easily accessible. Moreover, while movements of the lower lip are usually the sum of the component jaw and lip movements, those of the upper lip can be considered completely independent of the movements and positions of other articulators, and so directly reflect articulatory and coarticulatory motor commands. The visibility and accessibility of the lips and their greater freedom from physiological constraints as compared to the tongue articulator, explain why early speech production models were based on the observation of lip gestures and their temporal organization (Kozhevnikov and Chistovich 1965) and why studies of labial coarticulation and the lip or jaw system are fundamental to shedding light on speech motor control and the function of synergistic and compensatory strategies of interarticulator coordination.

Labial articulation
Phonological description and articulatory measures
Vowels

The configuration of the lips in vowel production (represented in phonology by the feature *Round*) is one of the three primary dimensions along which vowels are classified, the other two being related to tongue configuration (represented by the features *High* and *Back*). The majority of languages do not make phonological use of the feature *Round*, since lip rounding is associated with tongue backness (Ladefoged and Maddieson 1990). In

Front   Back

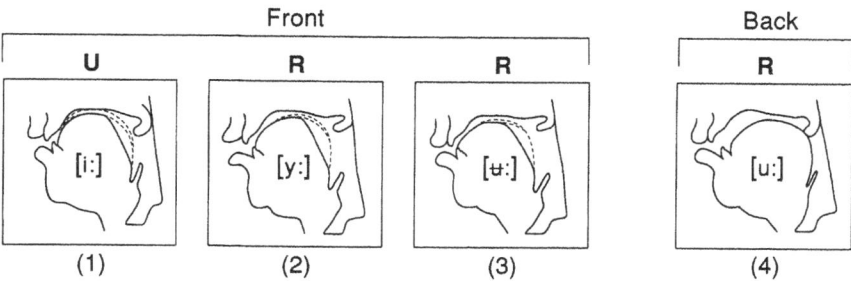

Figure 6.1   Tongue and lip profiles for the three high front vowels and the high back vowel of Swedish. U = unrounded; R = rounded (from Fant 1973).

a number of languages lip rounding has a distinctive phonological function, i.e. is the only feature distinguishing pairs of vowels. In French high and mid-high front vowels may be unrounded (/i, e/) or rounded (/y, ø/); a similar phonological patterning is observed in other languages, such as Finnish and Cantonese (Linker 1982). Swedish has three contrastive types of lip rounding: the three high front vowels /iː/, /yː/ and /ʉː/ are distinguished by a different lip configuration. According to standard phonological descriptions of Swedish, /iː/ is unrounded, /yː/ outrounded and /ʉː/ inrounded.

A number of investigations have been carried out to determine what the feature *Round* implies in articulatory terms (Fromkin 1964, for American English; Abry and Boë 1980 and Zerling 1992, for French). Linker's cross-language study (Linker 1982) addresses the issue of whether the articulatory parameters associated with lip rounding differ among languages, in particular among those where the feature has different phonological functions. The overall results of these investigations indicate that a parameter used in all languages for distinguishing rounded from unrounded vowels is lip width (i.e. horizontal lip opening), which correlates inversely with all lip protrusion parameters (Abry and Boë 1986): rounded vowels have less horizontal lip opening than unrounded vowels. The second dimension is vertical lip opening: rounded vowels tend to have less vertical opening than unrounded vowels. However, different languages make different use of these dimensions: in English, where lip rounding is redundant, only lip width is necessary and sufficient to separate rounded from unrounded vowels, while in French, Cantonese and Finnish, where rounding is phonological, speakers seem to make use of more elaborated lip gestures for realizing the rounding distinction (Linker 1982). As for Swedish, Linker's data agree with both X-ray data (Fant 1973) and kinematic data (McAllister 1980). Figure 6.1 (from Fant 1973) illustrates how the two parameters, lip protrusion and vertical lip opening interplay in the implementation of the rounding distinction in the three high front vowels of Swedish (the high back vowel /uː/ is also shown for comparison).

It can be seen that inrounded [ʉː] (3) is distinguished from unrounded [iː] (1) by a larger protrusion of lips and a smaller (vertical) lip opening and that back [uː] (4) is very similar in lip configuration to front inrounded [ʉː]. Outrounded [yː] (2) is distinguished from inrounded [ʉː] by much larger protrusion and opening of the lips. So, while inrounding is implemented by protruding and approaching the lips, as is lip rounding in general, outrounding exploits the two parameters in quite a different way, by combining maximal lip protrusion with a substantial lip separation.

If, as these studies indicate, the articulation of rounded vowels can vary across languages, two questions arise concerning coarticulation: are there cross-language differences depending on how rounding is implemented? Are there cross-language differences depending on the phonological function of rounding (distinctive versus redundant)? In other words, how is coarticulation related to the intrinsic articulatory component and to phonology?

Labial, labialized and neutral consonants

With the contribution of the jaw, the lips act as primary articulators in the production of bilabial stops, fricatives and trills; the lower lip is the active articulator for labiodental fricatives and approximants. The gesture associated with labial and labiodental consonants is a constriction of various degrees, ranging from a wide constriction for approximants, to a much narrower constriction for fricatives, to complete closure for stops.

The lips can also act as secondary articulators in the production of consonants: the consonants are then said to be *labialized*. In articulatory terms, labialization refers to an active deviation of lip configuration from a neutral shape (Lindblom 1966). Consonant labialization can be redundant or distinctive. Chomsky and Halle (1968) and Ladefoged (1964, 1975) report on a number of African and Asian languages in which labialization of lingual consonants has a contrastive function and on a West African language (Kutep) in which labialization is contrastive even for labial consonants.

Finally, consonants with no labial configuration of their own are said to be *neutral* or *unspecified* with respect to labiality. The lip shape of a neutral consonant is that associated with a relaxed lip musculature. Neutral consonants acquire the lip configuration of the adjacent segments.

Instrumental investigations on French carried out by the Grenoble group (among them Descout, Boë and Abry 1980) show that French alveolar and postalveolar fricatives are labialized: postalveolars /ʃ, ʒ/ are produced with lip protrusion, alveolars /s, z/ with lip retraction. Protruded fricatives have a degree of protrusion similar to that of rounded vowels (Benguerel and Cowan 1974) but are produced with much greater vertical lip separation than retracted consonants. Thus, the parameters distinguishing protruded and retracted fricatives are not the same as those distinguishing rounded and unrounded vowels. The lip configuration of protruded consonants is somewhat similar to that of the outrounded vowels of Swedish.

In English and in other languages in which lingual consonants are traditionally described as phonologically unspecified for labiality, there is evidence that they can be produced with a greater or lesser degree of protrusion also in a non-rounded environment, i.e. they can be articulatorily specified for a labial target. According to the consonant-rounding phonetic literature (reviewed by Brown 1981) postalveolar fricatives and affricates can be produced with lip protrusion and also alveolars (stops and approximants) can be produced with a certain degree of lip protrusion. A cross-language experiment by Faber (1989, 1990) on English, Italian, German and Polish, which aimed at determining whether or not phonologically neutral lingual consonants have a lip target of their own, showed that postalveolar fricatives are produced with protruded lips in any environment in all the languages analysed. Alveolar fricatives instead showed much more variability across speakers and languages; they were retracted in the German subject, protruded in one of the two English subjects and had no apparent lip positions in the other subjects. As for the phonetic role of such consonant-specific lip positions, the data by Faber suggest the possibility of a trading relation between location of lingual constriction and lip retraction/protrusion, tending to preserve the acoustic contrast between alveolars and postalveolars in any vocalic environment. Postalveolar and alveolar fricatives are distinguished acoustically by a low versus a high frequency frication noise. Lip protrusion, by lengthening the cavity in front of the constriction, causes a further lowering of the centroid frequency of postalveolars and thus increases the acoustic differences between the two consonants. The relative contribution of lip protrusion to the centroid frequency of postalveolar fricatives was assessed by Faber (1989) through regression analysis: the data show that the lip protrusion and the tongue constriction parameters together account for more variance in the centroid frequency than the tongue parameters alone.

Upper lip protrusion peaks associated with intervocalic consonants in /iktli/ utterances were observed in the coarticulation study by Boyce (1990) for one of the four English-speaking subjects examined.

Studies of Swedish (McAllister 1978; Engstrand 1981) approach the problem by examining the extent to which a consonant resists labialization in a labial context: a neutral consonant would have to fully acquire the feature *Round* from a rounded environment. The data show that in /uC$_n$u/ sequences where Cs are lingual obstruents, protrusion of the lips relaxes during the consonants, and the lip movement trace forms a 'trough' between the vowels. According to Engstrand (1981) such de-rounding manoeuvres may have the function of maintaining the lip area constant across rounded and unrounded contexts, which ensures an adequate noise level for the stop burst, and a high frequency level for /s/. This consonant, in particular, seems to be highly sensitive to perturbations of the mouth orifice area, and the troughs systematically observed in the lower lip movements in the context of /u/ may aim at counteracting the very high jaw position required by the fricative to achieve the appropriate tongue constriction.

These studies indicate that the presence or absence of labial targets in phonologically unspecified consonants depends on languages and often on individual subjects. So far, while postalveolar fricatives appear to be targeted for lip protrusion in a number of languages, alveolar fricatives are produced with retracted lips in French and German, show resistance to coarticulatory rounding effects in Swedish, but do not seem to have a consistent lip target in the other languages analysed. Much less is known for other lingual consonants: the available data on English (Boyce 1990) indicate that the presence or absence of a lip target for lingual stops strongly depends on individual production strategies.

It will be shown below that knowledge of lip configuration of non-labial consonants is crucial for a correct interpretation of the extent of anticipatory labial coarticulation and the studies just reviewed suggest that in lip coarticulation experiments, consonant-specific labial characteristics should have to be assessed for each subject.

Phonological neutrality and articulatory specification

The finding that phonologically unspecified features may be associated with articulatory targets concerns not only the lips but also the velum (Bell-Berti 1980; Bell-Berti and Krakow 1991) and the tongue (Engstrand 1983) and raises a number of general issues. First, how to reconcile phonological underspecification with target specification? The problem is the object of current debate among speech production theorists – see the proposal of the 'window' model by Keating (1988a) and see Boyce, Krakow and Bell-Berti (1991b) for general discussion on the matter. A second question concerns the function of these independent gestures. Do they aim at preserving or enhancing acoustic contrast between categories (as indicated by the behaviour of postalveolar fricatives), at ensuring that certain aerodynamic requirements are met (as proposed by Engstrand 1981, 1983) or are they idiosyncratic movements depending on production strategies, or circumstances and style, as suggested by the very high intersubject variability observed in a number of studies? These various accounts do not necessarily exclude one another, in the sense that different speakers and languages may exploit differently the free articulators, i.e. those not involved in the production of a given phone. According to Boyce, Krakow and Bell-Berti (1991b), underspecification, for the fact that it can be associated with various articulatory positions, is an important factor in cross-speaker and cross-dialectal variability. Underspecification is seen by Keating (1988a) as a source of cross-language variability owing to a different interpretation that language-specific phonetic rules give to unspecified features.

Motor commands for labial activity

Owing to the accessibility of the facial muscles responsible for labial articulation, quite a number of coarticulation studies are based on electromyography (EMG). According to the speech physiology literature (see chapter 13), at least twelve facial muscles can be involved in labial movements during speech. Electromyographic experiments during the 1960s and 1970s have made it possible to associate the activity of a number of facial muscles with the production of vowels and labial consonants (Öhman 1968; McAllister, Lubker and Carlson 1974; Hadding, Hirose and Harris 1976; for a detailed review see Gentil and Boë 1980). From these early experiments, carried out on Swedish-speaking subjects, we know that at least seven facial muscles can be activated for the production of rounded and unrounded vowels, as illustrated in figure 6.2 (adapted from Gentil and Boë 1980).

The main muscle responsible for lip rounding and protrusion is *orbicularis oris,* a sphincter-like muscle embracing the lips; its antagonist is *buccinator,* a deep muscle at the sides of the mouth, whose contraction determines the spreading of lips. A second lip spreading muscle, *risorius* (see figure 6.2), is probably less important than *buccinator* and its action does not appear to be constant (Gentil and Boë 1980).

A number of other muscles act in synergy with *orbicularis oris* and *buccinator: mentalis* and *depressor labii inferioris* (see figure 6.2) are synergistic with *orbicularis oris*: the effect of their contraction is to lower and protrude the lower lip. The activity of these two muscles seems to be especially important in the production of non-high rounded vowels. *Levator labii superioris* and *depressor anguli oris* may act in synergy with *buccinator* in the production of spread vowels: the former (which runs deeply from the lips towards the orbits) contributes to elevate the upper lip, while the latter seems to contribute to pull

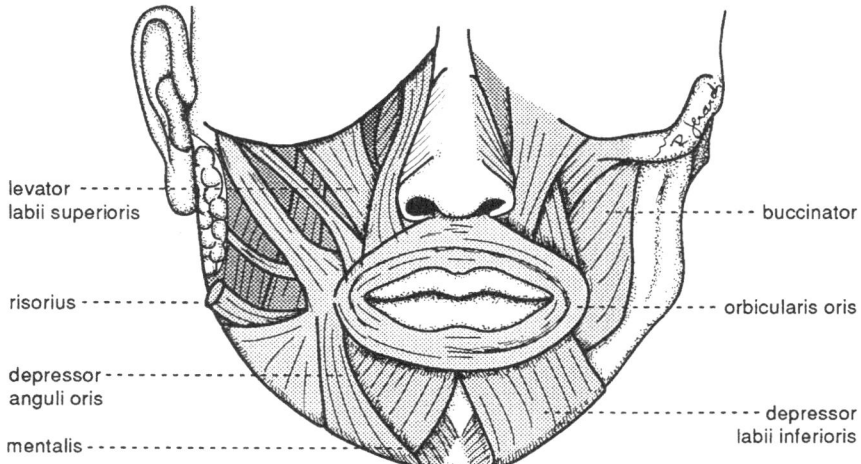

Figure 6.2   The facial muscles involved in the labial articulation for vowels (from Gentil and Boë 1980)

the corners of the mouth down and laterally especially for /i/ and /e/ (Öhman 1968). This complex picture is further complicated by the fact that antagonistic muscles can also be activated simultaneously with the agonistic and synergistic: such coactivation probably serves to check the reciprocal effects and achieve finer control of labial movements.

Taken together, these studies indicate that the production of lip rounding and spreading results from complex interactions among the lip muscles, whose details are not yet fully understood. Recent dissection studies underline the complexity and the relevant interindividual differences of the anatomical interconnections between the fibres of *orbicularis inferior* and the surrounding muscles (Blair 1986).

Lubker and Gay (1982) explored the correspondence between EMG activity of *orbicularis, buccinator, modiolus* (a tiny muscle at the corner of the lip, connected with *risorius* and *levator angulis oris*) and the lip movements and showed that this relation is often far from clear. Their findings indicate that inferences about coarticulation based on the activity of one or two muscles without simultaneous monitoring of lip movements have to be taken with caution.

The acoustics and perception of lip rounding
According to the acoustic theory of speech production (Fant 1960), a decrease in lip opening or an increase in length of the lip passage

causes a lowering in the frequencies of formants. Acoustic data on Swedish vowels (Fant 1973) indicate that rounded and unrounded vowels are separated by F2 and F3. For high front vowels the frequency of F2 and F3 decreases from /iː/ (unrounded) to /yː/ (outrounded) to /ʉː/ (inrounded). Linker's acoustic data on high front vowels in French, Finnish, Cantonese and Swedish agree with Fant's; the mid-high vowel pairs are also distinguished by F2 and F3 but F2 becomes more important. Acoustic data on French rounded and unrounded minimal pairs (Mantakas, Schwarz and Escudier 1988) agree with Linker's finding that the main acoustic discriminant for high vowels is F3 and for mid-high vowels is F2, confirming that the relevance of the different formants in the rounding distinction depends in large part on the configuration of the tongue (Fant 1973c).

According to Stevens, Keyser and Kawasaki (1986), the redundant lip rounding associated with back vowels in various languages, by inducing a lowering of the higher formants of back vowels, functions as an 'enhancement' of the front/back distinction (cf. Faber 1989, for a compatible account of the role of lip protrusion in postalveolar fricatives).

Despite the important acoustic consequences of lip configuration, most labial coarticulation studies focus on articulation and/or motor commands and there are no specific studies exploring the relation between the articulatory and the acoustic level of labial coarticulation.

The studies by Benguerel and Adelman (1976) and Lubker, Lindgren and Gibson (1984) concern the perceptual function of coarticulation. The aim of the two investigations was to assess whether listeners make use of coarticulatory lip rounding information contained in the acoustic signal. These experiments were based on the gating technique, i.e. listeners had to identify a vowel which had been gated out from the signal together with various portions of the preceding consonants. The data indicated that listeners can indeed use coarticulatory information to identify the missing vowel. There were no differences between English and French subjects listening to French utterances (Benguerel and Adelman 1976), whereas in the experiment by Lubker, Lindgren and Gibson (1984) the Swedish subjects identified Swedish vowels better and earlier than the American English speakers identified English vowels. The authors showed that the differences in perceptual behaviour between the two groups are due to the differences in coarticulation between the two languages: Swedish is characterized by larger and longer anticipatory lip rounding gestures than English (Lubker and Gay 1982), hence acoustic information on the incoming vowel is conveyed and perceived earlier.

Spatio-temporal aspects of labial coarticulation
Coarticulatory spatial effects of lip rounding

The study of reciprocal interactions between adjacent segments with different specifications for a feature (e.g. $-/+$ *Round*) is of great theoretical interest because it permits us to establish the extent to which coarticulatory effects are blocked by contradictory requirements and to assess the role of the phonological function of a feature (e.g. the feature *Round*) in coarticulatory processes.

Systematic work of this kind on labialized vowels and consonants has been carried out for CV syllables in French (Abry, Boë and Descout 1980; Descout, Boë and Abry 1980) by measuring the reciprocal anticipatory and carryover vowel-consonant effects at the mid-point of each segment. In French, vowel rounding is a phonological feature, while consonant protrusion (also represented by the feature *Round*) is a redundant feature. The vowels in the CV syllables were either front rounded or front unrounded and the consonants were either the spread /s, z/ or the protruded /ʃ, ʒ/. The results indicated that rounded vowels are never affected by the preceding spread consonants, which were assimilated to the following rounded vowel for four of the five subjects analysed; unrounded vowels, on the other hand, were affected to some extent by the preceding protruded consonants, showing increased protrusion and vertical opening, while in the preceding consonants protrusion was reduced. Thus, when V is rounded, V-to-C coarticulation is maximal and C-to-V coarticulation is blocked; when V is unrounded, there are reciprocal V-to-C and C-to-V effects, i.e. a blending of vocalic and consonantal influences. Rounding or protrusion gestures appear to overwhelm in strength retraction gestures and vowels resist coarticulatory influences more than consonants. According to the authors, the finding that distinctive lip rounding associated with vowels is less liable to be neutralized than redundant lip protrusion associated with consonants could reflect a phonological constraint. This hypothesis should be tested by comparing French with a language where rounding in vowels and protrusion in consonants are both non-phonological.

Temporal extent of anticipatory coarticulation

The temporal aspect of labial coarticulation, and in particular its anticipatory extent, has been the focus of most experimental research on labiality. Its theoretical interest lies in the fact that anticipatory coarticulation may reveal how linguistic units are temporally organized in speech. Temporal organization, in turn, can reveal much of the nature of the process (phonological or phonetic) and of the units themselves (static or dynamic).

Look-ahead

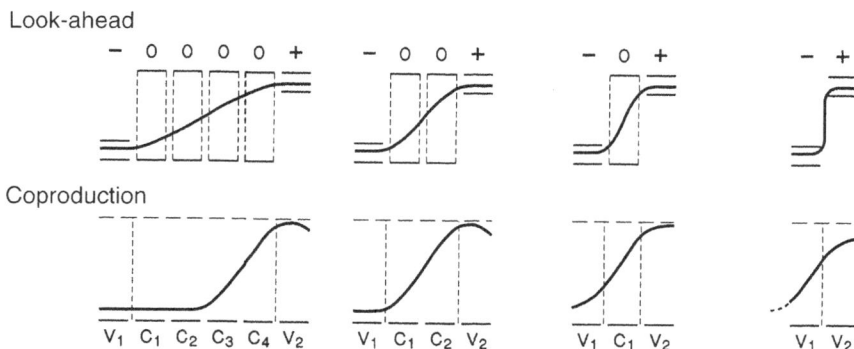

Coproduction

Figure 6.3   The look-ahead and the coproduction (or time-locked) models of anticipatory labial coarticulation. $+ 0 -$ indicate rounded, neutral and unrounded segment, respectively

The look-ahead and the time-locked models

Data on anticipatory coarticulation can be interpreted in light of two alternative theories of speech production, the featural and the gestural (or coproduction) theories. The models expressed by the two theories predict different coarticulation strategies, the look-ahead and the time-locked strategy respectively (for a comprehensive account of the two theories see Farnetani and Recasens, chapter two of this volume).

Figure 6.3 shows the patterns of anticipatory movements predicted by the two models; here the predictions of the look-ahead model are illustrated within the 'window' framework (Keating 1988a, 1988b), the most recent account of coarticulation within featural phonology.

While the traditional featural account assumes that anticipatory coarticulation is the output of phonological feature-spreading rules (Daniloff and Hammmarberg 1973), the window model views coarticulation as the output of low-level phonetic implementation rules. In this new account, the anticipatory rounding movement is seen as a smooth trajectory connecting the segment specified as [−round] with the one specified as [+ round] (both represented by quite narrow windows), across any number of unspecified segments (represented by wide windows). The rounding movement starts as soon as the [− round) feature has been implemented and ends at the acoustic onset of the [+ round] segment. Consequently the trajectories will have shorter durations and steeper slopes as the number of neutral segments decreases (compare top panels 1, 2 and 3 in figure 6.3). Since the segments are concatenated one after the other in a non-overlapping manner, in no instance will there be any interaction between the two specified segments. When they are adjacent to each other (see the sequence – + in figure 6.3), 'the entire transition will take place quickly between the windows' (Keating 1988a: 10).

According to Keating (1988b), in some languages anticipatory coarticulation can be governed by phonological rules, in this case the [+ round] feature will spread to all intervening consonants and the anticipatory rounding movement will not be a smooth V-to-V transition but will take a plateau-like shape (as predicted by the feature-spreading model of Daniloff and Hammarberg 1973).

In the coproduction model (Bell-Berti and Harris 1981; Boyce *et al.* 1990; Fowler and Saltzman 1993) the observed rounding movement reflects an underlying gesture of constant duration (independent of the number of consonants), which is 'time locked' to the rounded vowel and overlaps in time with the lingual gestures for the consonants. Thus, the temporal interval between the onset of the rounding movement and the onset of the rounded vowel will be constant, while the interval between the offset of the unrounded vowel and the onset of rounding will vary, decreasing as the number of consonants decreases (see bottom panels 1 and 2 in figure 6.3). If the consonant interval is short or the vowels are adjacent, the rounding movement will start well within the unrounded vowel, as a result of the spatio-temporal overlap of the underlying gestures for the two vowels.

Thus the two models make different predictions not only for the main variable, *viz.* the duration of the rounding movement, but also for the velocity and shape of the movement and for the coarticulatory spatial effects between the rounded and the unrounded vowel.

Most of the data in support of one or other model are based on temporal measures, i.e. the relation between the duration of the rounding movement and the duration of the intervening consonants (or the number of consonants). The studies on English by Bell-Berti and Harris (1979, 1982), Gay (1979), Gelfer, Bell-Berti and Harris (1989) are in support of the time locked model. The parameters used were EMG activity while Gelfer, Bell-Berti and Harris (1989) used both EMG activity and lip kinematics. Other studies on various languages are instead in agreement with the look-ahead model: Daniloff and Moll (1968), for English; Lubker, McAllister and Carlson (1975), McAllister (1978), Lubker (1981) for Swedish; Benguerel and Cowan (1974) for French; Magno-Caldognetto *et al.* (1992) for Italian. The parameters used were EMG activity and/or lip movements. These studies support the idea that the longer the consonantal interval, the earlier will be the onset of the labial activity associated with the rounded vowel. This relation has often been expressed as a linear correlation between the duration of the consonant interval and that of the anticipatory rounding interval (e.g. Lubker 1981).

A study by Sussman and Westbury (1981) on three English-speaking subjects is also in substantial agreement with the look-ahead model. The authors point out, however, that this model cannot explain some of their findings, such as why the EMG *orbicularis oris* activity starts earlier when V_1 is /i/ (here the [− round] specification should delay the rounding command) than when V_1 is /a/ (whose lip configuration does not conflict with a rounding command). Moreover, in the one subject for whom both EMG activity and labial movements were measured, the authors observed a rather peculiar relation between the timing of the two parameters: lip protrusion was found to start before the onset of *orbicularis oris* activity. This suggested to the authors that in this subject the onset of lip protrusion could be a mere consequence of the cessation of *risorius* activity and thus a passive return of the lips from a spread to a neutral position. This interesting hypothesis, however, has not been further tested on other subjects.

The study on Swedish by Abelin, Landberg and Persson (1980) reveals that the anticipatory strategy is not the same in children and adults: the onset of EMG activity appeared to be time locked to the production of the rounded vowels for five of the six children examined (aged seven to ten years); only one child showed an anticipatory look-ahead pattern comparable to that of a control adult speaker. The data indicated that anticipatory coarticulation is a *learned* behaviour and that its achievement depends on the physiological/linguistic maturity of the child. The authors propose language-specific 'temporal windows' for anticipatory coarticulation as part of the learning of any language.

A cross-linguistic study by Lubker and Gay (1982) compares Swedish and American English-speaking subjects and shows that the upper lip targets for rounded vowels are different in the two languages: the rounded vowels of Swedish were systematically produced with more extensive and more precise lip-protrusion movements than the rounded vowels of English. Also the timing of labial movements was found to differ in the two languages: for the same number of consonants, the onset of the movement occurred earlier for the Swedish than for the American subjects (which would explain the perceptual results in Lubker, McAllister and Carlson 1975 – see above). An unexpected finding concerned the anticipatory strategies: the values and the significance of the correlation coefficients (describing the relation between number of consonants and movement interval) indicated that only three of the five Swedish subjects and two of the three American subjects used the look-ahead strategy. The Swedish subjects who appeared to use a time-locked strategy (and consequently shorter movements) did not exhibit, however, higher variability than the look-ahead subjects. Overall, these data are consistent with the notion that in languages where lip rounding has a phonological function, speakers learn to make more accurate and extensive gestures than in languages where lip rounding is redundant and that this is independent of the coarticulatory strategy used. From the authors' conclusion it is not clear, however, what factors might underlie the differences in coarticulatory strategies within and across languages. Probably, besides the constraints proposed in the paper, some other factors deserve to be considered: individual speech rate and style, and/or different realization of the word boundaries occurring within the series of consonants.

The hybrid model

Perkell and Chiang (1986) and Perkell (1990) were the first to take into account both the onsets and the trajectories over time of lip movements. Al-Bamerni and Bladon (1982), in a study of anticipatory velar coarticulation in $(C)V_nN$ sequences, had observed that the temporal patterns of velum opening differed across subjects and repetitions: sometimes it was a single gesture aligned with the onset of the first vowel and smoothly increasing in amplitude, sometimes it was a two-stage gesture, whose onset was aligned as previously with the first vowel but whose second-stage velocity peak was linked with the oral closing gesture for the nasal consonant.

Perkell and Chiang (1986) observed similar two-stage patterns in the labial gestures in $/iC_nu/$ utterances, where the onset of lip rounding was temporally linked to /i/ (as predicted by the look-ahead model), but the onset of the second phase of the gesture (detectable from the point of maximum acceleration) was linked to /u/ (as predicted by the time-locked model). The authors proposed a hybrid model of anticipatory coarticulation, a compromise between the look-ahead and the time-locked strategies, as shown in figure 6.4.

Perkell's data on three English speakers (Perkell 1990) indicate that the coarticulatory strategy for two of the subjects is compatible with the hybrid model. As predicted by the model, very high correlations were observed between consonant duration and the total duration of the rounding movement and no significant correlations were found between consonant duration and the second phase of the movement. A subsequent study with four English speakers (Perkell and Matthies 1992) confirmed that the two-stage movement pattern is the preferred coarticulatory strategy. However, for three of the subjects, the second phase of the movement was not as closely

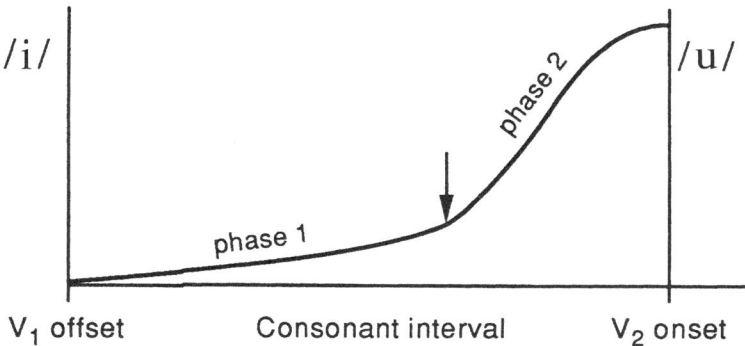

Figure 6.4   The two-phase or hybrid model: the low velocity phase and the higher velocity phase of the rounding gesture are separated by an inflection point (marked by an arrow), which is caused by the peak of acceleration.

linked temporally to the rounded vowel as the hybrid model would predict. In fact, for these subjects, the protrusion interval (from the maximum acceleration point to the acoustic onset of /u/) was also correlated significantly with consonant duration (though the variance accounted for by this relation was very low). According to the authors, none of the three existing anticipation models in their strong versions can account for the temporal relations observed in the data. It is proposed, instead, that the two-stage anticipatory movements may reflect the simultaneous expression of two competing constraints: (a) that of initiating the rounding gesture as soon as possible under the constraint that the vowel /i/ be preserved unrounded; (b) that of using and maintaining the preferred kinematics of the rounding gesture. A third constraint is that of ending the gesture as close as possible to the rounded vowel. The authors attribute intersubject and within-subject variability to the different degrees to which the two competing constraints are expressed.

   The role of consonants and of speech rate
   Gelfer, Bell-Berti and Harris (1989), Boyce *et al.* (1990) contest the claim that early initiation of lip activity (or of the protrusion movement) reflects the onset of the gesture associated with the rounded vowel, as the look-ahead and the hybrid models propose. According to the authors, the various studies on anticipatory lip rounding have been based on the assumption that phonologically neutral consonants are also articulatorily neutral; consequently these studies have attributed the onset of the rounding movement to an antic-ipatory strategy, without first testing whether or not the neutral segments are

specified for a lip target.[1] This can be tested in sequences of unrounded vowels: the presence of labial activity in /iC$_n$i/ is a clear indication that some of the medial consonants have a lip target position. Gelfer, Bell-Berti and Harris (1989) propose a subtraction procedure for ruling out any lip movement associated with a consonant and for determining the *actual onset* of the vocalic gesture. Superimposition of the /iC$_n$i/ on the /iC$_n$u/ patterns allows the subtraction of the consonant contribution to labial activity and thus the detection of the onset of anticipatory coarticulation. The application of this procedure to two English-speaking subjects (using EMG data from *orbicularis oris inferior* and lower lip kinematic parameters) showed that the coarticulatory strategy, though apparently hybrid, was in fact time-locked.

A cross-linguistic study by Boyce (1990) on lip rounding in Turkish and English also applied the subtraction procedure for identifying the onset of anticipatory coarticulation. The results indicate that anticipatory labial coarticulation is time-locked in English, while the coarticulatory plateau patterns in Turkish seem to support the look-ahead model in its phonological version (as proposed by Daniloff and Hammarberg 1973). The different coarticulatory patterns observed in the two languages throw some light on the relation between phonological structure and coarticulation and suggest that the former may influence the latter. Turkish is a vowel harmony language and has strict rules for sequences of rounded and unrounded vowels; words with mixed rounded and unrounded vowels are exceptions. These phonological constraints seem to exert a pressure to reproduce, in asymmetric /i–u/ and /u–i/ sequences, the typical V-to-V strategy used in the language, where vowels harmonize in the majority of words (e.g. /i–i/ or /u–u/ sequences), i.e. a pressure to start the lip gesture for the following vowel as soon as possible and to reproduce the plateau-like patterns that characterize sequences of harmonized vowels. Perkell and Matthies (1992) tested the hypothesis of consonant contribution to the onset of lip-protrusion movements on four subjects: they did observe some consonant-related protrusion associated with /s/ in /iC$_n$i/ utterances but the correlations between the duration of the consonants and that of the rounding movement interval were significant both for the non-/s/ utterances and for those containing a leading /s/. This indicated that the beginning of the rounding movement can indeed be influenced by a consonant-specific lip target (in agreement with Boyce *et al.* 1990) but that the protrusion movement tends nonetheless to be longer in longer consonant intervals.

According to Boyce *et al.* (1990), a second factor that can modify the shape of the coarticulatory movements and give rise to alternations between one-stage and two-stage patterns is speech rate. According to the authors, these alternations do not reflect different coarticulatory strategies (the look-ahead for one-stage movements and the hybrid for the two-stage movements) but rather the component consonantal and vocalic gestures which overlap to different degrees as a function of speech rate. For example, in /iC$_n$u/-type utterances produced at a fast rate, the underlying gestures for /u/ and the lip-targeted consonants overlap more than at a normal rate, and their effects can sum up and blend into a single rounding movement that starts within or around the end of /i/ (one-stage patterns). When the same utterance is produced at a slower rate, the overlap between the consonantal and the vocalic gestures decreases and the consonantal and vocalic components of the movement re-emerge distinctly (two-stage patterns). The hypothesis that a change in rate alone can give rise to different movement patterns was tested and confirmed for velar coarticulation by Bell-Berti and Krakow (1991).

The movement expansion model

The anticipatory lip rounding model proposed by Abry and Lallouache (1995) is the result of systematic research on the upper lip kinematics of French subjects. The research began with a study of within-subject variability across repetitions and recording sessions (Abry and Lallouache 1991a, 1991b). The test utterances were /iC$_5$y/ embedded in Noun + Verb phrases, with the word boundary after C$_3$. The results indicated that the shape of the lip movement trajectory was quite stable in the session where the subject had realized the word boundary, while in the session where the phrases had been produced as a whole (and at faster rate) the lip profiles were extremely variable and exhibited both one-stage and two-stage patterns. A detailed analysis of the stable profiles of the first session indicated that there was a first phase characterized by no movement, followed by a protrusion movement whose duration was proportional to the consonantal interval. This finding indicated that protrusion gestures are one-phase movements which expand in time as the consonant intervals become longer.

The corpus analysed for one subject by Lallouache and Abry (1992) and for three subjects by Abry and Lallouache (1995), consists of /iC$_n$y/ utterances with varying numbers of consonants as well as /iy/ utterances with no consonants in between. The parameters were all the kinematic points and intervals proposed by Perkell, as well as measures of the protrusion amplitude. The overall results can be summarized as follows.

First, protrusion appears to be a one-phase movement. Second, points of maximum protrusion and maximum amplitude occur around the rounded vowel, indicating that there are no plateau-like patterns. Third, the relation between consonant duration and the protrusion interval (as well as between consonant duration and the intervals of maximum acceleration and

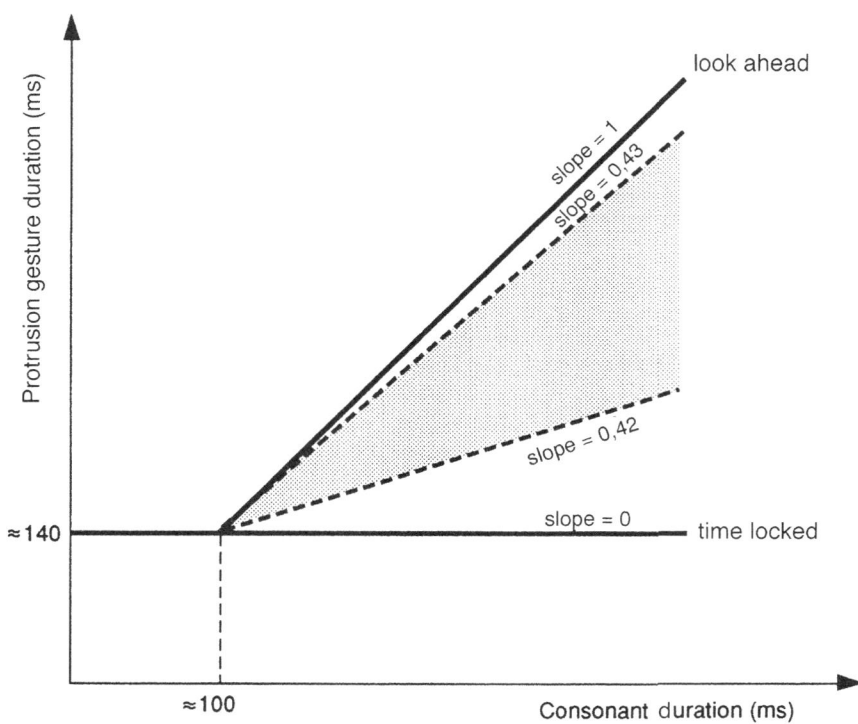

Figure 6.5   The movement expansion model of anticipatory labial coarticulation proposed by Abry and Lallouache (1995). See text for explanation.

maximum velocity) is not linear but is better described by a hyperbolic function. This is because the protrusion movement tends to expand in longer consonant intervals, but cannot be compressed below a certain duration in shorter intervals. In /iC$_1$y/ as well as in no-consonant /iy/ sequences, protrusion duration remains fixed at around 140–150 ms, indicating that the protrusion gesture strongly modifies the upper-lip configuration for the vowel /i/. There is much greater movement stability within and across subjects in the shorter than in the longer consonantal sequences. The temporal expansion of the movement does not mean that the protrusion movement is linked to the unrounded vowel: it can start before, within or after it and has temporal limits (as was observed for anticipatory coarticulation in Swedish by McAllister 1978). The conclusion of the authors is that the French data cannot be accounted for by any of the three current models of anticipatory rounding. A new model is illustrated in figure 6.5 (adapted from Abry and Lallouache 1995).

The filled area between the steeper and the shallower slopes comprises the individual slopes of the three subjects and indicates that, at longer consonantal intervals, protrusion gestures become longer and intersubject variability becomes greater. It can be seen that the positive slopes meet the 0 slope at short consonant durations and this reflects the hyperbolic function that relates the two coordinates. It can also be seen that at the shortest V-to-V intervals the protrusion movement does not decrease in duration below about 140 ms (intercept value). Hence such short movements might be accounted for by the coproduction model, which assumes a blending of conflicting influences rather than a blocking of coarticulation. The look-ahead model would predict much lower values for the intercept, since the conflict would block coarticulation, forcing the rounding movement to be much faster (see Keating's model in figure 6.3).

The data of the three French subjects are strikingly similar to the upper-lip protrusion data analysed so far for an Italian subject (Farnetani in preparation). This study examines the coordination of lip and tongue gestures in the production of /u/ and /i/ using the Selspot technique and electropalatography. The data indicate no difference in protrusion duration between the /iu/ and /iC$_1$u/ sequences and suggest that for that given speech rate the protrusion movement cannot be compressed below 120–140 ms for the Italian subject examined. Also for Italian, longer consonant intervals induce an expansion of the protrusion movement but its onset is not necessarily associated with the acoustic offset of /i/.

Carryover coarticulation

Very few data on carryover labial coarticulation are available in the literature. The only investigation on the carryover extent of lip movements is the study of Benguerel and Cowan (1974) for French. The authors compared the temporal extent and the velocity of upper lip protrusion movements after /y/ in /yC$_6$i/ utterances with the anticipatory movements towards /y/ in mirror utterances. It was found that carryover movements tend to be slower and longer than anticipatory ones.

McAllister (1978), on the other hand, studying the onsets and offsets of EMG activity in Swedish C$_n$yC$_n$ monosyllables, found that the carryover temporal extent of coarticulation is much shorter and more variable than the anticipatory extent. The data of Bell-Berti and Harris (1982) – also based on EMG activity – agree with McAllister's: they show that in both /uC$_n$i/ and /uC$_n$u/ utterances the offset of *orbicularis oris* activity occurs very soon after /u/ and is thus more limited in temporal extent than anticipatory EMG activity. The results of the two EMG studies appear to contradict the movement study. However, the two sets of data cannot be directly compared, since – as seen above – very little is known on the timing relations between EMG activity and onset/offset of movements (see chapter thirteen of this volume). Since the theoretical issue concerning carryover movements is whether they are actively controlled or merely passive consequences of mechanico-inertial factors, a better procedural approach to the problem would be the simultaneous use of EMG and kinematic techniques.

General comments and conclusion

Despite the vast experimental literature on labial articulation in various languages, we still know very little about the relation between coarticulation and cross-language differences in vowel articulation, in phonological rules or in the phonological function of lip rounding. Two cross-language experiments (Lubker and Gay 1982; Boyce 1990) indicate that labial coarticulation does differ across languages in a direction that complies with language-specific rules but much more research is needed for a better understanding of the relation between phonology and coarticulation.

A second theoretical issue concerns how conflict is resolved when adjacent segments are characterized by contrasting labiality features. Much of the work on this topic has been carried out by the Grenoble group. Their studies on mutual C-to-V and V-to-C spatial effects indicate that both blocking of coarticulation and blending of influences can occur, depending on whether the feature is + or − *Round*: rounded vowels exert much stronger effects on retracted consonants (and block their effects) than unrounded vowels do on protruded consonants (where blending occurs); C-to-V effects appear to be weaker than V-to-C effects, presumably because the feature *Round* is constrastive in vowels but not in consonants. The issue of V-to-V spatial effects between adjacent rounded and unrounded vowels, though of great theoretical interest, has not been addressed in a systematic way. In a number of anticipatory coarticulation studies it has been noticed that the rounding movements may start during or even before the unrounded vowel (e.g. Benguerel and Cowan 1974) but this fact was not thoroughly explored until the recent work by Abry and Lallouache, who found that unrounded vowels can be heavily affected by the following rounded vowels.

As for the temporal extent of coarticulation, a number of factors can explain, at least in part, the contradictory results of the studies of anticipatory coarticulation, including the use of different experimental techniques and of different procedures, such as the choice of the upper lip in some studies and of the lower lip in others. Since the lower lip movement in a VCV utterance results in part from the rising movement of the jaw for the consonant constriction, appropriate use of the lower lip for investigating labial coarticulation would require recording of jaw movement as well, and subtracting the jaw component.

The review shows that contextual factors, such as an inherent lip protrusion or retraction in supposedly neutral consonants, have important effects on the patterns and the timing of labial movements. Moreover, the various studies reviewed clearly indicate that the presence or absence, and/or the degree of labialization of lingual consonants may vary across subjects and languages. The important effects of speaking rate on the global patterns of labial movements have been shown by Boyce *et al.* (1990). Prosodic factors, such as the degree of stress on the syllable containing the rounded vowel, seem to affect the extent and velocity of protrusion gestures in a significant way (Benguerel and Cowan 1974). A factor recently identified by Abry and Lallouache (1991a, 1991b) is word boundary. All the experiments with real word corpora have to combine words into short phrases in order to get a high number of consonants between vowels. Abry and Lallouache have shown that coarticulatory patterns vary importantly depending on whether a word boundary is or is not realized. Each of these factors, if not carefully controlled, may lead to different results and different interpretations.

But even the data of the latest, carefully conducted studies by Perkell and colleagues for English and by Abry and Lallouache for French evidently contradict some of the assumptions of both the look-ahead and the coproduction models in their present versions. The new models proposed for English (the hybrid model) and for French (the movement expansion model) call for important theoretical revisions of both theories of speech production.

Acknowledgments

I thank Michael Studdert-Kennedy, Jim Flege and Bill Hardcastle for insightful comments and suggestions on an earlier version of the manuscript. This research was supported in part by the European ESPRIT/ACCOR project WG 7098.

Note

1 A notable exception is the study by Benguerel and Cowan (1974), who excluded from analysis all the consonants showing an inherent lip position.

7

Lip and jaw coarticulation

JANET FLETCHER and JONATHAN HARRINGTON

Introduction

Lip and jaw or mandibular movements in speech production have been extensively studied (see e.g. Lindblom 1967; Perkell 1969; Lindblom and Sundberg 1971; Kelso *et al.* 1985; Ostry and Munhall 1994; Vatikiotis-Bateson and Ostry 1995; Ostry, Gribble and Gracco 1996), partly because they are more amenable to direct instrumental investigation than other speech articulators which often require invasive techniques. The types of investigations are numerous and include movement and kinematic studies (using e.g. cinefluorography, the X-ray microbeam system, strain-gauge and optoelectronic devices and electromagnetic midsagittal articulatory tracking devices), studies of the mandibular and labial muscle systems (using electromyography) and numerous acoustic analyses.

Briefly, the jaw is a large and relatively sluggish articulator compared to the tongue tip or blade, for example. Extensive studies of jaw motion by Ostry and Munhall (1994) and Vatikiotis-Bateson and Ostry (1995) among others, suggest that during jaw opening in a CV sequence the jaw rotates downwards and moves forward, whereas during closure (i.e. VC) the jaw rotates upwards and translates backwards. The jaw also provides a framework for both lingual and labial gestures (e.g. Perkell 1969). For example bilabial closure is achieved via contribution of the jaw and upper and lower lips. The jaw is connected to both the hyoid bone and tongue. Consequently, movement of the jaw alters the position of the tongue and to a lesser extent overall tongue shape (e.g. Linblom and Sundberg 1971).

The jaw is therefore involved in both the production of consonants and vowels and can be associated with left to right (carryover) and right to left (anticipatory) coarticulatory effects – although these effects are not as pronounced temporally as other forms of coarticulation. According to Fowler

(1985: 249) 'coarticulation of tongue and jaw gestures is less extensive anticipatorily than lip rounding or nasalisation . . . these are gestures that achieve the acoustic consequences identified as segment onset. If they were anticipated more, the segment itself would be anticipated.'

Similar questions relating to whether coarticulation is the result of 'central planning' or of overlapping control signals to different articulatory organs emerge in studies of the jaw and associated articulators (see Fowler 1995 and Ostry, Gribble and Gracco 1996 for a discussion). Furthermore, studies of the jaw (and lip aperture – see below) have been important to the so-called 'timing control debate', i.e. whether observed timing properties of articulatory movements are the result of mechanical constraints of the system or are regulated by some kind of external clock (see Saltzman and Munhall 1989; Fowler 1995; Saltzman, Löfqvist and Mitra in press, for a discussion of these issues). Recent empirical and simulation studies of jaw movements by Ostry, Gribble and Gracco (1996) also consider the contribution of jaw musculature, musculo-skeletal geometry and inherent jaw dynamics to anticipatory and carryover coarticulation in VCV sequences. Their findings suggest that the latter must be taken into consideration in any discussion of the origins of coarticulation.

The patterning of jaw and tongue movements, often referred to as movements of the lingual-mandibular complex, also shows evidence of 'functionally organized goal-oriented behaviour' during the articulation of consonant–vowel sequences (Abbs and Gracco 1984). To achieve a particular articulatory goal, for example, the jaw and tongue may exhibit motor equivalence and compensatory behaviour. In this section, the term *gesture* will be used to refer to a movement that belongs to a group of movements that are functionally equivalent ways of achieving the same goal (Saltzman and Munhall 1989; Browman and Goldstein 1993). The jaw also forms part of the labial–mandibular sub-system or articulatory complex, comprising the jaw and upper and lower lips. Movements consist of raising, lowering, protrusion and retraction – these are all actions that are readily measurable in the vertical and horizontal dimensions.

This review will be mainly concerned with movement of the mandible and lips in the vertical dimension. Whilst these organs can be thought of as relatively independent, their movements during speech production often illustrate compensatory and coordinative behaviour, like the lingual–mandibular system. For example, the jaw and both lips contribute to lip aperture, measured as the vertical difference between the upper and lower lips. Lip aperture is one of the gestures that is thought to be under active control, with the contributions of the lip and jaw combining in different ways to achieve this goal depending on contextual factors (Lindblom 1967; Browman and Goldstein 1993). For example, both /aba/ and /ibi/ are characterized by the same goal of lip closure (for the medial consonant) but the way in which lip closure is achieved is different: in /ibi/ the jaw, which is in a more raised position (due to the close vowel context), can make a greater contribution to lip closure than in /aba/. The exact nature of these articulatory tradeoffs in the spatial and temporal domain, together with a summary of the segmental and prosodic factors that influence lip–jaw articulation (and to a lesser extent jaw–tongue articulation) will be discussed in the following sections. *Spatial effects* refer to the vertical position of the jaw and lip aperture, and *spatio-temporal effects* to the relative timing of successive gestures and related spatial modifications. This review summarizes some of the major findings of earlier studies but is in no way an exhaustive account of the literature.

Spatial effects

Jaw position covaries with tongue body height during the production of vowels (e.g. Perkell 1969; Lindblom and Sundberg 1971; Sussman, MacNeilage and Hanson 1973; Gracco 1993) although there can be a degree of inter-speaker variability (e.g. Johnson, Ladefoged and Lindau 1993). English close vowels such as /i/, /ɪ/ and /ʊ/ are associated with less jaw opening than open vowels like /æ/. Swedish vowels exhibit similar jaw patterning, open vowels showing jaw displacement differences of the order of 8–9 mm compared with close vowels (Lindblom 1967; Lindblom and Sundberg 1971; Keating, Huffman and Jackson 1994). Kiritani and colleagues (1977, 1983) also note correlations between jaw position and vowel height for Japanese.

Lindblom and Sundberg (1971) suggest that there may be very few basic tongue shapes, with further differences in vowels coming from degree of jaw lowering. They suggest that 'the degree of openness of a vowel reflects a position of the jaw that is optimised in the sense that it cooperates with the tongue in producing the desired area function . . . such cooperation prevents excessive tongue shape deformation' (Lindblom and Sundberg 1971: 34). However, Farnetani (1991, after Kiritani 1977) notes potential language-specific tongue body and jaw coordination – the tongue body and jaw position contribute to vowel height contrasts in English, whereas the jaw makes more contribution to vowel height differences in Japanese. Maeda and Honda (1995) note a high degree of compensatory behaviour between jaw and tongue body position of /i/ and /a/ for French. In their subsequent synthesis model, they propose an 'optimum jaw–tongue compensatory rule' (p. 82) in which tongue body position for a given vowel remains invariant and subsequent observed differences can be modelled as a function of actual jaw position.

With respect to lip–jaw coordination, Gracco (1993) and Macchi (1988) note that the jaw, and not the lower lip, is largely responsible for oral opening differences in both the pre- and post-consonantal vowels in VCV sequences, where C is a labial consonant. Likewise, in /bVb/ sequences the jaw contributes more to open the lips into a following vowel, while the lips contribute more to form the final bilabial closure. Lindblom (1967) interprets this as evidence for temporal compensation, due to the larger and slower movement of the jaw. The movement requirements for the slow mandible are related to vowel height differences. High vowels are associated with faster and shorter opening and closing movements than low vowels (Gracco 1993; Harrington, Fletcher and Beckman in press).

Lindblom (1983) suggests that jaw height is influenced to a much greater extent by vowels than consonants. The position of the jaw may therefore be marginally influenced by anticipatory coarticulation with a following consonant in VCV sequences (Perkell 1969; Tuller, Harris and Gross 1981) and, in their comparative study of English and Swedish, Keating, Lindblom, Lubker and Kreiman (1994) found no significant influence of intervocalic consonant on flanking vowels, reflecting similar results to those of Farnetani and Faber (1992) for Italian. At the same time consonants can marginally influence jaw position: for example, Tuller, Harris and Gross (1981) found that the consonants /f/, /p/, /t/, and /k/ exerted the strongest to weakest influence respectively on the jaw position for the final vowels /a/ and /i/. Studies have shown that when consonant-induced coarticulatory effects are present, they tend to influence low vowels to a greater extent than high vowels (Abbs, Netsell and Hixon 1972; Westbury 1988; Keating, Lindblom, Lubker and Kreiman 1994).

There is a degree of consensus in the literature that bilabial and velar consonants seem more prone to influence of flanking vowels than alveolars although there is some disagreement concerning the directionality of these coarticulatory effects. The height of the jaw during the bilabial closure is influenced by the phonetic height of the preceding vowel (Sussman, MacNeilage and Hanson 1973; Tuller, Harris and Gross 1981; Macchi 1988), i.e. there are strong carryover effects, even though anticipatory effects of the final vowel on a medial /p/ are not necessarily evident in some studies (e.g. Tuller, Harris and Gross 1981). By contrast, other studies have found strong anticipatory lowering of the jaw in anticipation of a following vowel during the closure of the initial /b/ in /bVb/ sequences (Fujimura 1961b). Schulman (1989) also found strong anticipatory coarticulatory effects correlated with vocal effort, in the medial bilabial in Swedish /i'bVb/ sequences where V is one of twelve Swedish vowels. The relatively more open vocal tract during the stressed syllable in loud versus normal speech resulted in an absolute lower jaw position of the preceding bilabial stop.

Both anticipatory and carryover effects of V_1 and V_2 are evident in the characteristic jaw positions of velar stops in V_1CV_2 sequences (Tuller, Harris and Gross 1981; Kiritani *et al.* 1983). The classic example of tongue body–jaw coarticulation in this respect is the fronting of velar consonants in the context of high front vowels. However Tuller, Harris and Gross (1981) found that /f/ and /t/ did not exhibit jaw height variation, unlike /p/ and /k/. Other studies have shown that preceding and following vowels influence tongue blade and jaw position for alveolars in VtV sequences (Edwards 1985). The height of the tongue blade varies with the height of the preceding vowel, tending to be higher when the preceding vowel is high and conversely lower when the vowel is low. Anticipatory effects of V_2 in VCV sequences on blade height were also observed by Edwards (1985) and Parush, Ostry and Munhall (1983).

Jaw perturbation studies provide further evidence of covariation and coordination between the lips, jaw and tongue body (see Löfqvist 1990 for a summary). In many of the so-called *static perturbation* studies, the upper lip is shown to compensate for the jaw which is artificially held in a fixed position due to a bite-block and, as a result of this compensation, normal lip closure for the bilabial consonant is achieved (e.g. Lindblom, Lubker and Gay, 1979; Gay, Lindblom and Lubker 1981; Folkins and Linville 1983) although it has been suggested that the absolute jaw position for bilabial closure in these cases presents an articulatory setting that is akin to loud speech (Schulman 1989) and vice versa.

Similar findings are reported in dynamic perturbation studies in which responses are recorded to a load applied to the jaw, upper and lower lip and tongue (e.g. Abbs, Gracco and Cole 1984; Shaiman, 1989). According to Löfqvist (1990), compensatory responses reflect the goal-oriented nature of speech production. If the jaw is loaded during the transition from vowel to bilabial stop, the compensatory responses are evident in the lip activity relating to bilabial closure. If the load is applied during the transition from a vowel to dental fricative or dental stop, for example, responses are noted for tongue activity (Kelso *et al.* 1984; Shaiman 1989). Tongue body gestures have similarly been shown to compensate for a fixed mandible position to achieve the same, or nearly the same, acoustic vowel target in some studies (e.g. Gay, Lindblom and Lubker 1981). However, Löfqvist points out that not all perturbation studies have examined the acoustic consequences of compensation and perfect compensation should not be expected – merely sufficient compensation to 'maintain the integrity of the acoustic signal' (Löfqvist 1990: 312).

Coproduction and spatio-temporal effects

Investigation of the kinematics of jaw and lip articulation has contributed a great deal to the understanding of temporal patterning in speech and in particular to coproduction theories of coarticulation (Fowler 1980, 1983a; Fowler and Rosenblum 1989). A central aspect of coproduction models, which is taken from the earlier acoustic studies of Öhman (1966) and which has strongly influenced the more recent task dynamic model of speech production (e.g. Saltzman and Munhall 1989), is that consonants and vowels are associated with independent articulatory strategies that overlap in time. An important prediction of this theory is that there should be evidence of coarticulatory influences between the flanking vowels, across a medial consonant in VCV sequences. Compatibly, Öhman's (1966) spectrographic data show that the closing transitions into the medial consonant are influenced by *both* flanking vowels (see also Butcher and Weiher 1976; Recasens, Pallarès and Fontdevila 1997, for related evidence from electropalatographic data). With respect to jaw articulation, Sussman, MacNeilage and Hanson (1973) note that the degree of opening of V_1 influences the jaw position of V_2, in spite of the jaw raising for the intervening consonant. By contrast however, Harrington *et al.* (1997) found that additional factors such as degree of accentual prominence, can result in *less* coproduction of V_1 and V_2, i.e. dissimilation.

As Fowler (1983a) suggests, if it is the case that vowels and consonants are controlled by autonomous production strategies, then it is likely that they can be timed, or phased, relatively to each other in different ways. In the last few years, some jaw movement studies have considered *truncation* as a source of evidence for the variable phasing of vowels and consonants. A simple illustration of the effects of a closer phasing of the vowel and consonant on jaw movement (in the production of Australian English 'barb', phonetically [bäːb]), resulting in truncation, is shown in figure 7.1. As the temporal overlap increases between successive opening and closing jaw movements, vowel duration will also decrease (figure 7.1b, 7.1c), assuming that the velocity of the gestures does not change. In producing /bab/ for example, the vowel and consonant make competing demands on the jaw trajectory: the jaw needs to be lowered for /a/ but raised for the following /b/. Since the vowel and consonant are timed to occur closer together, the raising gesture for the final /b/ overlaps to a greater extent with the lowering gesture. As a result, the full displacement for the /a/ vowel is never attained in more extreme forms of truncation because it is cut off, or *truncated*, by the gesture for the final /b/ (figure 7.1b, 7.1c). This theory of truncation due to gestural overlap (Saltzman and Munhall 1989; Munhall and Löfqvist 1992), is similar in many respects to

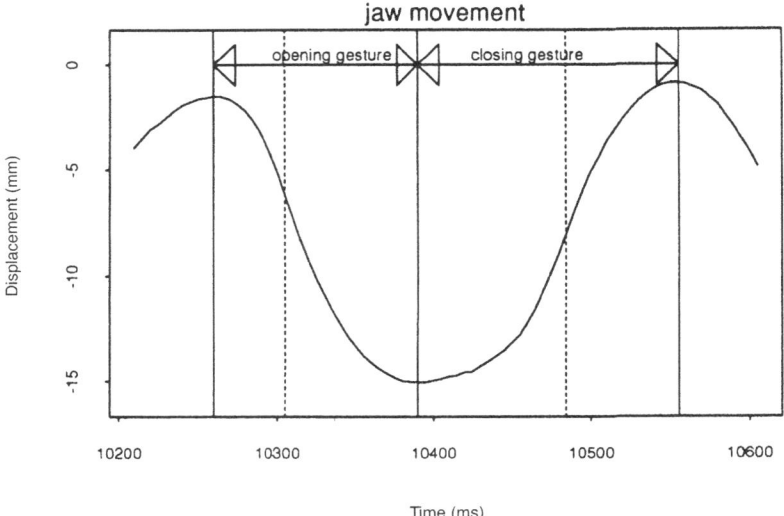

Figure 7.1a   Jaw displacement trajectory for a production of [bab] showing the peak displacements associated with the consonants and vowel (solid vertical lines) and the times of the peak velocities in the opening and closing gestures (dotted vertical lines).

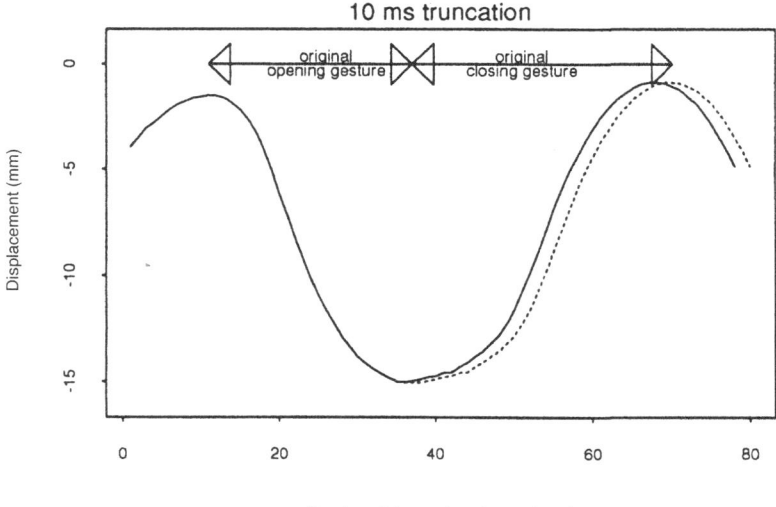

Figure 7.1b   The opening gesture, from the time of the peak vowel displacement to the end of the trajectory, is moved 10 ms closer to the closing gesture. The resulting trajectory is shown by the solid line, with the original trajectory indicated by the dotted line.

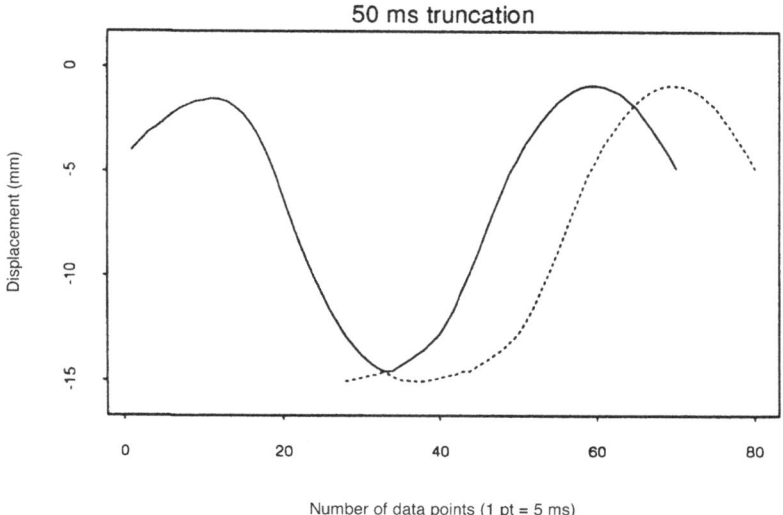

Figure 7.1c   The temporal displacement of the opening gesture is greater than in figure 7.1b, causing a reduction in the peak displacement for the vowel. The resulting trajectory is shown by the solid line, with the original trajectory indicated by the dotted line.

Lindblom's (1963b) earlier model of target undershoot because both models are characterized by a form of articulatory invariance. In the gestural-overlap model, the gestures themselves do not change, only the phasing between them, while in Lindblom's model, the articulatory commands are presumed to be invariant (in changing from e.g. a stressed to an unstressed vowel), but the duration changes (resulting in target undershoot).

Several phonetic and phonological phenomena effect the measured acoustic duration of a vowel. Observed vowel shortening has been attributed to many different kinds of articulatory changes that can often be interpreted in terms of increased coarticulatory overlap of competing gestures. These include: vowel duration changes due to a final coda (Munhall *et al.* 1992); post-vocalic voicing (van Summers 1987; de Jong 1991; Gracco 1993); accentuation (Edwards, Beckman, and Fletcher 1991; Bretonnel Cohen *et al.* 1995; de Jong 1995b; Harrington, Fletcher and Roberts 1995; Beckman and Cohen in press, Harrington, Fletcher and Beckman in press), vowel quantity differences (Kroos *et al.* 1996; Hertrich and Ackermann 1997) and tempo (Gay 1981; Wieneke, Janssen and Belderbos 1987). A summary of the above findings together with any examples of counter-evidence are presented below.

Vowel changes due to the coda

A well-known finding is that vowel duration decreases with an increasing number of consonants in a syllable coda (e.g. Umeda 1975). A possible explanation for this finding in coproduction models is that the articulation of the vowel and coda overlap to a greater extent when there are multiple consonants in the coda: since the acoustic duration corresponds to the part of the vowel which is *non*-overlapping with flanking consonants (Fowler 1983a, 1984), a consequence of the closer phasing of the vowel and coda is a decrease in acoustic vowel duration. In order to investigate further the articulatory correlates of this decrease in acoustic duration, Munhall *et al.* (1992) examined jaw kinematics in various syllables that differed in the number of consonants in the coda (see also de Jong 1991 for a related study on tongue body articulation). Their general finding was that jaw raising associated with the movement from the vowel to the following consonant started earlier in CVCC compared with CVC syllables. In deriving averaged jaw trajectories for CVC and CVCC syllables, the observed difference was attributed to a marginal change in the phasing of the coda relative to the vowel: if the extent of earlier phasing of the coda is less than the duration of the relatively steady-state jaw trajectory associated with vowel production, then the peak displacement (for the vowel) is minimally changed. This is illustrated in figure 7.1b: although the opening gesture is truncated by the closing gesture, the extent of truncation is not sufficient to bring about a change in peak vowel displacement. Munhall *et al.*'s interpretation of their data is that the shorter vowel duration in CVCC syllables is due to the truncation of the vowel by the following consonant cluster.

Changes due to post-vocalic voicing

Studies of the articulatory basis of the duration changes associated with postvocalic voicing also provide some evidence that closing gestures for voiceless segments begin earlier than for voiced segments. De Jong (1991) compared tongue body and jaw trajectories in tokens like 'tote/s' versus 'toad/s' and found that vowel shortenings before the voiceless consonants was due to greater gestural overlap or truncation. In other words, the difference due to voicing of the following consonant is realized in much the same way as an accentuation related duration contrast (see above). Van Summers (1987) found that the degree of jaw lowering was no greater in /bab/ versus /bap/, although closing gestures in voiceless tokens are shorter, faster and occur earlier than in voiced tokens. Van Summers also investigated the effects of stress on jaw lowering and raising gestures and concluded that the effects of stress on spatial characteristics of jaw trajectories were much greater than the effects of voicing. Rather than the two vowel duration effects being realized by different articulation strategies it may be more a question of degree of articulatory overlap. It is possible that deaccenting results in greater gestural overlap than devoicing. Gracco (1993) also suggests the later, longer and somewhat slower closing gestures observed in /CVb/ sequences compared to /CVp/ sequences not only indicate greater intra-articulator coarticulation (jaw) in the voiceless sequences but also a complex accommodation between jaw and laryngeal gestures to effect devoicing.

Changes due to accentuation

Words in languages like English can have an intonational event (pitch accent) associated with the rhythmically strongest syllables that makes the word accentually prominent relative to other words in a phrase. There are non-tonal attributes of accent that, broadly speaking, can be associated with a greater deflection of the vocal organs from a neutral position (e.g. Kelso *et al.* 1985; van Summers 1987; Beckman, Edwards and Fletcher 1992). At least two acoustic correlates of these supralaryngeal modifications are longer acoustic duration and greater loudness in accented versus unaccented syllables (Harrington, Fletcher and Beckman in press). Greater jaw lowering or 'sonority expansion' in low vowels (Beckman, Edwards and Fletcher 1992) results in an overall more open vocal tract and greater loudness in the vowel which enhances the percept of accent. Alternatively de Jong (1995b) interpreted these affects as evidence of localized hyperarticulation and the greater sonority expansion is actually due to the same process as the greater tongue backing observed in accented back vowels, with the end result being a more peripheral vowel. This model therefore implies that segments are more likely to attain more extreme targets when accented, and that there will be diminished evidence of coproduction.

These two theories of accentual prominence are not necessarily unrelated. The greater gestural magnitude observed in these studies can in most cases be directly linked to a decrease in coarticulatory overlap between segments. For example, the kinematic studies of jaw movement in Edwards, Beckman and Fletcher (1991), Harrington, Fletcher and Roberts (1995) and Bretonnel Cohen *et al.* (1995) all show that the jaw lowering gesture for a low vowel is cut off or truncated by the jaw raising gesture for the following bilabial consonant in CVC or CVCə sequences (i.e. figure 7.1c), where C is a bilabial consonant, implying that a *less* peripheral low vowel is articulated in this case. The link between 'stress' or accentuation, diminished coproduction and increased gestural magnitude can also be linked to potential sound changes as discussed by Beckman, Edwards and Fletcher (1992). They suggest that in Old Irish, truncation of the closing gesture associated with neighbouring vowels could explain spirantization of stops in 'prosodically weak' contexts.

Vowel quantity and tempo effects

Hertrich and Ackermann (1997) examined vowel quantity contrasts in German by analysing the kinematics of lower lip–jaw articulation in /gepVpe/ sequences. They found that intergestural timing or phasing differences accounted for longer deceleration portions (i.e. the time period between moment of peak velocity and onset of closing gesture) in long versus short vowels. However, in closing gestures into the final syllable they found that the longer acceleration phase (moment of closing gesture onset to point of peak velocity in closing gesture) did not necessarily reflect either a change in intergestural phasing or change in the peak velocity – amplitude relationship. They suggest rather that it might be accounted for by a general slowing down during the initial stages of consonant closure in much the same way that Edwards, Beckman and Fletcher (1991) accounted for final lengthening. They further suggest that their findings together with those of Edwards, Beckman and Fletcher might be evidence of some kind of specified time representation that is not purely a consequence of specific control mechanisms like stiffness or phasing in the task dynamic model, for example. On the other hand, they claim their results might reflect the relative lag of the jaw (i.e. the inherent physical constraints of the articulator) relative to the lips in effecting bilabial closure, referred to earlier in this review. The timing lag of the jaw relative to the lips during bilabial closure is reportedly shorter in fast relative to slow speech (Gay 1981).

In general, studies of tempo effects on coarticulation provide less clear-cut support for this view of coarticulation as truncation and blending. On the one hand, findings suggest that there is greater CV than VC coarticulation with reduced opening versus closing jaw displacements at fast tempo (Kuehn and Moll 1976; Gay 1981). Other findings (e.g. Wieneke, Janssen and Belderbos 1987) suggest that the extent of spatio-temporal blending of gestures is reduced at slower rates of speech.

This is supported by Edwards, Beckman and Fletcher's (1991) finding that opening gestures in slow accented syllables show no evidence of truncation. At fast tempo, Kroos *et al.* (1996) note tighter coupling of CV to VC movements in their German corpus but no intragestural modifications particularly in lax vowels. An important issue in these studies and all papers cited in this review, however, is the high level of inter-speaker variability (e.g. Westbury and Moy 1996).

Conclusion

Clearly further data from tongue body gestures are needed to augment articulatory studies of lip and jaw coarticulation. Increasing use of magnetometer and other articulator tracking devices will enable broader analysis of the spatio-temporal patterning of tongue–body and jaw articulation under the influence of contextual effects. Most studies have been restricted to analysing a handful of subjects and have generally used corpora based on nonsense sequences. One notable exception is the study by Westbury and Moy (1996) based on jaw, lip and tongue movements of twenty-two speakers. Also, recent developments in both the technical and theoretical domains have resulted in more studies using less artificial corpora (e.g. de Jong 1995; Harrington *et al.* 1997; Harrington, Fletcher and Beckman in press). It is clear, nevertheless, that the development of coproduction and other theories of coarticulation, speech dynamics, and articulatory phonology has been greatly influenced by the accessibility and measurability of lip and jaw data.

Part III
Wider perspectives

Cross-language studies: relating language-particular coarticulation patterns to other language-particular facts

SHARON MANUEL

Introduction

This chapter focuses on cross-language studies of coarticulation. It addresses, in part, the question of why coarticulation patterns appear to be different in different languages. I will concentrate mostly (but not exclusively) on studies of non-Indo-European languages. For related discussion of cross-linguistic aspects of coarticulation, focusing more on Indo-European languages, the reader may wish to consult Farnetani (1990). In addition to referring to some of the classic works on cross-language studies of coarticulation, I have chosen to emphasize several recent studies, many of which are based on doctoral dissertations or conference papers. The rationale behind this choice is two-fold. First, much of the work which specifically addresses the question of cross-language aspects of coarticulation and which evaluates non-Indo-European languages has been completed by doctoral students. Second, precisely because some of these works do not yet appear in widely available formats, they may be unfamiliar to many readers.[1]

Often the term coarticulation is restricted, at least implicitly, to clear cases of contextual variation in the way a segment appears to be produced, such as nasalization of vowels before nasal consonants. In this chapter coarticulation is defined rather more broadly, as *patterns of coordination, between the articulatory gestures of neighbouring segments,*[2] *which result in the vocal tract responding at any one time to commands for more than one segment.* Of course, according to this definition, it is almost impossible to produce an utterance that is more than one segment long without engaging in coarticulation. The implication of this broader definition is that phenomena captured by the narrower definition are simply special cases of the more general phenomena of intra- and inter-segment coordination.

Since Öhman's (1966) classic study of coarticulation in three languages

(Russian, Swedish and English) it has been clear that languages differ in their coarticulatory patterns. Öhman's work raised the following question: 'What is the basis for cross-linguistic differences in coarticulation?' We want to know if the language-particular coarticulation facts are *independent* facts about the languages in question or are somehow *derivative* of other properties (such as differing use of distinctive features) of the languages. That is, if we knew X, Y and Z about a language, could we predict its coarticulation facts? The latter possibility has been explored most aggressively with respect to the role that linguistic contrast (the crucial fact being that systems of contrast are language-particular) plays in limiting coarticulation. The relationship between phonological contrast and coarticulation is explored in the following section. We then examine the role that other language-particular parameters (such as prosody and vowel harmony) might play in determining patterns of coarticulation.

The role of contrast in coarticulation

The idea that contrast (or distinctiveness) affects coarticulation is well known and has been discussed at least briefly in a variety of places. The basic idea is that while the articulatory commands for adjacent segments may overlap in time, the patterns of overlap are affected by speakers' efforts to maintain distinctions among segments. Precisely because what counts as contrastive or distinctive varies both from language to language and for different segments within a language, we would expect to find differences in coarticulatory patterns in different languages, and within a language depending on what segments are being considered.

This general hypothesis rests on certain assumptions, some of which are not very controversial while others are more problematic. A basic assumption is that segmentally distinct words in a language are distinct primarily because they are composed of different strings of segments. Furthermore, the segments themselves are differentiated in terms of their patterns of articulatory movements and the acoustic consequences of those articulatory patterns. If speakers want listeners to understand them (and presumably that is the main reason for talking), it is reasonable to expect that speakers make some effort to ensure that the acoustic consequences of their articulatory gestures remain distinct (see also Martinet 1952, 1957; Lindblom 1983; Lindblom and Engstrand 1989; Stevens 1989).

Manuel (1987, 1990) tried to capture these ideas with the concept that there are 'output constraints' (or tolerances) on segments which set limits on how much the articulatory–acoustic patterns of a segment are allowed to deviate from an ideally distinctive pattern. For example, a speaker who intends to say the English word *tick* must be sure to make a tight constriction between the tongue tip and the palate somewhere in the general region of the alveolar ridge, as a too weak constriction might result in frication and the word being heard as *sick* or *thick*. Coarticulation can introduce contextual variability in the way a segment is produced, by effectively altering or apparently deleting articulatory gestures that are normally associated with that segment or by introducing 'alien' (to the 'host' segment) articulatory gestures. Thus, in a sequence ABC, if unchecked in temporal extent and in strength at initiation, commands to make the articulatory gestures appropriate for segment B could potentially have the effect of obliterating[3] phonetic contrasts needed in segment A or segment C. If speakers are to maintain contrasts, we might expect them to coarticulate segments in such a way as not to destroy the distinctive attributes of those segments (see also, for example, Martinet 1952, 1957; Schouten and Pols 1979a; Manuel and Krakow 1984; Tatham 1984; Engstrand 1988; Keating 1990b). That is, speakers might limit the temporal and spatial extent of coarticulation so that the output constraints on a segment are not violated.

As noted above, which articulatory gestures count as distinctive depends both on the segment and on the language. Let us first consider language-internal differences in whether or not a particular gesture is distinctive for a given segment. English distinguishes voiced oral and nasal stop consonants, so if the oral tract is completely closed and the vocal folds are vibrating, it matters if the velar port is appreciably open – this is the major difference between /g/ and /ŋ/. Consequently, we do not expect speakers to substantially lower the velum during the oral closure for the /g/ in *big man* – the velum lowering for the /m/ will have to wait till the /g/ has been made as an oral segment. But, for English, how much does it matter if the velar port is appreciably open or not during production of vowels? After all, English normally does not distinguish between oral and nasalized vowels. Thus we are not surprised to find that in /VN/ utterances, the velar lowering movement for the nasal begins rather early in the vowel. So even within a language, because what counts as contrastive varies from segment to segment, we expect coarticulation to vary for different segment strings.

Some classic studies of language differences in contrast

Beginning with Öhman (1966), several well-known studies reflect on language-particular patterns of contrast and coarticulation. Öhman showed that for V_1CV_2 utterances in English and Swedish, the articulators began moving toward configurations appropriate for V_2 toward the acoustic end of V_1, before the consonant occlusion was achieved. Apparently the tongue body was free to begin assuming positions appropriate for the second vowel before and during the intervening consonant. However, Öhman did not find similar effects in Russian. He attributed the relative weakness of V-to-V coarticulation in Russian to the fact that Russian generally contrasts palatalized and nonpalatalized consonants and suggested that because the position of the tongue body is used to distinguish these two sets of consonants, Russian speakers are not free to let the tongue body be manipulated by V_2 before the intervening consonant has had its chance to control tongue body position. Support for this basic explanation comes from Choi and Keating (1991), who find very limited[4] V-to-V coarticulation across relevant consonants in Russian as well as in two other Slavic languages (Polish and Bulgarian) which have a palatal–nonpalatal contrast for consonants.

As noted above, English does not have an oral–nasal contrast for vowels and we might assume that this is why English vowels allow extensive coarticulation of the velar-lowering gestures for neighbouring nasal consonants. Of course, in some languages vowels are distinguished with respect to the feature [*Nasal*] and it is of interest to see how much velar coarticulation is found for vowels in those languages. Clumeck's (1976) work on velar opening during vowels in /VN/ sequences in American English, Swedish, French, Amoy Chinese, Hindi and Brazilian Portuguese is an attempt to do just that. Clumeck found language differences in the timing and amplitude of velar opening during the vowel. Of significance here is that the latter four languages have an oral–nasal contrast for vowels, whereas the former two do not.

Unfortunately, it is not exactly clear what predictions these patterns of contrast would make with respect to coarticulation of a nasal consonant and preceding vowel. One *might* expect that the languages *without* an oral–nasal vowel contrast would allow and exhibit greater amplitude of (or earlier) velar lowering during the vowel in a /VN/ context than would the languages *with* an oral–nasal vowel contrast. However, in Clumeck's subset of languages with a oral–nasal vowel contrast, that contrast is said to be neutralized just in case the vowels occur before a nasal in the same syllable.[5] Of possible relevance is the assumption of the underlying nature of vowels in nasal contexts. For French, Amoy Chinese and Hindi the usual assumption is that these vowels are underlyingly oral. Clumeck points out that there is some evidence (Brito 1975) that at least some vowels in Brazilian Portuguese /CVNCV/ sequences are actually stored in the mental lexicon as nasal vowels.

Clumeck's (1976) results indicate that the velum lowered early (with respect to V onset) for American English and Swedish short vowels but relatively late in Swedish long vowels. The data for American English and the Swedish short vowels are not unexpected, on the premise that vowels in these languages could tolerate large amounts of nasalization. The relatively late nasalization of the Swedish long vowels is more problematic. Clumeck suggests that while nasalization is not distinctive in Swedish, the Swedish vowel space is otherwise generally crowded, and heavy nasalization of its long vowels might lead to perceptual confusion of the vowels (see Wright 1986). As Clumeck points out, this account leaves the heavy nasalization of Swedish short vowels unexplained. Following the coproduction model of coarticulation (e.g. Bell-Berti and Harris 1982; Fowler 1981b, 1983a; Boyce *et al.* 1990) we conjecture that the velar-lowering gesture is timed with respect to the oral gestures for the nasals, and this temporally fixed 'advanced' lowering of the velum simply occurs later in the long Swedish vowels because the long Swedish vowels *start* earlier with respect to the oral movement for the nasal consonant.

For three of the languages (French, Hindi and Amoy Chinese) that have systems of oral and nasal vowels, the velum lowered relatively late in the vowel. Such patterns would be expected if these vowels are underlyingly oral, and if speakers generally avoid nasalization on underlyingly oral vowels. Brazilian Portuguese, the fourth language with distinctive nasalization of vowels, had relatively heavy nasalization of vowels in the environment of nasal consonants. As noted above, because these vowels may be stored as underlyingly nasal, it is not clear that the nasalization observed by Clumeck is actually coarticulatory in nature. In summary, Clumeck's study revealed cross-linguistic differences in velar coarticulation, some of which could plausibly, but not conclusively, be related to systems of contrast in the respective languages. In fact, more recently, Farnetani (1990) reported very restricted contextual nasalization of vowels in Italian, a language which does not have distinctive nasalization of vowels. Furthermore, Solé (1992, 1995) finds that the temporal extent of nasalization of vowels before tautosyllabic nasal consonants varies as a function of speaking rate for English but not Spanish. Based on the patterns she finds, she argues that in English, nasalization of vowels which precede tautosyllabic nasal consonants is not due to coarticulation at all, but due to their being *intrinsically* nasalized (presumably due to a phonological rule).

Lubker and Gay (1982) also used the notion of contrast to explain differences they found in anticipatory lip rounding in English and Swedish V_1CV_2 utterances. They found that Swedish speakers had a tendency to begin rounding for V_2 earlier in the C than did English speakers. Lubker and Gay suggested that precisely because rounding is contrastive for Swedish (but not for English) vowels, Swedish speakers begin rounding early, to make sure that adequate rounding is achieved in V_2. In other words, Lubker and Gay implicated the role of contrast in the *influencing* segment as a factor which led to that segment being initiated early, resulting in relatively strong coarticulatory effects on neighbouring segments.

Recent studies of V-to-V coarticulation, with emphasis on non-Indo-European languages

We now turn to several studies which are more recent and which focus at least in part on non-Indo-European languages. Manuel and Krakow (1984) and Manuel (1987, 1990) sought to explicitly test the hypothesis that the system of contrast in a language would affect the magnitude of coarticulation. Manuel and Krakow (1984) compared acoustic effects of V-to-V coarticulation in English, which has a relatively crowded vowel space, and two Bantu languages, Shona (spoken in Zimbabwe) and Swahili (spoken in Kenya and Tanzania), which have typical five-vowel systems (/i, e, ɑ, o, u/). The authors began by assuming that because the vowels in English are more crowded[6] in the articulatory or acoustic space, the range of production for each one would be rather small so as to maintain distinctions among them. On the other hand, as the vowels of Shona and Swahili are more spread apart, they could presumably tolerate larger ranges of production (equivalent to looser output constraints) without running the risk of encroaching on each other's distinctive space. On the basis of these assumptions about how relative spacing[7] would affect the size of acceptable 'target areas' for vowels in the three languages and a further assumption that speakers would coarticulate as much as possible while still making an effort to retain distinctiveness, Manuel and Krakow then predicted that there would be larger V-to-V coarticulation effects in Shona and Swahili than in English. The results were largely as predicted. In contrast to Öhman's study of English and Swedish, in which V-to-V effects were reported only at the edges of vowels, both Shona and Swahili showed coarticulatory effects which extended from V_1 into the middle of V_2, and vice versa. The English speaker in Manuel and Krakow did exhibit V-to-V effects which were temporally so great that they too extended into the middle of neighbouring vowels. However, the magnitude of the effects was considerably smaller in English than in Shona and Swahili. Similarly, Magen (1984a) found smaller V-to-V coarticulatory effects in English than in Japanese (whose phonemic vowels are /i, e, ɑ, o, ɯ/).

As noted by Manuel and Krakow, their study was limited in that the data came from one speaker of each language. The possibility remained that what appeared to be language differences were simply speaker differences. Furthermore, in addition to distribution of vowels, the vowel systems of the languages differ in that the English vowels are more diphthongized. However, the pattern of data was as predicted by the two-part hypothesis: that speakers

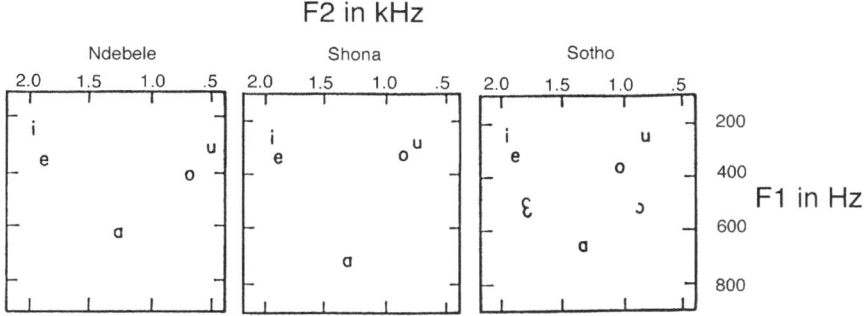

Figure 8.1 Examples of phonemic vowels of Ndebele, Shona and Sotho. Data are from one speaker of each of the languages.

try to maintain distinctiveness, and that patterns of distinctiveness are defined in the phonology (in this case by the distribution of vowels).

In a subsequent larger study, Manuel (1987, 1990) compared V-to-V coarticulation from three speakers of each of three Southern Bantu languages. Phonetically, the languages are all characterized as having primarily open syllables, monophthongal vowels, and phonemic tone (Doke 1954; Cole 1955). Two of the languages (Shona and Ndebele, spoken in Zimbabwe) have five-vowel systems (i, e, ɑ, o, u) while the third (Sotho, spoken in Lesotho, South Africa, and parts of Zimbabwe) has seven distinctive vowels (ɑ, e, ɛ, i, o, ɔ, u). As shown in figure 8.1, the vowels are more crowded in the low and mid vowel region in Sotho than they are in Shona and Ndebele. For example, in Sotho the vowel /ɛ/ intervenes between /e/ and /ɑ/. On the assumption that this crowding affects the output constraints on /e/ and /ɑ/ and that coarticulation is limited by output constraints, Manuel expected to find /e/ and /ɑ/ to be less susceptible to anticipatory coarticulatory effects from transconsonantal vowels in Sotho than in the other two languages.[8] The test data were acoustic measures of F1 and F2 in the middle and toward the ends of the target vowels /e/ and /ɑ/ in either the first vowel in /pepV₂pV₃/ and /pɑpV₂pV₃/, or the second vowel in /pɑpepV₃/ and /pɑpɑpV₃/. The independent variable was the quality /i, e, ɑ, o, u/ of the vowel which followed the target vowel.

The results were basically as predicted for the target vowel /ɑ/. The anticipatory V-to-V coarticulatory effects were greater in Shona and Ndebele than in Sotho, particularly in the F2 dimension, as can be seen in figure 8.2. It appeared that even in the middle of Shona and Ndebele /ɑ/, the tongue was moving toward a front position if followed by /i/, and toward a back position if followed by /u/. For Sotho, a following vowel appeared to exert a substantial influence only near the end of the target vowel /ɑ/ and even there the

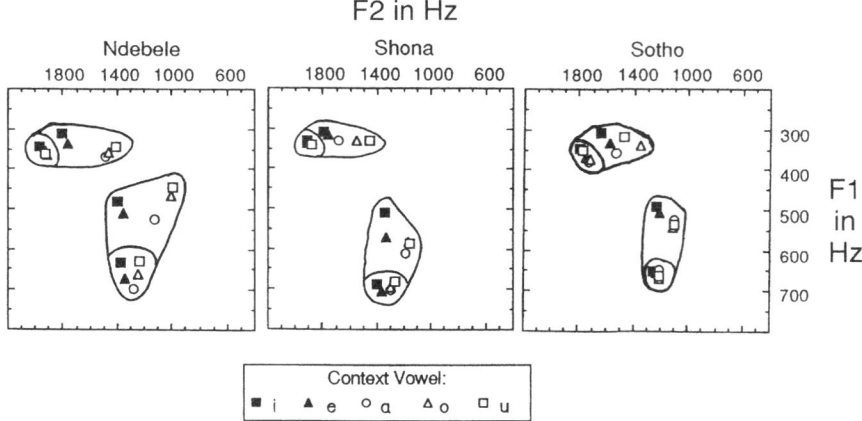

Figure 8.2   Acoustic effects of following context vowel on the target vowels /ɑ/ and /e/ in the three languages. Inner loops enclose data from the middle of the target vowels, outer loops enclose measurements made at the end of the target vowels. Data are averaged over three speakers of each language.

effects were smaller in magnitude than what was observed at the end of /ɑ/ in Shona and Ndebele. A somewhat surprising result was that target /e/ did not appear to move toward the /ɛ/ space as a function of a following low or back vowel in any of the languages. Possibly the flanking /p/ consonants led the speakers to keep a rather high jaw position, limiting or even cancelling any lowering effects of a following low vowel.

Manuel points out that the three Southern Bantu languages do not differ greatly in their respective spacing of phonemic vowels, but that all three of the languages studied might be expected to exhibit large coarticulatory effects when compared to English. A direct comparison of the relative magnitudes of anticipatory coarticulation on the vowel /ɑ/ can be seen in figure 8.3, which shows a single token each from English, Sotho and Ndebele. The coarticulatory influence of the following vowel is much clearer in both of the Bantu languages than it is in English.[9]

The data in Manuel (1987, 1990) and Manuel and Krakow (1984) are consistent with the idea that there are output constraints on segments, that these output constraints are determined (at least partially) by the distribution of contrastive segments in the phonetic space, and that coarticulation 'respects' the output constraints. Obviously more studies need to be done on more languages and with more speakers to determine if the coincidence of the results and the predictions occur purely by chance. Until such work is completed, the possibility still remains that the patterns found in Shona, Ndebele, Swahili

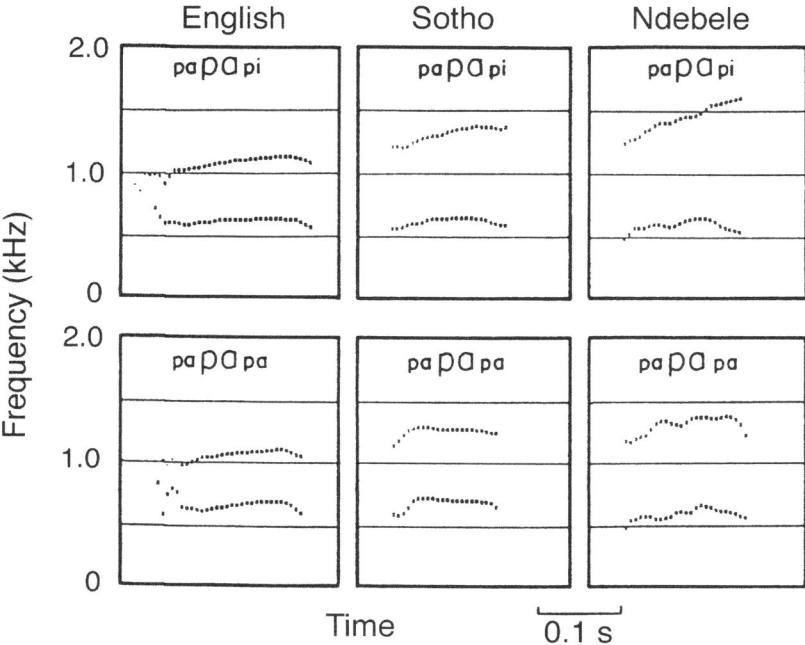

Figure 8.3   First and second formants for the middle vowel /ɑ/ in a single token of /pɑpɑpɑ/ and /pɑpɑpi/ from a speaker of each of the languages indicated. The rising F2, in anticipation of following /i/, is particularly striking for the Ndebele speaker.

and Sotho are actually unrelated to the distribution of contrastive vowels in the languages. Some support does come from the work of Choi (1992, 1995), discussed below, and Magen (1984a), noted above.

Recently, Choi (1992, 1995) has studied the production of vowels in Marshallese (spoken in Java). Marshallese has an unusual vowel system: vowels contrast for height, but not for front–back or rounding. The front–back and rounding qualities of Marshallese vowels are apparently determined by neighbouring consonants. The consonant system itself has front–back (palatal–velar) and rounding contrasts. Expanding on Keating's 'windows' model (see further discussion below), Choi models the vowels as phonologically and phonetically unspecified for front–back features. Because F2 is well-known to be affected by the front–back position of the tongue, and as that is not a distinctive feature for vowels in Marshallese, Choi predicts that F2 trajectories for vowels will be dependent on the F2 target values for surrounding consonants. The acoustic data Choi examines largely support this hypothesis. In general, the F2 trajectory through the vowels of Marshallese is dependent on target F2 values for surrounding consonants. Choi elegantly models deviations from such dependencies as largely a function of the partial dependence of vowel F2 on vowel height.

Studies such as Manuel and Krakow (1984), Manuel (1987, 1990) and Choi (1992, 1995) focus on the susceptibility of a segment to coarticulatory influences as a function of constraints on the *influenced* segment itself. In a study of anticipatory lip rounding on Mandarin fricatives, Xu (1989), like Lubker and Gay (1982), takes into account the role of contrast for the *influencing* segment. A number of earlier acoustic studies of English (e.g. Soli 1981) indicate that lip rounding for a following rounded vowel can begin during the production of a fricative in a fricative–vowel sequence. Xu's work is a particularly appropriate addition to this corpus of studies because it addresses the question of amount of anticipatory coarticulation as a function of the role of contrast for the feature [*Round*] for the influencing vowels and looks at the course of rounding through the duration of the fricative. Xu examines acoustic and perceptual data for the Mandarin voiceless fricatives [s], [ʂ] and [ɕ] followed by high rounded and high[10] unrounded vowels. The fricative [s] can be followed by [u] and a high central[10] unrounded vowel and [ʂ] can be followed by [u] and a high retroflexed unrounded vowel. Both [s] and [ʂ] can also be followed by non-high vowels. Crucially, the voiceless fricative [ɕ] can only be followed by the high front vowels [i] and [y], which are distinguished solely by rounding. Xu[11] finds perceptual evidence that anticipatory rounding begins earlier in [ɕ] than in the other two fricatives. His results are compatible with the notion that speakers accentuate the rounding of [y], in part by initiating it early and during the preceding fricative, because rounding is the only feature which distinguishes [y] from [i].

Limitations of the role of contrast in determining coarticulation

The studies described here are certainly consistent with the hypothesis that the extent of coarticulation is generally sensitive to the system of phonological contrast in a language. This does not necessarily mean that simply knowing what features (or articulatory gestures) are contrastive for certain segments in a given language will allow us to totally predict the degree of coarticulation for those segments. Several reasons for this will be discussed in this section; other reasons will be presented later.

First, while a lack of contrast might *allow* speakers to coarticulate extensively, there is no reason that speakers *must* coarticulate extensively. As Ladefoged (1983a) has pointed out, languages are free to be more or less particular in how they produce their phonemes. Certainly the inter-speaker differences we encounter when we study any one language suggest that speakers vary in how much they coarticulate: some speakers of a language do not seem to do so very much compared to their fellow speakers who show relatively extensive temporal and spatial coarticulatory effects. The role of contrast then, is more likely to set a maximum limit on coarticulation, but has little to say about how it is further limited.

Second, not all differences between the apparent resistance of various phonemes to coarticulatory variation are readily explainable by the notion of contrast. For example, several studies (Recasens 1984b, this volume; Recasens and Farnetani 1990; Recasens, Pallarès and Fontdevila 1997) suggest that lingual consonants which themselves entail more extensive dorsal–palatal contact are more resistant to coarticulation-induced variation than consonants with less extensive contact (but see Connell 1992). Thus, it may turn out that the amount of coarticulatory resistance of a given segment is predictable to some extent from knowledge about the phonetic implementation (e.g. how much tongue dorsum contact it entails) of a segment in a particular language, even though, as Disner (1983) has pointed out, the exact phonetic implementation of segments in a language is not entirely predictable from knowledge of its phonemic inventory (nor, presumably, from knowledge of other facts about the language).

Third, the idea that speakers limit coarticulation in order to maintain contrast assumes that contrast is never neutralized, at least by coarticulatory effects. However, to the extent that assimilation can be modelled as coarticulation, and to the extent that complete assimilation occurs, coarticulation often results in the loss of underlying distinctions. Similarly some (if not all) casual speech phenomena such as vowel and consonant reduction or deletion can be modelled as resulting from coarticulation (see Browman and Goldstein 1990a). While my colleagues and I have argued elsewhere (Manuel *et al.* 1992; Manuel 1995) that detailed acoustic analysis reveals that casual speech reduction is often less extreme than one might think, cases do exist where a very long string of segments is reduced to a syllable or two (Kohler 1990, 1991). If coarticulation is in some sense a strategy by which speakers reduce their overall effort, and limiting coarticulation is a way of responding to the need for listeners to get a clear and unambiguous signal (see Lindblom 1983), then it would seem that sometimes sloth wins out.

Even within a language, a given speaker may vary speaking style from very clear (as when speaking to the hard of hearing or giving formal lectures) to rather sloppy. This alone suggests two things. First, coarticulation can and does vary even within a speaker. Second, speakers seem to vary coarticulation at least in part as a function of what they perceive to be the needs of their listeners (see also Lindblom and MacNeilage 1986 and Lindblom and

Engstrand 1989). Manuel (1990) suggests that contrast does not play a *direct* role in limiting coarticulation. Rather, coarticulation generally respects output constraints on segments, and output constraints for a particular segment might vary partly due to contrast, but partly due to other factors, such as speaking style. In general, output constraints would be expected to tighten, resulting in less pervasive coarticulation, just in those situations where speakers are worried about the clarity of their speech.

Output constraints, windows and models of speaking

How can output constraints be worked into a model of coarticulation? Manuel and Krakow (1984) and Manuel (1987, 1990) proposed that speakers somehow find the most efficient path from, through, and to, a sequence of target areas.[12] Keating's (1990b) 'window' model is similar in many respects,[13] and assumes that a path is interpolated between target 'windows' of various sizes. More explicit models relating what are effectively output constraints ('don't care' and 'strongly care' conditions on outputs) and path-finding have been developed by Jordan (1997) and Guenther (1995).

One difference (and see note 13) between the 'target areas' and 'output constraints' concepts described by Manuel on the one hand, and the 'windows' model described by Keating on the other, is the assumptions each makes about whether or not all sub-regions of the target area or window are equally valued. Keating explicitly rejects the idea that particular regions within a window are more highly valued than other sub-regions and assumes that the path through a given window is determined solely by the values of neighboring windows. A similar assumption is implicit in Manuel and Krakow (1984). Manuel (1986, 1987) gives more credence to the idea that certain productions of a segment, and therefore certain sub-regions within a target area or window, are more highly valued than others. Evidence supporting this latter contention comes from perceptual experiments, such as in Manuel (1986, 1987). One finding was that when the /ɑ/ in a /ɑpV/ utterance was heavily coarticulated with a following /i/ or /u/ (in contrast to coarticulation with a following /ɑ/), perception of the /ɑ/ was degraded. An additional argument that certain sub-ranges are more valued comes from 'clear' speech data which can be modelled, at least in part, as a narrowing of range toward some specific part of the range (Picheny, Durlach and Braida 1985, 1986). Finally, while output constraints may be quite loose and the trajectories through them largely determined by context, in certain cases no context is available to help select a particular path. In those cases, productions do not vary randomly. For example, while English vowels may tolerate a great amount of contextual nasalization, in isolation they are never very nasal. Similarly, while English /d/ may be made more retroflexed or dental in certain phonetic contexts, presumably because it has a wide tolerance for place, it is normally alveolar.

In any case, neither the 'output constraints' notion nor the 'window' model alone is meant to be a complete model of speaking. Fortunately, rather good and more explicit models of speaking exist and it seems both desirable and possible to incorporate the idea of output constraints into these models. Examples are the coproduction models of Fowler (1981b, 1986), Bell-Berti and Harris (1982) and Browman and Goldstein (1986, 1990a, 1990b). These accounts of speech assume that surface paths or movements may sometimes reflect simultaneous input from distinct invariant commands (or 'gestures') to move to different targets. In these models, coarticulation occurs when the commands for neighbouring phonemes at least partially overlap in time. Thus the velum lowers during what we normally think of as the vowel portion of a VN sequence because the vocal tract is simultaneously responding to commands for the V and to some of the commands ('lower the velum') for the nasal consonant. Similarly, the tongue is more fronted just before /p/ closure in /ɑpi/ than it is in /ɑpu/ because at that point in time the tongue is responding to commands for both the /ɑ/ and the /i/.

The idea that the vocal tract responds to commands for several phonemes at once is not new nor is the idea that phonemes somehow overlap in time. What is especially attractive about the work of Browman and Goldstein (e.g. 1986, 1990a, 1990b) is that they have developed a very explicit model, drawing on Task Dynamics (e.g. Saltzman *et al.* 1988). Within their Articulatory Phonology framework, it is possible to test the relevance of various control parameters (such as phasing of gestures associated with neighbouring segments) and parameter settings. Varying degrees of apparent overlap of gestures can be modelled, as well as several different combinatorics to be applied when overlap occurs. Thus, overlapping gestures could sometimes essentially have additive effects, but in other cases one gesture could effectively suppress the other (Saltzman *et al.* 1988; Saltzman and Munhall 1989). It seems quite possible that output constraints, or something like them, could be built into this general model, possibly in the form of one segment's commands suppressing the effects of another which happen to overlap in time. The waxing of a following segment's effects, as its dominance in the signal becomes more imminent, could presumably be modelled by some function in which the suppression factor associated with the currently dominant segment wanes over time (see also Fowler 1993).

Coarticulation, prosodic structure and vowel harmony

Coarticulation is known to vary across languages in ways that do not seem at all related to phoneme inventory or contrast. For example, Manuel and Krakow (1984) found that anticipatory V-to-V coarticulation was stronger than carryover coarticulation in Swahili. Magen (1984a) found a similar result for Japanese. In both of those studies, the opposite pattern was found for English, as would be expected from the work of Fowler (1981b), who found more robust carryover than anticipatory V-to-V coarticulation in English. Of course, languages differ phonologically in ways that are not related to their phoneme inventory, and it may be that some of these phonological patterns are related to patterns of coarticulation. In what follows we will consider two other ways in which languages differ, and how those differences might be reflected in coarticulation.

Relation of prosody to coarticulation

We begin with the fact that languages differ in their global rhythmic structure, in ways that are not clearly related to phoneme inventory. For example, English has been characterized as stress-timed with a tendency for isochrony between left-dominant prosodic feet, French and Italian as syllable-timed, and Japanese and Finnish as mora-timed. Several studies have attempted to relate these prosodic structures to coarticulatory patterns.

Fowler (1981b) and Vayra, Fowler and Avesani (1987) note that in stressed-timed languages there is a coincidence in which (a) the stressed vowels are shortened by following (but not preceding) unstressed vowels and (b) the stressed vowels exert a substantial amount of coarticulatory influence on the following (but not preceding) unstressed vowels. Fowler and her colleagues explain this coincidence by positing that in stressed-timed languages like English, within the foot the production of unstressed vowels (and any intervening consonants) overlap to some extent with the production of the stressed vowel. Vayra, Fowler and Avesani (1987) predict less of a coincidence of unidirectional shortening and coarticulation in languages (such as Italian) which are less clearly stress-timed, and in which the foot plays less of a prosodic role, precisely because relatively little overlap is expected between neighbouring vowels. Indeed, Vayra, Fowler and Avesani found less unidirectional shortening and coarticulation in Italian than in English.

More recently, Smith (1992, 1995) has asked whether or not basic differences in the prosodic role of consonants are related to the way vowel and consonant articulatory gestures are coordinated. Smith's theoretical basis is the gestural models of speech production, and in particular Articulatory Phonology (Browman and Goldstein 1986, 1990a). In the general framework of Articulatory Phonology, the timing of a sequence of segments is based on coordinating a particular phase of one or more of the articulatory gestures associated with a given segment to a particular phase of some preceding segment. Within Articulatory Phonology, it is possible to incorporate Öhman's (1966) and Fowler's (1981b) suggestion that (stressed) vowels are produced in a continuous fashion with consonants superimposed on the vowels. This can be done for a V_1CV_2 by coordinating some phase of V_2, such as its onset, directly to some phase of V_1, such as achievement of the V_1 target. The consonant itself could be coordinated with either of the vowels. Smith points out that with this type of V-to-V coordination, the movement from V_1 to V_2 ought to be insensitive to the duration of any intervening consonants. At the same time, because the consonants are in some way superimposed on the V-to-V movement, a longer consonant would be expected to cover up, and therefore acoustically shorten, one or both of the vowels more than a shorter consonant would. An alternative coordination strategy is what Smith calls the 'combined consonant–vowel' model. In the combined consonant–vowel strategy, V_2 is coordinated with some phase of the C, and the C is coordinated with some phase of V_1. In this case, the onset of V_2, relative to various phases of V_1, might be expected to be more delayed if a longer consonant intervenes between V_1 and V_2. The longer consonant is not expected to necessarily differentially shorten either of the vowels – it simply pushes them apart more than a short consonant does.

In syllable-timed languages, each syllable tends to have the same duration and the time between successive vowels tends to be fixed, regardless of the number of intervening consonants. Smith predicts that these languages will be associated with V-to-V strategies by which successive vowels are coordinated directly with each other. However, in mora-timed languages the mora (which in Japanese may be a CV, a V by itself, the first C in a geminate CCV or a syllable-final nasal) has a tendency to have constant duration. As syllables can consist of one or more mora, syllables tend to vary in duration. Given the importance of at least some consonants in the basic timing unit, Smith predicts that mora-timed languages will exhibit combined consonant–vowel production strategies in which vowels are coordinated with preceding consonants, and not preceding vowels.

Smith's test cases are the production of singleton (short) and geminate (long) consonants in VCV and VCCV utterances in Italian and Japanese. Acoustic data provided a measure of relative acoustic shortening, if any, of the vowels as a function of consonant duration. Smith used x-ray microbeam data to track lingual movement throughout the utterances. The results for Japanese were largely as expected. Vowels were not shortened by geminate consonants.

Comparison of x-ray microbeam data for V_1 to V_2 movements in V_1CV_2 and V_1CCV_2 revealed that the movements for V_2 were delayed, relative to V_1, in the geminate utterances. The results for Italian, while somewhat complicated, were clearly different from those for Japanese and in the direction predicted by assuming Italians employ a V-to-V coordination. Italian speakers showed substantial acoustic shortening of V_1 in the geminate utterances and the movement from V_1 to V_2 was either unaffected or in some cases actually shortened, in the case of geminate consonants.

Having predicted and found a relationship between strategies of consonant and vowel coordination and whether or not a language is characterized by syllable or mora timing, Smith goes on to try to explicitly model the behaviour of her individual subjects, using the parameters available in the computational model of Articulatory Phonology. Perhaps not surprisingly, given the relative complexity of patterns found in the two languages, she is able to model the behaviour of Japanese geminate versus singleton utterances by changing only a couple of parameter values. On the other hand, modelling of Italian, which exhibited more complicated patterns, required manipulation of more parameters. Importantly, however complicated the Italian model was, phasing of two vowels was accomplished without direct reference to consonants.

Again, more work is needed on a variety of languages which differ in their prosodic structures. An example of the possible complexity of patterns to be uncovered can be seen by comparing Smith's work with a recent analysis of Finnish and Italian. Finnish, like Japanese, has short (singleton) and long (geminate) consonants, short and long vowels, and has been characterized as mora-timed. Dunn (1993) compared coordination of vowels with singleton and geminate consonants in Finnish and Italian VCV and VCCV utterances. Her study employed both acoustic and lip aperture data. Her data for Italian were generally consistent with what Smith found: geminates differentially shortened a preceding vowel. The Finnish data were similar to Japanese for Finnish short vowels: geminates did not differentially shorten preceding vowels. Thus, in some ways the Finnish data parallel Smith's Japanese data. Curiously (and eluding ready explanation) geminates did shorten preceding long vowels.

The studies discussed in this section are encouraging in that to a great extent they do show a connection between prosody and patterns of coordination of vowels and consonants. Assuming further work confirms these relationships, it will be interesting to see whether the coarticulatory patterns are driven by the prosodic character of a language, or the reverse. That is, as Browman and Goldstein (1992) have suggested in their Articulatory Phonology model, it may well be that prosody, as well as several other phonological patterns, are reflections of patterns of articulatory organization, with articulatory organizations being considered the primitives of the phonology. However, as Ogden (1995) suggests in his comments on Smith's work, the picture may be more complicated.

Vowel harmony and coarticulation

For our final example we consider the relationship between vowel harmony and coarticulation. Vowel harmony, like coarticulation, can be viewed as a type of assimilation. As Boyce (1988, 1990) notes, vowel harmonies have the effect of restricting all or most of the vowels in a word to having the same value for some feature, e.g. rounding harmony in Turkish words constrains a string of high vowels, uninterrupted by a non-high vowel, to have the same value for rounding. In contrast, English has no restriction whatsoever on combinations of rounded and unrounded vowels. Boyce speculated that these differences in the predictability of lip rounding may lead speakers of Turkish and English to employ different articulatory strategies. More specifically, she suggested that Turkish speakers might employ a strategy in which having once protruded the lips for a vowel, they keep the lips protruded throughout the string of rounded vowels, including while they are producing consonants. She examined lip-protrusion data for four speakers each of Turkish and English, producing strings like /kuktluk/, /kiktlik/, /kuktlik/, and /kiktluk/.

The results were superficially rather complicated for some English speakers, but Boyce was able to simplify the patterns after disentangling the effects of inherent rounding on some consonants from inherent rounding for vowels for these speakers. Having done so, she found rather clear differences between the two languages. Turkish speakers exhibited a 'plateau' in their lip rounding movement in words like /kuktluk/, whereas English speakers had 'troughs'[14] during the consonants. Boyce relates these different patterns to the current debate between look-ahead and coproduction models. She concludes that each of the models does a plausible job of explaining the data from one language (look-ahead for Turkish, coproduction for English), but that either model would have to be complicated to handle both data sets.

Conclusion

A number of studies have attempted to relate apparent language-particular aspects of coarticulation to other ways in which the languages studied are known to vary. Do we now know enough to say for sure that systematic relationships exist between independently motivated aspects of languages and their patterns of coarticulation? Probably not – the jury is still out on this, and more study is needed. How sanguine can we be about the possibility of ever answering the questions posed here? It probably depends on which relationships we are considering. For example, there probably is a tendency for coarticulation to be constrained so as to maintain contrast, but it is just that – a tendency. If there truly is only a tendency for coarticulation patterns to be derivative from patterns of contrast, then we would expect to find examples in which the principle of contrast maintenance makes the wrong prediction about coarticulation. On the other hand, prosody clearly has to do with timing, so it seems extremely likely that prosody and temporal coordination of articulatory gestures are strongly linked. The relationship between this aspect of coarticulation and prosodic organization is particularly interesting to pursue for another reason. Even if coarticulation and prosodic organization are found to be closely linked, there is still a question of whether prosodic organization is derived from patterns of gestural organization (Browman 1991; Smith 1992) or vice versa or whether they are both predictable from some third parameter. Finally, surely it is the case that even if we ultimately cannot completely resolve these issues, we will learn much by studying them.

Acknowledgments

Many thanks to Patrice Beddor, Rena Krakow and Kenneth Stevens for generously giving numerous helpful (and speedy!) comments on an earlier version of the paper.

Notes

1 However, several of these dissertations have been published, at least in part, and appropriate references are given.
2 I am making no special claim by using the term 'segment' rather than 'phoneme' or 'gesture constellation' – it is merely a convenient way to refer to a set of articulatory gestures or features which somehow cohere.
3 The assumption here is that coarticulatory-based variation can be so extreme that listeners are unable to recover the 'intended' segment. This is an arguable point. See Fowler and Smith (1986) and Krakow *et al.* (1988) which show that listeners can sometimes disentangle acoustic consequences of articulatory gestures or postures associated with one target phoneme from those gestures and postures imposed by neighbouring phonemes.
4 As Choi and Keating note, they did find statistically significant V-to-V coarticulatory effects in the Slavic languages they examined. However, the effects were much smaller than what they found for English, and what is reported for several other languages.

5 Some languages do maintain an oral–nasal contrast for vowels in nasal environments (Kawasaki 1986; Huffman 1987b; Beddor 1993).

6 It is important to emphasize here that the prediction of Manuel and Krakow is not based directly on the number of vowels in a system. Rather, the emphasis is on the relative spacing of the vowels. A hypothetical five-vowel system in which all of the vowels were crowded into the high front quadrant of the vowel space would be characterized as a crowded vowel space, and thus expected to exhibit relatively little V-to-V coarticulation.

7 See Keating and Huffman (1984) for a discussion of whether or not the total vowel space is actually phonetically filled, and whether or not variability of vowel articulation is dependent on the number and spacing of vowels.

8 It has been claimed that Sotho has a phonological rule which raises the mid vowels /e, ɛ, o, ɔ/ if the following syllable contains a higher vowel or a syllabic nasal, as well as certain palatal consonants. Note that if the Sotho speakers in this study *did* use such a rule, it would have the result of making them appear to have greater V-to-V coarticulation effects than if the rule did not apply. This possible confounding factor could only work to decrease any apparent differences between transconsonantal V-to-V coarticulatory effects in Sotho as opposed to in Shona and Ndebele.

9 Note that Russian, which like Shona and Swahili has only five or possibly six phonemic vowels (Jones 1959), appears to exhibit *less* V-to-V coarticulation than does English. Presumably, in Russian it is the *consonants* in VCV utterances which constrain V-to-V coarticulation, as discussed above.

10 The precise phonetic characterization of the high central unrounded and high retroflexed unrounded vowels is complicated. Cheng (1973) considers them to be context-conditioned variants of a phonologically high, central, unrounded vowel.

11 Xu (1989) concludes that there is acoustic evidence of earlier rounding for [ɕ] for his single speaker. Subsequently Xu (personal communication) suggests that his earlier conclusion may need to be modified, pending further additional acoustic data and analysis; his intuition as a speaker is that rounding does begin earlier for [ɕ].

12 Whether to specify targets and paths in the articulatory, acoustic or perceptual space is not clear. Manuel (1987) suggested that output constraints are ultimately based on perception, but that to speak, speakers translate these targets into articulatory dimensions.

13 Keating's model and its developments (Cohn 1990, 1992; Keating 1990b; Huffman 1990) are much more explicit than Manuel (1987) in explaining where contrast is determined and how it relates to target values. The general idea being developed is that some segments leave the phonological component of the grammar without any specification for their feature values and thus have wide windows, whereas other segments either start out with feature values or acquire them by virtue of participating in feature spreading or default fill-in rules. According to Keating (1990b), the exact phonetic 'width' of a window is determined empirically by looking at all of the contexts a segment appears in. This latter facet of the model, while in some sense appealing in that, relative to the 'output constraints' idea, it is more explicit about just how the windows are determined, can in fact be viewed as a serious weakness. If window widths are

empirically determined, then we will never find them violated – we can always claim that we have under- or over-estimated the width of the window.

14 For some English speakers, some protrusion was found during some consonant intervals. However, as similar protrusion was found for consonants in the contexts of unrounded vowels (/kiktlik/), Boyce attributed the consonant-interval protrusion to inherent rounding of the consonant themselves. See also Boyce *et al.* (1990).

9

Implications for phonological theory

MARY BECKMAN

Delimiting the phonological

The topic of this chapter subsumes two broad questions. First, what do phonological models and representations developed for other purposes imply for our understanding of the coarticulatory patterns described in the previous chapters? Second, what do the coarticulatory patterns imply about the shape of phonological models and representations? Implicit in these questions is the assumption that coarticulation is properly in the purview of something other than 'phonological theory', and hence, that we can delimit some aspects of sound structure that are not 'phonological' but merely 'phonetic'.

This assumption is not uncontroversial. For example, in the late 1970s and early 1980s, a series of articles in the *Journal of Phonetics* juxtaposed two diametrically opposed understandings of coarticulation, neither of which recognized this distinction between phonetic coarticulation and its phonological implications. First, Hammarberg (1976, 1982) proposed to define away the phonetics of coarticulation by ascribing the phenomena to phonological assimilation. That is, he described coarticulation as the accretion of context-dependent rewrite rules in the derivation of the surface representation of an utterance, the same mathematical formalism developed by Chomsky and Halle (1968) to account for morphological alternation and allophony. Fowler (1980, 1983b), on the other hand, rejected the phonological model of segmentation that Hammarberg's position required – namely, a serially ordered list of juxtaposed discrete alphabetic segments – along with the sequential derivational view that it required of the relationship between phonological and phonetic representations. That is, she proposed that speech production does not involve first assembling by rule an ordered list of phonological segments, then assigning details such as interval durations for each segmental unit, extent of coarticulatory spread between unit intervals, and so on. Rather, serial order is encoded directly in the phonological representation of prosodic organization, in which consonant gestures are phased relative to the cyclic rhythm of stressed and unstressed vowel gestures. Thus there can be no separable 'implications for phonological theory' because the phonetics of coarticulation is an intrinsic part of the prosodic specification in any viable phonological model.

The definition of what is phonological (or conversely of what is properly only phonetic) is no less controversial today. We can contrast, for example, the three quite different positions taken by Pierrehumbert (1990) and Local (1992), by Keating (1990a) and Kingston and Diehl (1994), and by Ohala (1990b), Browman and Goldstein (1990d, 1993) and Pierrehumbert (1994).

Both of the first pair of papers make a strict distinction between phonology and phonetics. Phonological representations are characterized by discrete symbolizable entities associated with different nodes in prosodic structures. These entities 'encode relational information' about the language's system of paradigmatic contrasts, and hence are mere 'algebraic objects appropriately formulated in the domain of set theory'. Phonetic representations, on the other hand, involve 'quantitative, non-cognitive' models of 'physical, temporal events'. The relationship between these two kinds of representation is a 'semantic' mapping; the phonetic events are the 'real-world referents' of the 'algebraic objects'. An important consequence of taking this position on the relationship between phonology and phonetics is that the different representations can be declarative and simultaneous, rather than procedural and sequential. That is, instead of positing a sequence of generative rules in modular rule components, the production of an utterance can be pictured as the act of invoking the phonological specification of the features in contrast and assembling them unchanged into a particular structural organization and simultaneously as marshalling and composing the phonetic specification of the physical events that instantiate the assemblage of features. Speech perception, conversely, then is an act of 'interpretation' which decomposes the utterance into its component features by 'parsing' the structural organization in which they are situated.

The authors of the second pair of papers also recognize something like the categorically different 'algebraic objects' and quantitatively specified 'physical, temporal events' differentiated in the first pair of papers. However, they do not use these characterizations strictly to distinguish between phonological and phonetic representations. Instead, they propose that there are discrete symbolizable phonetic categories such as 'voiced stop' versus 'voiceless unaspirated stop', which function as an 'intermediate device' in the 'phonetic implementation' of phonological contrasts. That is, this second position says that there is something like the countable sounds distinguished in the International Phonetic Alphabet. These categories come into play at a stage in the derivational chain where the symbolic categories of the phonological component of the grammar 'interface' with the continuously variable values of parametric representations such as Voice Onset Time. Thus, speech production is viewed in terms of derivational rules – rewrite statements that change or build representations. Speech perception, conversely, then must be stated as the inverse of the rewrite statements, e.g. as an online process of 'analysis-by-synthesis' (see Halle and Stevens 1964), so that this second position contrasts with the first also in necessitating a sequential 'generative phonetics' view of the relationship between phonological and phonetic representations, rather than a simultaneous 'declarative' one.

In this regard, the position stated in the last set of papers is more like the first position. It is amenable to a non-procedural view of language sound structure. Indeed, it requires such a view, since it differs from the first position in recognizing no clear division between phonology and phonetics. Instead, these papers emphasize the physical and perceptual constraints that shape common patterns of phonological organization and contrast, and they highlight the only 'quasi-categorical' nature of knowledge of sound structure even at the innermost core of phonology – generalizations over forms in the lexicon. The authors of these papers insist that if the division of labour between phonology and phonetics is to be equated with the place where the algebraic representations of invariant categorical knowledge 'interface' with quantitative descriptions of variable real-world performances, then 'there is no interface between phonology and phonetics'. That is, there can be no interface because phonetics simply is (one face of) phonology. Theories of phonological representation then can be (indeed must be) evaluated directly for their plausibility as models of human speech production and perception.

These three different viewpoints suggest rather different representations of what coarticulation is in relationship to possible phonological representations. An important implication for phonological theory, therefore, is that the phonetic patterns described in previous chapters might be used as a benchmark to test the adequacy of phonological models which assume one or another point of view. For example, can some phonological models or an entire class of models be ruled out because the phonological representations cannot be implemented as input specifications to speech synthesis programs to generate commonly observed coarticulatory effects in an illuminating way?

The most rigorously formulated phonetic representations for the second view described above emerged in the context of developing formant-based text-to-speech systems using a feature matrix of allophone segments as input (e.g. Holmes, Mattingly and Shearme 1964; Carlson and Granström 1975; Hertz 1982; Allen, Hunnicutt and Klatt 1987). For example, in synthesizing a language like English, Danish or German, the input would be strings of feature bundles, which are first processed by a phonological rule component that modifies the feature matrices for the voiceless stops /p/, /t/, /k/ to denote categorically distinct aspirated allophones in stressed syllable onsets as compared to other contexts. The feature matrix is then input to duration rules that specify a sequence of interval durations for the string of allophones and other parametric rules that specify independent target values for, e.g., F2, F3, amplitude of voicing and the like, to occur at some time within the segments. For example, rules for source parameter might specify a sequence of target values to generate a sudden spike of aperiodic energy and then a sharp rise in voicing amplitude for all intervals associated with the features of a stop–vowel sequence. The aspirated stops in stress syllable onsets would then be differentiated by specifying the voicing amplitude targets to occur later with respect to the segment boundary when the consonant has the feature [+ spread glottis].

The problems that coarticulation poses for this class of phonological models were recognized quite early (see e.g. Mattingly 1981). The two main problems are the difficulty of modelling larger prosodic organization and its relationship to the strictly alphabetic segmentation, and the question of how to specify categorical features for segments in a way that translates neatly into sequences of parametric target values in time. For example, in English, Danish and German, there are tightly controlled but continuously variable patterns of temporal coordination between laryngeal abduction and different sets of oral constrictions (see e.g. Hoole, chapter 5 in this volume). These patterns are extremely difficult to capture in any general way in a system that first categorically specifies that an 'aspirated stop' segment in stressed-syllable onset alternates with an 'unaspirated stop' in other positions, and then uses an independent rule component to specify the course of formant transitions over the longer or shorter aspiration phase in different stop–vowel and stop–glide–vowel sequences. In a model like the one specified above, the duration of the aspiration interval might be included in the consonant segment or the vowel segment or it might be inserted as a 'segment' in its own right. By any of these solutions, however, it is difficult to capture the effect of prosodic position on the closure duration and the shape of the formant transitions that generalizes across voiced and voiceless stops in different places of articulation, at different speech tempi, and in different positions relative to word and phrase boundaries.

The other two classes of phonological model described above are also beginning to inform the development of speech synthesis systems (e.g. Browman *et al.* 1986; Coleman 1992; Kröger 1993). The input representations for these systems accommodate much more plausible general phonetic models of coarticulation – as should be expected, given that features common to their designs were prompted by the implausibility of the model of coarticulation in the earlier synthesis systems – but this serves to highlight another class of problems with the input specification. That is, if specific features of categorical segmental contrast and a prosodic organization are provided as input, it is possible to generate the coarticulatory patterns using quite general principles of coordination and movement dynamics. However, there is as yet no comparably general model of how actual speakers learn to provide this input; the feature categories and their prosodic organization are simply stipulated by the phonetician *ex cathedra* (see Pierrehumbert and Pierrehumbert 1990; Johnson 1994).

The recurrence of these two issues, i.e. how to achieve plausible models of prosodic organization and category specification, suggests that coarticulation is a problem not only because of difficulties in understanding the phonetic (inter)face but also because of difficulties in our understanding of the other faces of phonology. A fully adequate phonological theory must account for not just those aspects of language sound structure that are the way they are because speech is sound wave patterns produced by the human articulatory apparatus. It must also illuminate those aspects of sound structure that are the way that they are because speech is a system of communication and cultural transmission among highly social, intelligent, tool-using animals.

Hockett (1960) lists thirteen such 'basic design-features' for human language. Some of these features (e.g. 'broadcast transmission and directional reception', 'rapid fading' and 'total feedback') are trivially true of any vocal communication system. Several other features are found in rudimentary form in the vocal communication systems of other primates. For example, the decade's worth of research summarized in Cheney and Seyfarth (1990) shows that the vocalizations of vervet monkeys have 'semanticity', 'arbitrariness' and 'discreteness'. The vervets have a repertoire of alarm calls in which different spectral transients arbitrarily denote different dangerous real-world referents – eagles versus snakes versus unfamiliar humans and so on. Vervet social vocalizations likewise divide a continuously variable timbre space into discretely differentiated grunts associated with different acts – appeasing a dominant monkey in the same group versus challenging an encroaching monkey from another group versus signalling other vervets to be watchfully alert as some member of the group ventures into open ground and so on. Thus the monkeys' meaningful vocalizations clearly have a phonology; the alarm calls and social grunts are a system of signs partaking of categorical paradigmatic contrast, just like any human lexicon.

However, there is one striking difference between the vervet communication system and human languages. By contrast to the thousands or tens of thousands of words in any adult human lexicon, the vervet inventory comprises only a half dozen or so alarm calls and somewhat fewer social grunts. This difference in inventory size is clearly related to two more of Hockett's design-features that are notably missing from the vervet's system of vocal communication, *viz.* 'productivity' and 'duality of patterning'. The vervets do not coin novel signs by recombining features of existing signs in new ways. There is no syntagmatic grammar internal to the vocalizations that allows this. There is no decompositional analysis of the meaningful forms into smaller meaningless components that can be prosodically organized in other ways, such as other serial orders. Thus, it is difficult to conceive of there being a much larger repertoire of signs than already exists, despite the evolutionary advantage that might accrue, for example, from having another social grunt for the function of quietly calling an infant away from danger (see Cheney and Seyfarth 1990: 119–20).

This phylogenetic difference is paralleled in the ontogeny of individual human phonologies. Behaviour strongly suggestive of a compositional re-analysis of first words emerges at the 'fifty-word stage' (see e.g. Ferguson 1986; Vihman and Velleman 1989). Thus, a crucially important design feature of fully formed human phonologies is that the meaningful vocalizations have internal patterns which recur across the lexicon, so that new signs can be acquired by analysing them into smaller components that can be equated with similar components of other, already familiar signs. The challenge to the phonologist is to identify the internal components of signs and the constraints on how they can be re-arranged. That is, first and foremost, a phonological theory must provide a way of describing the systematic similarities and differences observed across different word-forms in the lexicon and across different tokens of the same word-form when it occurs in the phrase-forms that result from well-practised or novel combinations of these word-forms. Moreover, this description must be a plausible model of human knowledge. It must accord with the behaviour of speakers when they produce various partially similar words or produce the same word in varying contexts.[1]

As in any science, a method fundamental to this enterprise is the careful observation of ingeniously controlled variation. Phonology aims at investigating cognition, i.e. the speaker's intent to produce a specific organization of specific word-internal components and his skill in realizing that pattern in such a way that the listener will recover the intent. The speaker's intent and the components that the listener recovers from the speaker's production are things that we cannot observe directly. We can only study something that we cannot observe directly by investigating how something we assume is constant behaves under systematic variation in something else. For example, to find the atomic weight of an element we observe the measured weight of the different compounds that result when the element is combined with varying amounts of various other elements. In the same way, phonologists investigate phonological intent by observing variability across a morphological paradigm, i.e. the different word shapes that result when a common morphological element (such as a particular inflectional affix) is combined with various other morphological elements (such as various verb roots). Such observation of systematic variation across morphological paradigms is the single most common tool used in building and testing theories of phonological representation today and many phonologists use this tool and no other. As a consequence, in many courses of phonology, languages with few or no revealing patterns of morphological alternation are relegated to the periphery of the students' attention. The language index of Kenstowicz (1994), for example, lists just two references to Cantonese alone among the Yue dialects, as compared to 69 references to 12 different Arabic dialects. It is not surprising, therefore, that phonologists often understand the implications of coarticulation only as it relates to this research tool. They think of coarticulation primarily in terms of its possible diachronic relationship to the sometimes extremely complex patterns of short- and long-range vowel or consonant harmony described for the inflectional and derivational morphologies of many languages (see e.g. Suomi 1983; Cohn 1990; Steriade 1990; Clements and Hume 1994: 258).

A potentially more important phonological implication of coarticulation, however, is that it provides another kind of controllable variation for the phonologist to use in uncovering the speaker's intent. Instead of neglecting languages like Cantonese, phonologists might study the invariants and changes in coarticulatory pattern across different discourse contexts that induce variation in tempo, prosodic phrasing, or intonational prominence (see *inter alia* Lindblom 1963b; de Jong 1995a). Speech synthesis then becomes a valuable test for phonological theories of representation. That is, if some representation of the speaker's knowledge of the internal composition of signs cannot be implemented as a workable input for a synthesis system that accurately models coarticulatory variation across different tempi and across different larger prosodic contexts, then the theoretical adequacy of the representation is in question.

In this light, it is telling that all of the synthesis systems mentioned above point to problems with our understanding of prosodic segmentation and feature specification. These also are two areas of controversy and flux in the current development of phonological theory and the rest of this chapter will concentrate on relating these developments in phonological theory to the phonetic models of coarticulation described in this volume.

Specifying features for segments

As Manuel (chapter 8 in this volume) points out, there is a long-standing notion that language-specific patterns of coarticulation can be explained in part by differences in the inventory and distribution of distinctive features, i.e. the named categories of paradigmatically contrasting sub-components of words in the language. As usually conceived, this notion depends on three assumptions that are rarely stated so explicitly as they are in Manuel's chapter. All of these assumptions are controversial.

The first assumption is that the named categories of contrast in the lexicon are in a fairly simple one-to-one or one-to-many correspondence with distinct articulatory patterns ('gestures'), which in turn correspond to distinct aerodynamic and acoustic consequences. This correspondence is assumed to be straightforward because the gestures (or their acoustic consequences) are the result of generative rules which rewrite 'underlying' specifications of categorical features as 'output' specifications for gestures (or for acoustic cues), as proposed by Keating (1990a) among others. As already discussed in the previous section, the nature of the correspondence between lexical contrasts and physical differences is a primary point of disagreement among the various views of the relationship between phonology and phonetics.

The second assumption is that words consist of linear strings of units of synchronously specified gestures, i.e. that the prosodic constituent relevant for specifying contrast is the alphabetic segment. This is the segmentation issue, to be discussed in the next section. This assumption is also controversial, as suggested by the review of new models of coarticulation in Farnetani and Recasens (chapter 2 in this volume).

The third assumption is the topic of this section – theories of contrastive specification and underspecification. Explanations of language-specific patterns of coarticulation that are based on the contrasts specified by the language require not just that there be differences in what features contrast in segment inventories across languages, but also that there be differences across classes of segments within a language. That is, these explanations rely crucially on models of phonological and phonetic representation in which one class of segments can be 'underspecified' or left unspecified for any of a set of feature values which differentiate among the segments in some other class in the language. As Manuel puts it in chapter 8 of this volume, 'what counts as contrastive or distinctive varies both from language to language and for different segments within a language' (p. 180).

To place this issue in its historical context, consider a classic example of language-dependent coarticulation cited in practically every textbook in Neo-Bloomfieldian Structuralist linguistics (e.g. Gleason 1961: 245 and 260). In many genetically unrelated languages, such as Arabic and Russian, there are categorically distinct stops made by raising the tongue body to contact the roof of the mouth at two different locations along the continuum from the soft palate to the uvula. In a language such as Swedish or English, where there is a contrast between stops made by the tongue tip versus tongue body but no contrast among dorsal stops, the point of contact for /k/ in the context of front versus back vowels varies across the regions distinguished by /k/ versus /q/ in Arabic or by /kʲ/ versus /kˠ/ in Russian. The neo-Bloomfieldians understood this variation in terms of allophony – a context-conditioned alternation between front and back dorso-velar stop allophone categories. The same understanding of the phenomenon was adopted in early Generative Phonology, where the characterization of front versus back allophones was embedded in a theory of binary distinctive features arranged in a matrix of boolean values. In Chomsky and Halle's (1968) model, lexical representations are minimally specified for only 'marked' feature values. However, at the stage in the derivation where the concatenated morphemes are passed to the phonological component, the matrix is fully specified, with each segment (a column of the matrix) being assigned the plus or minus value of each boolean feature (a row in the matrix). In this context, the binary feature value pair [+ back] versus [− back] is specified to represent the Russian contrast between velarized versus palatalized stops as well as the nearly universal contrast between back versus front vowels. Synthesis systems that implemented Chomsky and Halle's model naturally would characterize the coarticulation in Swedish or English as an alternation between two allophonic variants created by a phonological re-write rule that copies the value specified for an adjacent vowel segment onto the dorso-velar stop. The problem of contexts where preceding and following vowel segments disagree in backness was typically resolved by copying the value of the following vowel onto the stop, in keeping with the observation that the stop burst frequency is coloured more by it than by the preceding vowel.

A somewhat knottier problem was posed by Öhman's (1966) data showing that in VCV sequences, each vowel influences the transition into or out of the vowel on the other side of the intervening consonant in Swedish and English, but not in Russian. As already suggested by Manuel (this volume), this difference among the languages seems intuitively to be a consequence of the contrast between palatalized and velarized consonants being a property only of the Russian consonant inventory. Fowler (1980) uses Öhman's data for English and Swedish to argue against the alphabetic matrix for synchronizing feature specifications; that is she understands these data in terms of the segmentation issue and promotes a model in which the dorso-velar consonant gesture rides on top of the V-to-V transition rather than being discretely and linearly ordered between the two vowel gestures. She does not address the problem of the interlanguage difference. Keating (1985a, 1988b), by contrast, concentrates instead on the interlanguage difference. She argues for salvaging the alphabetic model by interpreting Öhman's data in terms of more recent models of phonological representation in which segment sequences need not be fully specified for all features. That is, contra Chomsky and Halle (1968), some columns in the matrix of distinctive features can be left underspecified for some features at the input to the phonological component and even (Keating argues) at the output of the phonological component, where the representation is passed to parametric phonetic rules. To evaluate Keating's arguments, then, we might begin by evaluating the proposal that phonological representations can be underspecified.

This turns out to be not one proposal, but several. As Archangeli (1988), Broe (1993) and Steriade (1994) among others have pointed out, there are several different kinds of phenomena that underspecification has been used to capture, and these uses are not all mutually compatible. Archangeli argues convincingly against one such use and Broe and Steriade argue cogently against several others that Archangeli advocates, proposing mechanisms other than underspecification to capture the same phenomena. We need to tease apart the different uses proposed for phonological underspecification to see which is implicated in Keating's (1985a, 1988b) underspecification-based analysis of Öhman's data.

The oldest use, considered as early as Halle (1959), is to leave some classificatory features temporarily unspecified at the earliest stages of phonological derivation in order to highlight distributional asymmetries in segment inventories and to minimize the information stored in lexical entries. For example, the most common inventory of vowel segments for languages with only five vowels is /i, e, ɑ, o, u/. In this inventory, the features [±high] and [±back] do not differentiate two [+low] vowels and the single [+low] vowel /ɑ/ contrasts with all other vowels except /o/ by having the opposite value of at least one other feature – [−high] in contrast to /i/ and /u/ and [+back] in contrast to /i/ and /e/. Therefore, in the lexical entries that are input to the phonological rules, the feature values [±low] could be left unspecified for all segments except /ɑ/ and /o/, and all other feature values also could be left unspecified for /ɑ/. The missing values then are filled in later by rules of the form:

(1)   [+low] → [−high]
        [+low] → [+back]

which should be motivated by universal principles of phonetic 'markedness' as well as by the contrasts available for morphemes in the lexicon.

Archangeli (1988) points out, however, that such 'contrastive underspecification' crucially depends on knowing what the segmentation of a word is. Thus, it precludes representing some inflectional and derivational morphemes as 'floating' specifications of a feature value, which can variably dock at different segmental locations in different stem morphemes. Since this kind of underspecified segmentation is necessary in many languages, Archangeli rejects 'contrastive' underspecification in favour of Kiparsky's (1982) 'radical underspecification', whereby 'all and only unpredictable features are specified' (Archangeli 1988: 190), with missing values again to be filled in by 'redundancy rules' that should be motivated by universal 'markedness' principles.

Broe (1993) points out, however, that the idea of leaving 'predictable' features unspecified conflates at least two more potentially incompatible uses. One is the use of underspecification to express 'default' or 'unmarked' feature values, i.e. expected specifications that occur frequently or without exception in some set of morphological or prosodic contexts. For example, in Russian, word-final obstruents do not contrast in voicing. A word-final obstruent either assimilates in voicing to the first obstruent in the following word or is predictably [−voice] if there is no following obstruent. The assimilation facts resemble sequential coarticulatory patterns. The notion of [−voice] as the 'default' value which surfaces when there is no following obstruent to trigger assimilation accords well with phonetic markedness. That is, it accords with the observation that the aerodynamic requirements of voicing are incompatible with the aerodynamic requirements of stop closure and frication noise – an incompatibility which also explains the order of acquisition that has been observed in languages that contrast phonetically voiced stops with voiceless unaspirated stops (Macken 1980; Gandour *et al.* 1986; Davis 1990).

The other use of radical underspecification is to express redundancy relationships. For example, in Russian the non-obstruent consonants, such as /lʲ/, /w/ and the nasals, are all voiced. (This is in keeping with the phonetic markedness of distinctively voiceless sonorants, see Ohala and Ohala 1993: 231–3.) Therefore, a classification value of [−sonorant] for a segment is predictable given a classification of [−voice], and conversely, a classification as [+voice] is redundant to a classification as [+ sonorant]. One phonological consequence of these redundancy relationships is that sonorant consonants do not undergo voicing assimilation. That is, since there is no contrast for voicing in sonorants, sonorants cannot change their classification from one category to the contrasting category in the presence of a following voiceless obstruent. A phonologist with a declarative bent might express the distributional fact by a 'filter' blocking the configuration:

(2) $*\begin{bmatrix} - \text{ voice} \\ + \text{ sonorant} \end{bmatrix}$

as the output of any rule. (Here the '*' means that the particular configuration of features is ill-formed in the language.) The attractions of this filter device are that it seems to allow the assimilation rule to apply across the board, thus making it more amenable to a non-procedural interpretation, and that it relates the morphological pattern to the phonetic markedness of voiceless sonorants.

On the other hand, the use of the filter is complicated by the fact that although they are voiced, the sonorant consonants do not trigger voicing assimilation in Russian. Nor do they block voicing assimilation when they occur between two obstruents. Kiparsky (1985) proposes to explain these facts by a radical underspecification that makes the only values of the feature stored in the lexicon be the [+ voice] specified for obstruents. All other values of the voicing feature are inserted by a redundancy rule:

(3)   [αsonorant] → [αvoice]

The phonological model is not completely amenable to a declarative interpretation, since the rule in (3) must be ordered relative to the assimilation rule to explain why nasals do not trigger or block assimilation, but this ordering might be viewed as intrinsic to the close relationship between redundancy rules and phonetic markedness and hence be less procedural than the phonetically arbitrary or 'extrinsic' rule orderings of earlier theories of Generative Phonology.

However, there is an ordering paradox. The redundancy rule needs to apply late in the derivation to be prevented from supplying the redundant value of [+ voice] to sonorants so as to avoid triggering assimilation on a preceding voiceless obstruent but it must apply early in the derivation in order to supply the default value of [− voice] for obstruents so that these can trigger assimilation in a preceding obstruent. Kiparsky resolves the ordering paradox by stating the markedness filter not as in (2) above, but as:

(4) $*\begin{bmatrix} \alpha \text{ voice} \\ + \text{ sonorant} \end{bmatrix}$

That is, rather than expressing the phonetic markedness of voiceless sonorants, the filter now is an arbitrary phonological statement that precludes any specification of the feature [±voice] for sonorants until after the derivation is complete. Unlike the filter in (2), this filter is not phonetically motivated. As Steriade (1994: 127) puts it, 'the filter is motivated only by the drive to generate an underspecified lexical component, not by independent considerations. To put it plainly, the argument for lexical underspecification in Russian based on [this filter] is circular.'

Steriade (1994) and Broe (1993) work through several other examples used by Kiparsky, Archangeli and others to motivate 'radical underspecification', showing how these uses all lead to phonetically arbitrary specifications and even to false predictions about the morphological alternations. They also both independently propose other mechanisms to handle the morphological patterns without underspecification. The mechanisms that Broe proposes have the added attraction of suggesting a way to accommodate the role of redundant features in robust speech perception. Steriade and Broe conclude that none of these three first uses of 'temporary' underspecification is warranted. However, they do not preclude the use of underspecification to express two other kinds of phenomena.

The first of these two other uses is related to the fact that classificatory features are not necessarily bivalent, i.e. that if the morphological alternations in a language provide arguments for grouping together a class of segments by a common specification of a value such as [+coronal] or [+round], there are not always arguments for grouping together all other segments by a common specification of a symmetrically opposite classificatory value [−coronal] or [−round]. Some of the strongest arguments against Chomsky and Halle's (1968) model involve their classification of place of articulation for consonants in terms of the bivalent features [±coronal] (for differentiating constrictions made with the front of the tongue from constrictions made with the lips and tongue body) and [±anterior] (for differentiating labials, dentals, and alveolars from palatals, velars, uvulars). One argument is that morphological alternations often single out [+coronal] sounds, but rarely single out [−coronal] sounds. Moreover, the features [+anterior] and [−anterior] never seem to occur in rules except in conjunction with some value of [± coronal]. In particular, one of the most common patterns of morphological alternation – assimilation of a nasal to the place of a following obstruent – is impossible to express in Chomsky and Halle's model without an awkward notation for making the nasal and obstruent agree in value for both the features [coronal] and [anterior].

In more recent phonological theories these phenomena of non-binary valence have been modelled by two different representational mechanisms. One is simply to say that the feature is monovalent, i.e. to stipulate that phonological rules can refer to all segments specified for the feature but that they cannot refer to all segments that are not specified for the feature. For example, if the feature *Round* is stipulated to be monovalent, then phonological rules can pick out segments that are *Round* but they are not allowed to pick out segments that are not *Round*. Underspecification comes into play here because the usual mechanism is to stipulate that there is no feature value to name a class of all segments that are not named as *Round*, so that such segments are not fully specified for all features.

The other mechanism that has been used to capture patterns of non-binary valence is to set up superordinate features which pick out not classes of segments but classes of features. For example, phonologists have found it useful to posit a blanket feature *Place* dominating features *Labial, Coronal, Dorsal* and *Radical* to capture the intuition that these subordinate features are essentially alternate values from the set of consonant place specifications. The usual notion for this idea is the feature tree; features are arranged in a branching structure with the node for *Place* dominating nodes for *Labial, Coronal, Dorsal* and *Radical*. The tree notation expresses the idea that *Place* is a multivalent feature whose possible values are the specification of monovalent features, so that the common patterns of nasal place assimilation can be described simply as agreement in the value of this superordinate feature. This treatment fits much better with phoneticians' intuitions about the valence of the consonant place feature and makes it easy to relate consonant-to-consonant place assimilation to the coarticulatory patterns and aerodynamic requirements of serially ordered closure gestures (see e.g. Ohala 1990a).

Treating *Place* as a multivalent cover feature also provides an easy way to express the idea of /h/ and /ʔ/ as 'defective' segments, inherently and permanently unspecified for any value of *Place*. This is the fifth use of underspecification in current phonological theory and it is the use invoked by Keating (1985a) to salvage the segmental model in the face of Öhman's (1966) data showing V-to-V coarticulation across stops in English and Swedish, but not in Russian. The Russian dorsal stops come in contrasting pairs that are distinguished by having a secondary palatal versus velar articulation. If these secondary articulations are represented by contrasting specifications of the bivalent vowel feature [±back], then the English and Swedish stops are different from the Russian ones by being inherently unspecified for the feature. That is, they are 'defective' for [±back] in the same way that /h/ and /ʔ/ are defective for *Place*. V-to-V coarticulation in these two languages can then be stated quasi-alphabetically by positing a phonetically determined interpolation function through the unspecified consonant between the target gestures for the specifications of the feature in the neighbouring vowels. The Russian stops, on the other hand, block the interpolation by providing their own specifications for this feature.

Steriade (1994) classifies both of these last two uses of underspecification together as examples of what she calls 'trivial' or 'permanent' underspecification, in contradistinction to the 'nontrivial' or 'temporary' uses of underspecification, which she and Broe (1993) dispute. She is careful to note that by 'trivial' she does not mean unworthy of study: 'Although there are important issues involved in the study of permanent underspecification, they have to do more with the relation between phonology and phonetics than with . . . assessing the validity of derivational scenarios . . . which invoke temporary underspecification' (Steriade 1994: 177). As an example of these issues, consider again the first method for representing non-binary valence. In the absence of relevant morphological alternations in a language, how can phonologists determine whether there is a bivalent feature [±round] or a monovalent feature *Round*? The published studies on language-specific patterns of labial coarticulation suggest that phoneticians have strong intutions about this question. The literature typically speaks of 'anticipatory lip rounding' and not of 'anticipatory lip spreading', as shown by Manuel's discussion of studies such as Lubker and Gay (1982) or by Farnetani's discussion of this and the many other studies reviewed in her chapter in this volume. It is possible that this practice merely reflects the limitations of the particular phonetic representation of labial configuration typically used in kinematic studies, *viz.* vertical and/or horizontal movement of the lips in the midsagittal plane.[2] On the other hand, it is also possible that the phonetic intuition reflects the greater acoustic consequences of changes in cross-sectional area at points of constriction, such that lip spreading and labial opening are less 'audible' gestures than lip protrusion and labial constriction (Böe, Badin and Perrier 1995). More extensive cross-linguistic studies of labial coarticulation using simultaneous articulatory and acoustic representations might help us to understand better the phonetic bases of the intuition, so as to suggest a principled answer to the question of whether *Round* is necessarily monovalent (there is no phonetically coherent class of *Spread* segments to be singled out in any language) or just monovalent by default (the class of *Spread* segments is phonetically not robust enough to be singled out for morphological generalizations across much of the lexicon or in many languages). In either case, a better understanding of labial coarticulation promises to provide phonetic arguments for this kind of 'permanent underspecification' of the logically possible opposite value to the feature *Round*, either universally or on a language-by-language basis.

Keating's (1988b) description of the very simple 'target-and-transition' pattern for the time-course of the second formant through the consonant in V-/h/-V sequences is an example of a different kind of argument from coarticulation for the other kind of permanent underspecification of features. That is, she interprets the smooth linear F2 transition through the /h/ as a simple interpolation between neighbouring vowel targets, in keeping with a universal permanent underspecification of any value of multivalent *Place* for this intrinsically *Place*-defective consonant. The same kind of analysis of the transition function between known specification points is invoked by Pierrehumbert and Beckman (1988) to argue for a language-specific permanent underspecification of tone features for potential tone-bearing constituents after the second mora in long unaccented phrases of Tokyo Japanese. That is, contra the predictions of the usual autosegmental account, which inserts a [+ H(igh)] tone specification on each subsequent mora (cf. Haraguchi 1977), there is a smooth fundamental frequency fall from the [+ H] on the second mora to the [− H] tone at the beginning of the next phrase, very similar to the smooth F2 transitions through the consonant in the V-/h/-V sequences examined by Keating. Choi (1995) models F2 transitions in CVC sequences to make a similar argument for permanent underspecification of [± back] for vowels in Marshallese.

In all three of these cases, the phonological implication of coarticulation is that a simple linear interpolation model of the transition pattern can provide positive evidence for permanent underspecification of some distinctive feature for some segments. But what would be the implication of not having such an interpolation function? A first question to consider is whether there are possible phonetic reasons for the more complex interpolation shape. For example, Beckman and Pierrehumbert (1992) suggest that the scooped shape of the fundamental frequency rise in unaccented low-beginning phrases of Osaka Japanese reflects the different physiological mechanism associated with the low tone at the beginning of these phrases as compared to the not so very low tone at the beginning of the next phrase in the Tokyo Japanese data. By the same token, if some V-/h/-V transitions in some languages are not simple interpolation lines, e.g. if the F2 often is higher than predicted by a simple model during the latter part of the consonant in /ahi/ sequences, we might want to consider how the F2 values along a simple transition function would be affected by coupling to sub-glottal resonances (Fant 1972). Given the many phonological reasons for defining /h/ as defective, a phonetician should be cautious about imputing a value of [− back] to the consonant unless there is an independent explanation for a phonological reinterpretation of the consonant as having a permanent underlying specification for *Place*. One such explanation might be language contact, as in younger speakers' productions of Taiwanese /h/, which apparently is being reinterpreted as an underlying /x/ under influence from the Mandarin fricative system (Peng 1993). This sort of phonological explanation would be another way of accounting for a nonlinear interpolation function without resorting to any of the controversial uses of temporary underspecification.

However, Keating (1988b) uses the time-course of the second formant during intervocalic consonants as evidence for another analysis which does invoke one of these other kinds of underspecification. After describing the patterns for /h/, she proposes that patterns of V-to-V coarticulation across the Russian voiceless velar fricative /x/ can be taken as evidence of a phonological specification of [− back] for a categorically front allophone for /x/ before /i/. Since there is no phonological contrast between velarized versus palatalized dorsal fricatives in Russian, and apparently no other morphological evidence supporting an underlying specification of any value for [± back] for this segment, Keating proposes that the feature is inserted by a phonological rule very late in the derivation. That is, in order to account for the phonetics of the time-course of F2 coarticulation in /axi/ sequences, she proposes that an underlyingly underspecified /x/ gets a late specification of [− back], making this a case of the controversial 'nontrivial' or 'temporary' underspecification of segments which Broe (1993) and Steriade (1994) dispute. Thus, accepting Keating's explanation of the coarticulatory pattern in this case would have important implications for current phonological theories of specification and underspecification, and it behooves the phonologist to examine the logic of the explanation especially carefully.

In this regard, one question to ask is whether Keating's account casts the burden of explanation in the right direction. That is, rather than resort to a categorical specification of [− back] to explain the time-course of the spectral band associated with F2 in the /axi/ sequences, perhaps we should look for a more complete model of coarticulation to explain the apparition of a categorical specification. For example, perhaps the /x/ only appears to be assimilated to the following /i/ because of two other phonetic phenomena: first, the existence of a very large quantal region for /i/ in the mapping from constriction place to second formant (Cohen 1994), and second, the aerodynamic (or other) causes of the forward 'loop' trajectories for the dorsum observed during dorso-velar constrictions even in languages that do not differentiate phonologically between front and back dorsal stops (Mooshammer, Hoole and Kühnert 1995). One test of such a phonetically grounded model of the time-course of coarticulation then can be how well it explains cross-linguistic patterns of velar palatalization. In particular, we should look for a model that can explain why morphological alternations between dorso-velar stops around back vowels and dorso-palatal stops or palatal affricates around front vowels are much more typically conditioned by a following tautosyllabic vowel than by the preceding vowel or by a heterosyllabic vowel. (Here see for example Rialland's 1994 interpretation of Zerling's 1981 data for /g/–V versus V–/g/ transitions in French and Nolan's 1994 commentary.) In other words, it seems likely that an explanatory model of CV coarticulation for dorsal consonants will need to refer to syllable structure and other prosodic units larger than the segment. What is less clear is whether an explanatory model will need to refer to the alphabetic segment as a discrete sequential (prosodic) component in the phonology. This is the other main issue in understanding the phonological implications of coarticulation.

Differentiating components from segments

As Kühnert and Nolan (chapter 1 in this volume) point out, the phenomenon of coarticulation as it is traditionally conceived depends crucially on a phonological model in which words are composed of linear strings of smaller, phoneme-sized alphabetic constituents. They suggest two arguments for accepting this model. Without some such representation of the sub-morphemic components common to sets of words such as 'caw' and 'caught', or 'key', 'Keith' and 'keen', it is difficult to account for the coarticulatory regularities observed in productions of these words. Moreover, without implicit knowledge of such smaller morpheme-internal elements it is difficult to explain the demonstrated efficiency of lexical storage and access. Indeed, sub-morphemic 'componentiality' and the larger lexicon that it allows is probably the single most important difference between monkey and human phonologies, or between infant and adult phonologies within the species.

However, in order to use this design-feature of human language as an argument for the phonological model underlying the traditional notion of coarticulation, it is necessary to assume not just that there are phonological components internal to words but also that these internal components come packaged into synchronous specifications for alphabetic segments that are arranged one after another as serial constituents in composing lexical representations. That is, if paradigmatic specifications of features (or 'gestures') are the component 'atoms' of speech, then phoneme-sized segments must be the smallest 'molecules' and these 'molecules' must combine in only one basic arrangement – as a chain of minimal prosodic units to be realized sequentially in time when a word is uttered.

Under the assumption of such an alphabetic model, coarticulation constitutes a mismatch between the sound pattern of an actual utterance of a word and its stored representation in the mental lexicon, a mismatch which seems to preclude a theory of the relationship between phonology and phonetics of the sort advocated by Ohala (1990b) or Pierrehumbert (1994). One of the most important phonological implications of coarticulation, then, is that it urges a reconsideration of the alphabetic model, as already suggested by Fowler (1980). Browman and Goldstein's (1989) Articulatory Phonology is one proposal for a model that does away with alphabetic constituents, but it is not the first (see e.g. Firth 1948; Fujimura and Lovins 1978). Moreover, although Chomsky and Halle's (1968) rigorous formulation of the alphabetic model made it the dominant paradigm in Generative Phonology for many years, phonologists trained in this tradition have argued more recently for 'nonlinear' models of morphological alternations in many languages, i.e. models that do not make the alphabetic segment the basic or even a necessary prosodic constituent. To pursue the phonological implications of coarticulation, therefore, it is useful to consider the phenomena that are used to argue for and against the alphabetic model.

The strongest argument for the alphabetic model comes from the prevalence of simple affixation as the dominant morphological pattern in the inflectional paradigms of many languages, and the very common appearance in these paradigms of root or affix morphemes that can be represented as segment strings that are not well-formed syllables on their own. The argument is essentially one of parsimony of representation, i.e. that since these roots and affixes can be represented as bare sequences of feature bundles, segments should be the minimal constituent, with syllables and other higher-level prosodic organization left unspecified in the lexicon. For example, in Japanese the nominal form or general connective base stem, the plain present form, and the plain negative present form of a large class of verbs all can be described by positing an underlying consonant-final verb root, onto which is appended /i/ in the connective base, /u/ in the plain present, and /-a.nai/ in the plain negative present, as in the examples in (5):

(5)	root[3]	nominal	polite present[4]	plain present	negative	gloss
	ojo.g-	o.jo.gi	o.jo.gi.ma.su	o.jo.gu	o.jo.ga.nai	'swim'
	ka.k-	ka.ki	ka.ki.ma.su	ka.ku	ka.ka.nai	'write'
	to.b-	to.bi	to.bi.ma.su	to.bu	to.ba.nai	'fly'
	no.ɾ-	no.ɾi	no.ɾi.ma.su	no.ɾu	no.ɾa.nai	'board'
	sa.s-	sa.ʃi	sa.ʃi.ma.su	sa.su	sa.sa.nai	'point'
	ma.t-	ma.tʃi	ma.tʃi.ma.su	ma.tsu	ma.ta.nai	'wait'
	ka.w-	ka.i	kai.ma.su	ka.u	ka.wa.nai	'buy'

None of the root-final consonants in these examples is a legal coda consonant for the final syllable of a prosodic word in Japanese. However, they can be syllabified as legal onsets when concatenated with a vowel-initial affix.

There is some variation in the surface form of the root-final consonant in the last three verbs. However, this variation is very amenable to procedural alphabetic models such as classical linear Generative Phonology, because it can be stated as the result of locally conditioned processes affecting only the target segment – palatalization of /s/ and /t/ before /i/, assibilation of /t/ before high vowels, and deletion of /w/ before non-low vowels. Further justification for such a model comes from the phonetic naturalness of the stipulated processes, all three of which are documented sound changes in the history of Japanese (see e.g. Miller 1967). Because they are the residue of regular diachronic changes, these processes also account for synchronic phonotactic constraints that hold more generally between onsets and rhymes. In the modern Japanese lexicon, [s] never occurs before [i], [t] never occurs before [u] or [i] except in recent loans such as /ɾemontiː/ 'lemon tea', and [w] only occurs before [a]. Moreover, these constraints hold in both major dialects, the Tokyo-based national standard and the Osaka-based Kansai regional standard. If we adopt the procedural alphabetic model to describe the patterns in (5), then the primary phonological implication of coarticulation is that the mismatch between coarticulatory overlap and the posited sequence of discrete feature bundles can help us understand the diachronic processes that lead to such phonotactic constraints on neighbouring segments and that result in such regular segmental alternations when morphological paradigms are based simply on affixation.

The strongest arguments against the alphabetic model come from morphological paradigms where the variant forms cannot be described completely by segment deletions and other simple local manipulations of segments that come to abut each other when elements such as roots and affixes are concatenated together. For example, the Japanese verb roots listed in (5) undergo more drastic changes in the plain past:

(6)

root	polite past	plain past	(Osaka)	gloss
ojo.g-	o.jo.gi.ma.ʃi.ta	o.joi.da		'swam'
ka.k-	ka.ki.ma.ʃi.ta	kai.ta		'wrote'
to.b-	to.bi.ma.ʃi.ta	ton.da		'flew'
no.ɾ-	no.ri.ma.ʃi.ta	not.ta		'boarded'
sa.s-	sa.ʃi.ma.ʃi.ta	sa.ʃi.ta		'pointed'
ma.t-	ma.tʃi.ma.ʃi.ta	mat.ta		'waited'
ka.w-	kai.ma.ʃi.ta	kat.ta	koː.ta < kaw.ta	'bought'

Here, the polite /-ma.s-/ forms and the plain form of 'pointed' can be accounted for by the same phonotactically motivated segmental processes operating in (5), which make the connective bases [-maʃi-] and [saʃi-] onto which the past tense suffix /-ta/ is simply appended. However, none of the other plain forms can be accounted for in this way. The segment sequences [ka.ki.ta] and [to.mi.ta], that by analogy with [sa.ʃi.ta] should be the plain forms for 'wrote' and 'flew', are by no means phonotactically ill-formed. Indeed, they are attested as the perfectly ordinary surnames Kakita and Tomita. Likewise, the form [kai.ta], that should be the past tense of 'buy', actually does occur in the list in (6) – as the past tense of 'write'. Thus, segmental processes that might be posited to derive the attested plain forms for 'wrote', 'flew', and so on, cannot be justified in terms of phonotactic constraints on segment sequences attested more generally in the lexicon. Moreover, when understood merely as changes to abutting segments, there is no unifying thread that might be stated as the dominant or prototypical phonological pattern for the simple past tense. In 'swam' and 'wrote' the root-final consonant segment is deleted (except for the trace of [+ voice] on the tense suffix in 'swam'), whereas in 'flew', 'boarded', and 'waited' it is the vowel segment of the connective base that is deleted, and both disparate deletions are attested in the different forms for 'bought' in the two dialects.

When we look at prosodic structure above the segment, however, there is a unifying thread. In all plain past forms other than that for 'point', the last two (short) syllables of the connective stem are replaced by a single (long) syllable. Moreover, this higher-level prosodic alternation between two moras that are independent syllables and two moras that are syllabified as daughters to the same syllable node is reminiscent of alternations attested elsewhere in the lexicon, as in the following nickname forms:

(7)   ha.na.tʃaN ~ haː.tʃaN ~ hat.tʃaN[5] < Hanako
        mi.do.tʃaN ~ miː.tʃaN ~ mit.tʃaN < Midori

Poser (1990) discusses these examples and other phenomena to support a bimoraic prosodic constituent called the 'foot' in Japanese, which Itô (1990) then posits as the basic minimal prosodic structure for a well-formed word. When the common pattern is stated in this way, as an alteration to the syllabic organization of the last foot in the connective base, the other modifications can all be motivated in terms of very general phonotactic constraints on the features that can occur on the second mora of a long syllable. In other words, these alternations are captured far more informatively if the phonological representation of the common morphological element includes not just a list of the segments of the past tense suffix but also some specification of the prosodic structure required for the preceding base morpheme.

Inflectional paradigms in some other languages offer even stronger arguments against alphabetic segments as the only, or even the primary, sequential constituents of morphemes. For example, the genitive plural morpheme for neuter-class nouns in Slovak can be described as the insertion of a second mora to make a long stem-final syllable, as shown in the examples below, from Rubach (1994):

(8)	nominative singular	genitive plural	gloss
	pivo	piːv	'beer'
	puto	puːt	'chain'
	lano	laːn	'cable'
	tʃelo	tʃ'el	'forehead'
	kolo	kᵘol	'wheel'
	mæso	m'æs	'meat'

This alternation cannot be described as a segmental process that simply copies the vowel of the stem, since in the forms with non-peripheral vowels /e/, /o/, and /æ/, the underlying diphthongal nature of the syllable nucleus surfaces when the syllable is lengthened.

The derivational and inflectional paradigms of Semitic languages are rife with such morphological elements that require the phonological specification of some prosodic structure. For example, the usual analysis of Standard Arabic content words is to posit a root consisting only of a series of (typically three) sets of consonantal features, which map onto successive syllable edges in the segmentless prosodic templates which are the derivational morphemes. Thus, in the forms in (9), the root for words with the core meaning of 'write' is /ktb/, the perfective tense morpheme is the vowel /a/, the plain verb stem is a /CV.CVC/ template, the causative stem is a /CVC.CVC/ template, and so on:

(9)	katab	'write'	(perfective)	ħamal	'carry'	(perfective)
	katːab	'teach/make write'	(perfective)	ħamːal	'make carry'	(perfective)
	kaːtib	'writing'		ħaːmil	'carrying'	

The discontinuously distributed consonant features of the root morphemes and the segmentally empty prosodic nature of the derivational stem morphemes are awkward to represent in older alphabetic models. Many Austronesian languages have reduplicative paradigms which are similarly awkward to capture in an alphabetic model because the common morphological element is an affixed feature-less syllable or larger prosodic constituent which takes its features from a partial copy of segmental material of the root (see Broselow 1994, for a succinct review). In all of these cases, it is not clear that the alphabetic segment is necessary at all except possibly to express what features are bundled together when the feature specifications of the root morpheme interleave with those of the inflectional morphemes or when root features are copied to fill the empty prosodic positions of the reduplicative affix.

Another (essentially opposite) kind of evidence that phonological componentiality does not necessarily involve discrete segmental sequence comes from morphemes with featural content but no structural organization. For example, the feminine form of the imperative in the Ethiopian Semitic language Chaha involves a 'floating' palatalization feature that is realized on the last consonant of the root morpheme (examples from McCarthy 1983):

(10) masculine feminine gloss
       nəmæd   nəmædʲ   'love'
       wətˀæq   wətˀæqʲ   'fall'
       bætət   bætʲətʲ   'be wide'
       nəqəq   nəqʲəqʲ   'take apart'

The description of this segmentless feature cannot be shoe-horned into a concatenative alphabetic model because the docking site is specified in reference to the underlying feature bundles of the root morpheme and not the surface segmental slots of the stem. That is, the last root consonant is palatalized whether the particular set of features surfaces only once on the coda of the stem-final syllable (as in 'love' and 'fall') or surfaces twice on both the onset and the coda (as in 'be wide' and 'take apart').

The representational demands of morphemes such as these, which consist either of prosodic structure but no featural content or of featural content but no inherent segmental organization, prompted the development of 'nonlinear' Generative theories such as 'CV Phonology' (Clements and Keyser 1983), 'Moraic Phonology' (Hayes 1989) and 'Prosodic Morphology' (McCarthy and Prince 1990a, 1990b). Since such theories are so clearly necessary to capture the specification of syllabic and higher-level prosodic organization for morphemes such as the Arabic causative stem, the argument from parsimony for underspecification of syllable and higher prosodic structure is no longer so compelling. The classic linear Generative Phonology picture of the lexicon as containing only bare strings of segments now warrants the same scrutiny as all other theories of temporary underspecification. The phonemic code that accounts for efficient lexical storage and retrieval does not require alphabetic segments *qua* minimal sequential constituents. Is there then any phonological evidence for alphabetic segments as discrete units of sequential organization, i.e. as countable prosodic constituents below the syllable? The best answer at this time is a tentative 'no' (see Broselow 1994). One of the most important implications of coarticulation for phonological theory today is that phonetic evidence for the segment as the basic unit of prosodic organization is even less likely to be forthcoming.

Another is that we need to frame new questions about coarticulation in terms of what the phenomenon might mean for the specification of syllables, feet, and so on. Here are two examples. First, Bladon and Al-Bamerni (1976) introduce the notion of 'coarticulatory resistance' to describe the variability in degree of influence of a context segment on different allophones of /l/ in English. How much of this variability can be accounted for by the role of these allophones in cuing prosodic structure? Are some positions within the syllable or stress foot more resistant to coarticulatory effects, as suggested by Recasens in his overview of lingual coarticulation in chapter 4 of this volume? Second, Künhert and Nolan in their chapter summarize the current state of our understanding of the development of coarticulatory precision in children by concluding 'that it is premature to derive any general statements about the acquisitional process of coarticulation'. Would the developmental literature make more sense if we considered also the child's developing control of the prosodic structures of the ambient language? To address these questions, it will be important to make cross-linguistic comparisons which are sensitive to the very large prosodic differences across languages, as demonstrated for example in the work of Cutler and colleagues (e.g. Cutler and Norris 1988; Otake *et al.* 1993) or Beckman and colleagues (e.g. Beckman 1986; Edwards, Beckman and Fletcher 1991; Fletcher and Vatikiotis-Bateson 1991). Phonologists, conversely, need to relate typologies of morphological alternations to typologies of prosodic hierarchies.

A final (and perhaps the most important) implication of coarticulation for non-linear phonological theories is the light it might shed on the actual role of segments as phonological components. The phonological arguments against the alphabetic model do not speak to the status of the segment as the basic 'molecule' for combining feature specifications at different positions in prosodic structures such as the syllable. Indeed, many of the morphological patterns that provide the strongest evidence against segments as minimal prosodic constituents provide equally strong evidence for segments as coordinated feature bundles. For example, although an Arabic root morpheme clearly cannot be represented as an orderly sequence of three abutting alphabetic time intervals, it must be specified as a series of something like three feature 'bundles' to account for the invariant tri-consonantal pattern across the different prosodic templates. That is, if the laryngeal or velic features of the two root morphemes in (9) were not coproduced in a particular way with the sequence of oral constriction features, how could the child learn that the roots are /ktb/ and /ħmn/ rather than, say, /kdb/ and /ʔmn/? In non-linear phonological representations, then, the implication of coarticulation cannot be simply that some gestures *may* be overlapped with other gestures when segments are strung together. Rather the true import of coarticulation is that in many cases some gestures *must* be coordinated with others in a precise way to ensure the correct interpretation of the prosodic affiliation of any opposing specifications for a given feature, i.e. for the language learner and perceiver to know the molecular arrangement of the atoms within the representations of contrasting syllables or other constituents.

A converse challenge to speech scientists, then, is to build and test theories about the phonetic exigencies underlying this fundamental organizational principle in the phonology. One such theory is the idea that some gestures in some prosodic positions must be coordinated with other gestures in order to make them audible. This is trivially true of the most basic gesture – the asymmetrical sustaining of the expiratory phase of breathing – which must be coproduced with some constriction upstream of the lungs in order to be audible as phonation or as turbulent noise. This basic 'audibility' theory informs Mattingly's (1981) proposal that the 'sonority' ranking that describes syllabification encodes aerodynamic constraints on which segment specifications will be audible if various constrictions and release gestures are coproduced. While Mattingly's model refers to the syllable, it is essentially a model of the audibility of segmental feature bundles. Stevens' (1994) notion of acoustic 'landmarks' is a similar theory about audibility constraints that makes no reference to syllable structure. Goldstein (1989, 1994), on the other hand, argues that segmental audibility does not completely constrain patterns of coordination, and that coproduction routines must be stated in reference to syllabic position. In this same vein, Browman and Goldstein (1990d) review a large body of evidence suggesting that preservation of segmental feature specification or even of entire feature bundles is not a strong constraint on patterns of consonant coproduction in connected or casual speech. See de Jong (1995b) for related evidence concerning the preservation of vowel feature specifications at different levels of the stress hierarchy in English, and a model which relates both the consonant and vowel patterns to local requirements for more or less salient segmental feature specification in prosodically strong versus weak syllables.

A not incompatible alternative theory is that coarticulatory patterns might be specified to preserve acoustic correlates of syllable count. Beckman (1996) reviews evidence suggesting that the audibility of syllable structures may be at least as strong a constraint on coarticulation as the audibility of segmental features. For example, in Standard Japanese, a voiceless obstruent typically overlaps with a following high vowel to the extent of aerodynamically hiding the vowel's specification of [+ voice], so that the disyllabic word /sita/ 'tongue' might sound like a monosyllable with an initial [ʃt] cluster to a native speaker of German. However, in words where the obstruent could be re-interpreted as a legitimate coda consonant, gestural timing is constrained to ensure that there is no such re-interpretation. The consonant constriction for the palatal fricative in the first /si/ of /kasisitu/ 'rented room' does not overlap completely with the somewhat lesser stricture of the vowel but has a 'release', an audible brief dip in amplitude not seen in the geminate palatal fricative of /hassja/ '(train) starting'. On the other hand, syllable preservation is not universally inviolable. Steriade (1990) describes a class of sound changes in which a less constrained coarticulatory pattern for an onset consonant apparently has led diachronically either to a re-ordering between the consonant and the tauto-syllabic vowel or to an increase in the syllable count (the alternations in the Slavic languages among *-gord, -gorod* and *-grad* being the best known of these). It is suggestive that the first result seems to have occurred only in lan-guages with the more complex syllable structures characteristic of stress-accent systems, whereas the second result seems to have occurred more often in lan-guages with only very simple CV syllables. Thus to understand these patterns fully, we probably need not only better phonetic models of the relationship between coarticulation and different syllable structures, but also better phono-logical models of the distribution of different syllable structures across typo-logically different prosodic systems.

Conclusion

This chapter has reviewed three general questions in phonological theory that are directly relevant to our understanding of coarticulation. The first, most basic question concerns the relationship between phonology and phonetics. The traditional notion of coarticulation is cast in a general frame-work that differentiates 'abstract, boolean' phonological representations from concrete phonetic events, and posits a procedural, derivational relationship between the two. Much of the data reviewed in earlier chapters of this book have been gathered within this framework, although the discussion hints at an increasing impetus to reinterpret these data within other representational frameworks which might allow the phonetic principles underlying coarticu-latory regularities to be integrated into a more declarative approach to spec-ifying phonological contrast and morphological variation.

The other two questions involve the role of segmental feature specification within the lexicon and the role of the segment in prosodic organization. These questions have become increasingly important as the dominant phonological theories gradually move away from the rigorously formulated alphabetic model of Chomsky and Halle (1968). Since coarticulation originated as a problem for the alphabetic model, it is important to re-assess the status of coarticulation as a coherent single 'problem' in non-alphabetic frameworks. Kühnert and Nolan (this volume, chapter 1) suggest that such a re-assessment of the phenomenon is necessary for current phonetic models of speech pro-duction. They call for 'further attention to the development of coarticulation in children, and to the variation exhibited by mature speakers'. Re-assessing coarticulation to see what it implies for 'nonlinear' models of phonological representation makes it clear that we also need more research into what aspects of coarticulation remain constant and what aspects vary across different inventories of phonological contrast and across different types of prosodic structure. Moreover, this research needs to aim at better models of the acoustic results of coarticulation and at more explanatory typologies of the prosodic structures available to the child in learning different languages. This in turn should lead to better phonological models which can be informed directly by the child's parsing of concrete articulatory 'events' and their acoustic consequences, as suggested by Browman and Goldstein (1989). These are issues where phonologists and other speech scientists might work hand in hand to develop phonological representations and phonetic models that can be related informatively to each other.

Notes

1 Of course, it must also accord with the behaviour of listeners when they parse these productions. However, there is not space in this chapter to explore fully the relevant literature on sentence processing and lexical access, and the implications of the perception of coarticulation for these topics and for how phonological models might inform machine recognition and understanding of speech (see e.g. Cutler 1994; Pierrehumbert 1994 and the many articles reviewed therein).

2 There are recording methods that allow better representations of lip spreading, such as horizontal lip opening measured from frontal photographs (see e.g. Fromkin 1964; Abry and Böe 1986), but these representations are more difficult to extract over time at comparable sampling rates.

3 Here and in (6), the syllable boundaries are marked in order to emphasize that the hypothesized root is not a prosodically possible word in Japanese.

4 The polite present illustrates the function of the nominal form as the general connective base onto which the polite ending /-ma.s-/ is appended to make a consonant-final stem. The full form for the polite present is then made by affixing /u/ onto this /-ma.s-/ stem. Other forms which are made from the connective stem include the durative (e.g. /ka.ki.na.ga.\a/ 'while writing'), the humilific (/o.ka.ki.su.\u/ 'I (humbly) write'), and the various donatives (e.g. /ka.ki.ku.da.sa.\u/ '(someone else) writes (for me)' and /ka.ki.ku.a.ge.\u/ '(I) write (for you)').

5 The last two forms could also be nicknames for Hatsune.

Part IV
Instrumental techniques

10

Palatography

FIONA GIBBON and KATERINA NICOLAIDIS

Introduction

Electropalatography (EPG) has become a widely used laboratory technique for recording and analysing one aspect of tongue activity, namely its contact with the hard palate during continuous speech. EPG in its present form developed from less sophisticated techniques of palatography which were able to record only the location of tongue–palate contact (for a review of earlier forms of palatography, see Hardcastle 1981). In one type of palatography, the surface of the palate is covered with a dark powder, usually a mixture of charcoal and chocolate. The speaker then produces a sound or sound sequence and the resulting area of 'wipe-off' on the palate is photographed (Abercrombie 1957). Records such as these provide useful spatial information about the location of tongue–palate contact, but the crucial dynamic dimension cannot be captured using this form of pala-tography. EPG, or dynamic palatography as it is sometimes called, has been devel-oped in order to do just this, and current models provide information relating to both temporal and spatial aspects of tongue–palate contact.

EPG as a technique in phonetic research has numerous attractions, which lie in a combination of practical features, such as conceptual simplicity, ease of operation and relative non-invasiveness. In the discussion which follows the first section describes the main features of current commercially available EPG systems. This is followed by an account of ways in which EPG raw data can be processed in order to extract useful measures for the investigation of lingual coarticulation.

Current EPG systems
Technical description

There are three commercially available versions of EPG in current use: a British system developed at the University of Reading (the latest version being the Reading EPG3 system, see Hardcastle, Gibbon and Jones 1991; Jones and Hardcastle 1995); a Japanese system manufactured by the Rion Corporation (the Rion DP01 described in Fujimura, Tatsumi and Kagaya 1973; Hiki and Itoh 1986), and an American 'Palatometer' marketed by Kay Elemetrics Corporation (described in Fletcher, McCutcheon and Wolf 1975; Fletcher 1983). All three systems share some general features, but differ in details such as the construction of the palates, number and configuration of electrodes and hardware/software specifications.

An essential component in all EPG systems is a thin custom-made artificial palate, sometimes called a pseudopalate, moulded to fit precisely the speaker's hard palate. Embedded in the artificial palate are a number of individually wired electrodes (also referred to as sensors) exposed to the lingual surface. These electrodes are scanned by electronic circuits, and when contact occurs between the tongue and any of these electrodes, a signal is conducted via lead-out wires, which exit at the corners of the mouth, to an external processing unit. A computer controls the real-time acquisition of tongue–palate contact data simultaneously with the acoustic signal from a microphone. These data are transmitted to a computer for storage, display and analysis.

EPG sampling rates vary from system to system, with both the Reading EPG3 and the Kay Palatometer sampling at 100 Hz, and the Rion DPO1 at 40 Hz. Obviously, slower sampling rates produce a less detailed record of tongue–palate contact. Sampling simultaneous acoustic information is essential for accurate segmentation and subsequent analysis of EPG recordings. The Reading EPG3 system samples the acoustic signal at 10,000 Hz, and the provision of a speech output facility makes it possible to play out the whole, or selected portions, of an utterance.

Some systems now have the facility to record simultaneous physiological data (such as aerodynamic, laryngographic and movement transduction data) on additional channels. A prototype multi-channel system has been developed by Reading University in collaboration with IBM, which allows simultaneous recording of up to six channels. EPG has been adapted for this system and, in order to obtain more detailed tongue palate information, the EPG data is sampled at 200 Hz (Hardcastle *et al.* 1989; Marchal and Hardcastle 1993). The importance of considering information from a number of sources in addition to EPG is illustrated in a later section.

The artificial palate

Artificial palates for use with EPG are made out of acrylic, polyester or similar non-toxic material. The Reading and Rion palates are made from a robust and relatively rigid acrylic and are held in place by a number of metal clasps, which fit over the upper teeth (see figure 10.1a and 1b). Palates

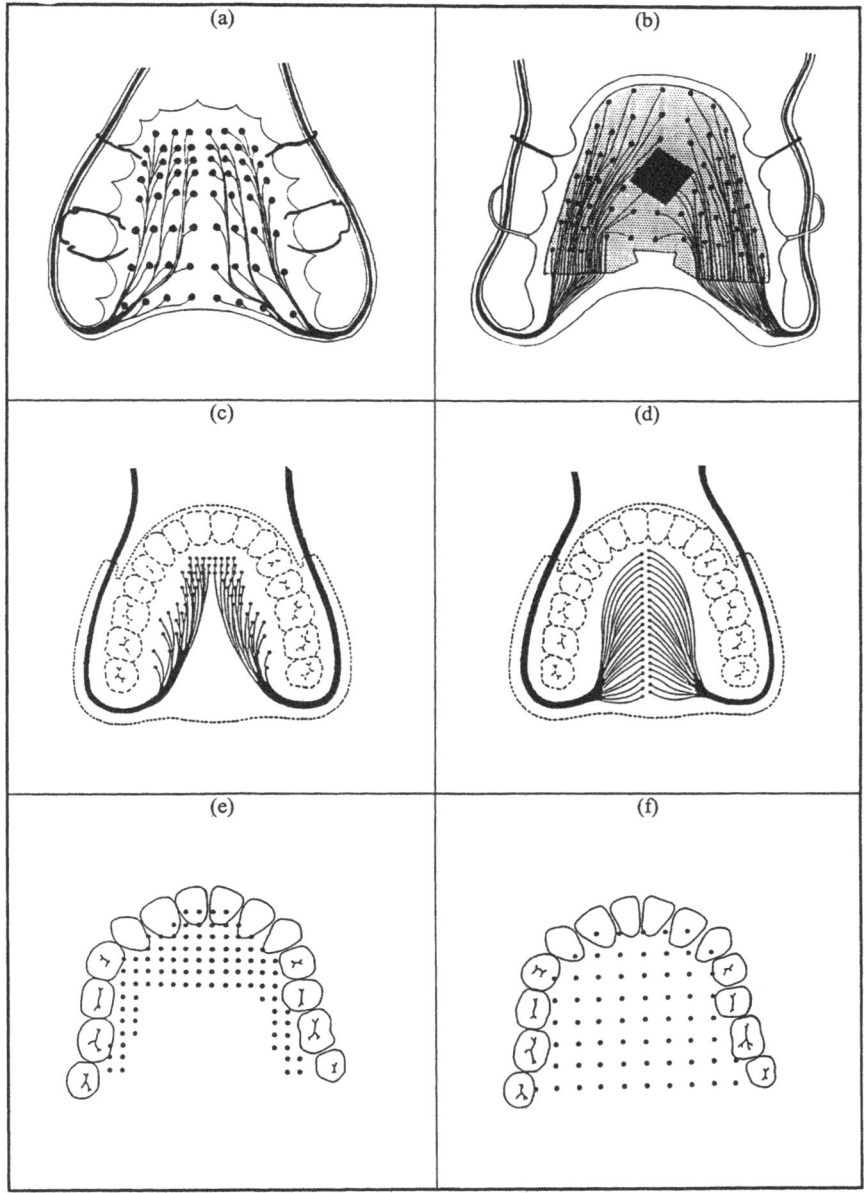

Figure 10.1   Electrode distribution on the (a) Reading, (b) Rion, (c–d) Kay
Palatometer (from Fletcher 1985), and (e–f) Kay Palatometer (from Fletcher 1988)
artificial palates. The number of electrodes varies from system to system: Reading
palates have 62, Rion palates 63, and although the Kay Palatometer palates vary, 96
is the usual number.

manufactured for use with the Kay palatometer are thinner and more flexible than those made for the other two systems. The Kay palates are made from polyester and do not have retention wires, but instead fit snugly over the hard palate and maxillary teeth.

The number and configuration of electrodes on the artificial palate differ in the various EPG systems (see figure 10.1). There are 62 electrodes in the Reading artificial palates, and these are placed according to well-defined criteria, such as identifiable anatomical landmarks (see Hardcastle, Gibbon and Jones 1991). The most posterior row is located on the junction between the hard and the soft palates, ensuring that production of velar gestures is registered. Lateral electrodes are located in the region between the upper teeth and gingival border, ensuring that lateral seal for alveolar obstruents is recorded. The electrodes are arranged in eight horizontal rows, with eight electrodes in every row except the most anterior, which has six (see figure 10.1a). There is a higher density of electrodes in the anterior (alveolar) region of the palate to ensure that important events such as tongue 'grooving' during sibilant production are captured in sufficient detail.

Rion produces six standard electrode configurations for their artificial palates, which are arranged in a series of hemispherical curves, following the contours of the palate (figure 10.1b). The standard number of electrodes on the Rion palate is 63, but if the size and shape of the hard palate requires a smaller number, it is possible to construct palates with 52 or 48 electrodes. The advantage of this type of palate construction is that the distance between electrodes is known and constant, regardless of the size or shape of the individual's palate. The drawback is that, since these electrodes are not placed according to an individual speaker's palate morphology, they do not always register lateral seal and/or velar gestures.

The location and distribution of electrodes on the artificial palates constructed for the Kay Palatometer vary but normally 96 electrodes are used and these are arranged in hemispherical curves in a similar arrangement to the Rion palates. However, for experimental purposes, the electrodes may be concentrated in specific regions of the palate or centred along the antero–posterior axis and the electrodes may extend along the lingual sides of the maxillary teeth (Fletcher 1985, 1988). In other studies, the electrodes have been distributed in 3 mm or 4 mm grid patterns (Dagenais, Lorendo and McCutcheon 1994; Dagenais, Critz-Crosby and Adams 1994; and see figure 10.1c–f).

Phonetic zoning schemes

Researchers have found it useful to divide up the artificial palate into reference zones, which relate in an approximate way to phonetically relevant regions of the hard palate. Based on the arrangement of the electrodes in the Reading system, two phonetic zoning systems have been proposed. In the first, four zones are identified (see figure 10.2a) and in the second, a more detailed zoning scheme has been adopted with the division of the palate in zones and sub-zones (see figure 10.2b and Recasens *et al.* 1993; Fontdevila, Pallarès and Recasens 1994).

With reference to these zoning systems and based on general knowledge of the anatomy of the tongue and speech production, inferences can be made about the part of the tongue involved in the production of particular sounds. For instance, the tongue tip/blade system is likely to be the active articulator where electrodes are contacted in the alveolar and postalveolar regions of the artificial palate, whereas the tongue body is more likely to be involved where contact is registered in the palatal and velar regions. A vocal tract representation (with articulatory zones, sub-zones and tongue regions) is shown in figure 10.2c and is based on the zoning system in figure 10.2b.

Various phonetic zoning schemes have been proposed for use with the Rion EPG system, following the arrangement of electrodes in hemispherical rows (see for example Recasens 1984b; Farnetani, Vagges and Magno-Caldognetto 1985, see also figures 10.2d and 10.2e).

EPG tongue–palate contact data

EPG records details of the tongue's contact with the hard palate and registers characteristic patterns for lingual obstruents such as /t/, /c/, /k/, /s/, /ʃ/, /ç/, /ts/, /tʃ/ (and their voiced cognates), the palatal approximant /j/, laterals /l/, /ʎ/ and nasals /n/, /ɲ/, /ŋ/. Relatively close vowels and diphthongs /i/, /ɪ/, /ɛ/, /eɪ/, /aɪ/ and /ɒɪ/ also show measurable degrees of contact, and this has allowed researchers to investigate the influence of vowel context on consonant production (see further below). There is little or no tongue contact during production of back or open vowels. In addition, articulations that have their primary constriction either further forward than the most anterior row of electrodes (e.g. labials) or further back than the most posterior row of electrodes (e.g. uvular, pharyngeal and glottal sounds) do not produce characteristic EPG patterns, although there may be some EPG contact present during these sounds due to the influence of surrounding vowels.

EPG raw data

EPG raw data are usually displayed as sequences of two dimensional representations, referred to as palatograms or EPG frames. Careful observation of raw data in this form is often informative, revealing relevant phonetic features of production, such as the location of tongue–palate contact (spatial information), the timing of tongue movement (temporal information) and also details of lingual coarticulation.

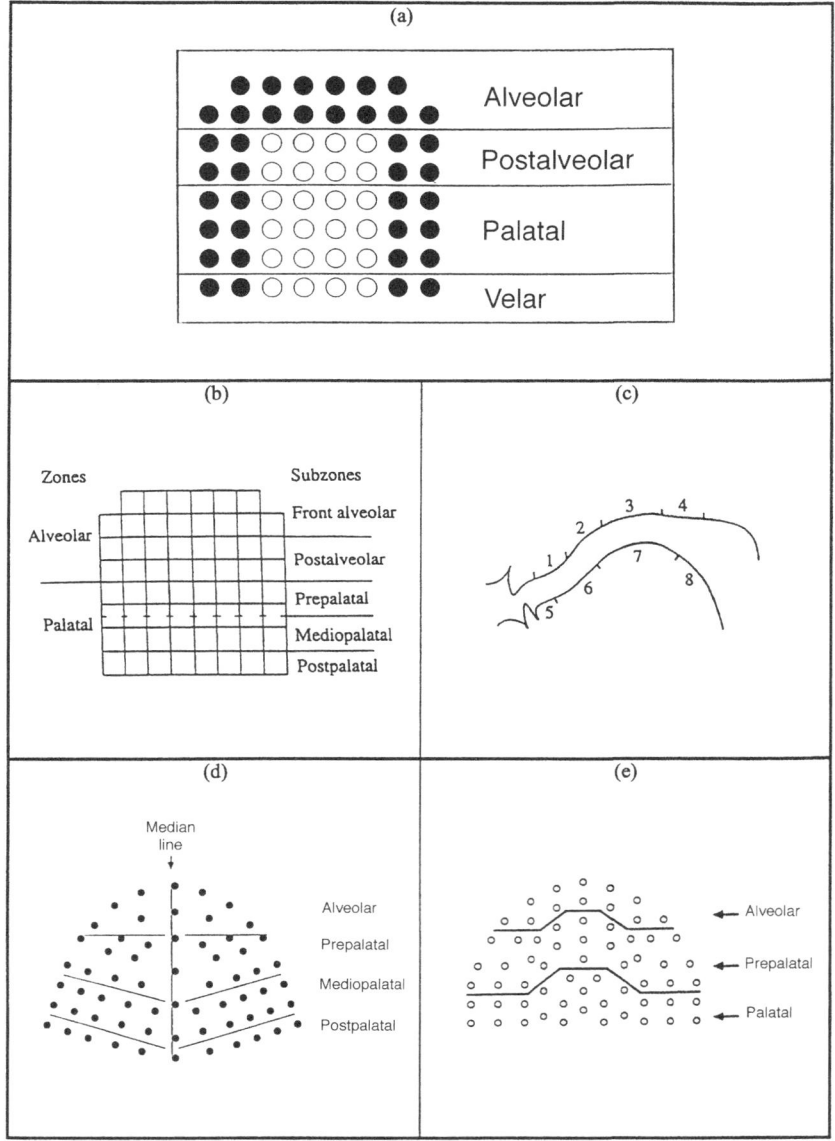

Figure 10.2   Phonetic zoning systems for (a–b) the Reading, (d–e) the Rion artificial palates, and (c) vocal tract representation with articulatory zones, subzones and tongue regions: 1 = alveolar; 2 = prepalatal; 3 = mediopalatal; 4 = postpalatal; 5 = tongue tip/blade; 6 = predorsum; 7 = mediodorsum; 8 = postdorsum (see Recasens 1984b, 1990; Farnetani, Vagges and Magno-Caldognetto 1985; Fontdevila, Pallarès and Recasens 1994).

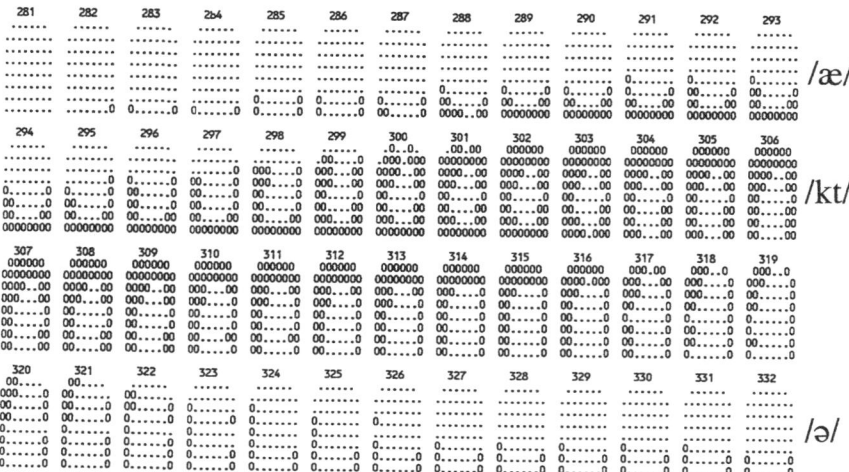

Figure 10.3   Computer print-out (Reading EPG3 system) of the /kt/ sequence in the word 'actor'. The palatograms are read from left to right. In each palatogram diagram, the alveolar region is at the top, the velar region is at the bottom and lingual contact is indicated by zeros. The sampling rate is 100 Hz, making the interval between individual frames 10 ms (see text for full details).

A full EPG printout of the word 'actor' is shown in figure 10.3. This illustrates an instance of *temporal coarticulation* involving two articulators (the tongue tip/blade and tongue body) during the production of the /kt/ sequence in this word. In figure 10.3 it can be seen that there is first a build-up of EPG contact in the velar region of the palate (frames 282–288), which represents the approach phase of the velar stop. The first EPG frame to show complete constriction across the palate occurs at frame 289, indicating the onset of /k/ closure. Following closure, complete velar constriction is maintained at the same time as lateral contact begins to build up (frames 290–300), in preparation for the upcoming /t/. Contact continues to extend from the lateral into the alveolar region until there is complete closure in the alveolar region (frame 301). A brief period of simultaneous alveolar and velar closure (i.e. double articulation) during frames 301 to 302 occurs, representing an overlap period of 20 ms. The velar gesture is released at frame 303, and a characteristic horse-shoe shaped configuration involving complete contact across the palate in the alveolar region and lateral contact for the /t/ ensues (frames 304–316). The closure phase of the /t/ ends at frame 316 (the last frame of complete contact across the palate) and following this there is a rapid decrease in tongue contact during production of the word-final schwa.

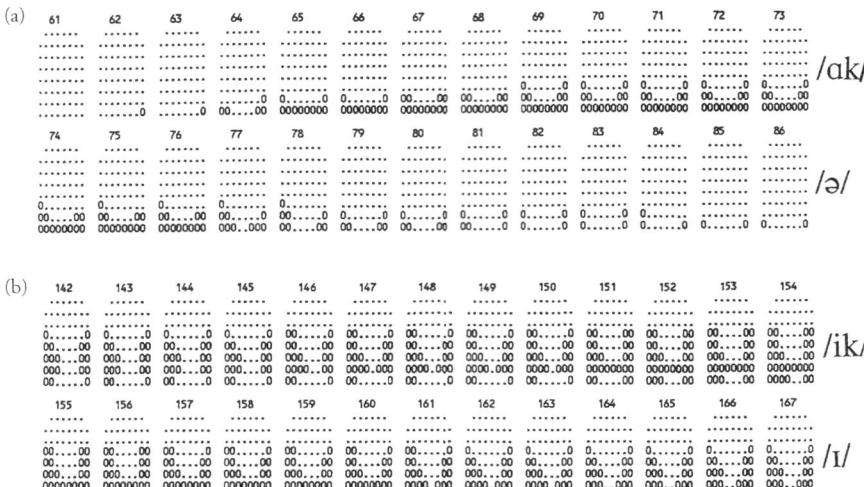

Figure 10.4   Computer print-out of velar segments in two different vowel environments. (a) shows the production of [ɑkə] (in the word 'darker') and (b) [ikɪ] (in the word 'squeaky'). Note the more posterior tongue placement in the context of the open back vowel compared to the close front vowel.

Spatial coarticulatory effects involving a single articulator can also be revealed by EPG. Figure 10.4 illustrates the different spatial characteristics of tongue body placement for the velar gesture /k/, which vary depending on the vocalic context. Figures 10.4a and 10.4b show the production of the velar segment in [ɑkə] (in the word 'darker') and [iki] (in the word 'squeaky'). A number of significant EPG frames that reflect important phonetic events can be identified as follows: the onset of closure for the stop (the first frame of complete constriction across the palate, frames 65 and 151 for [ɑkə] and [iki] respectively); the frame of maximum constriction (frames 71 and 157 for [ɑkə] and [iki] respectively); and the onset of the release of the stop (the last frame of complete constriction, frames 76 and 160 for [ɑkə] and [iki] respectively). The spatial configuration of the EPG data for all frames reveals a more posterior lingual placement for the /k/ in the context of the open back vowel compared to the close front vowel environment.

Data reduction methods

Whilst raw data provide detailed spatial and temporal articulatory information of lingual activity, they can be unwieldy for certain research purposes and so the need for data reduction methods and quantification of contact patterns arises. Such is the need for reliable and informative procedures that new methods of data reduction are constantly being devised for the different EPG systems (see for example Nguyen 1995; Holst, Warren and Nolan 1995 and reviews by Hardcastle, Gibbon and Nicolaidis 1991; Byrd *et al.* 1995). EPG data reduction methods can be divided into three major types. First, there are methods that capture spatial details about the location of tongue–palate contact, and this information may be combined with information about the frequency of electrode activation. Examples of this method are 'place of articulation' displays. Second, there are methods based on dynamic changes in lingual activity, and these provide information about lingual activity as a function of time (e.g. contact profile displays). Lastly, contact indices have been used to reduce the EPG contact information to a single value, giving an overall characterization of the contact pattern. These indices are valuable, especially when statistical analyses of the data are required. Indices are usually calculated for selected EPG frames (e.g. first or last frame of complete constriction, frame of maximum contact during a stop etc. see figure 10.4 for a description of these frames) but they can also be plotted as a function of time (see for example the centre of gravity index (COG) display in Hardcastle, Gibbon and Nicolaidis 1991).

Place of articulation measures

Several place of articulation measures have been proposed in the EPG literature. These are based on the identification of a relevant frame (e.g. the frame of maximum contact during the closure phase of an obstruent) and the schematization of the place of articulation of this frame in various ways, e.g. delimitation of its boundaries, shading etc. (Farnetani 1988; Recasens 1989). Various methods of quantification have also been used and place of articulation information may be combined with the frequency of electrode activation over a number of repetitions or over a longer stretch of speech (Matsuno 1989; Gibbon 1990). More detailed measures can be obtained for specific categories of sounds. For example, several measures have been proposed for sibilants, including groove width, groove length, location and dimension of constriction (Hardcastle and Clark 1981; Clark, Palethorpe and Hardcastle 1982; Fletcher 1985; Hoole *et al.* 1989).

Useful qualitative information can also be obtained by selecting specific EPG frames from the raw data, which correspond to important gestural events in the articulation of a sound. For example, many studies used the first and last frames of complete constriction across the palate for demarcating the beginning and end of the closure phase of stops (see Nicolaidis, Hardcastle and Gibbon 1993 for a review of EPG studies and the annotation points employed). This method provides a useful profile of tongue–palate contacts (Hardcastle *et al.* 1989) and allows for comparisons to be made between sounds at the various stages of their articulation.

Contact profile displays

The temporal evolution of tongue–palate contact in selected contact regions can be illustrated in contact profile displays. The dynamic changes are represented as the total number or percent of activated electrodes in a contact region expressed as a function of time. Qualitative information is obviously reduced in this type of display. Dynamic contact changes can be displayed for different regions of the palate and therefore the contact profile display depends on the EPG zoning system adopted (see figure 10.2). Contact profiles provide interesting quantitative information for different categories of sounds (e.g. alveolar versus postalveolar fricatives) as well as important timing relationships between contiguous segments (e.g. timing of gestures in consonant sequences) (Barry 1991; Hardcastle, Gibbon and Nicolaidis 1991; Byrd *et al.* 1995; Byrd and Tan 1996). Measures such as these have also been found to be particularly useful in the study of coarticulation in VCV sequences (Butcher 1989).

Contact indices

Various numerical indices have been used in phonetic research in order to capture different aspects of lingual contact and these are designed to elucidate specific areas of phonetic interest. Several indices have been proposed which aim to quantify the distribution of activated electrodes across the whole, or specific regions, of the palate. Such measures include the centre of gravity (COG) and anteriority, posteriority, centrality indices (for reviews of these methods see Hardcastle, Gibbon and Nicolaidis 1991; Fontdevila, Pallarès and Recasens 1994).

Centre of gravity indices

The COG index expresses the location of the *main concentration* of activated electrodes. The calculation assigns progressively higher values to electrodes contacted towards the anterior rows. The formula used to calculate the COG index for the Reading EPG system is described in Hardcastle, Gibbon and Nicolaidis (1991). This can be adapted to measure electrode concentration in selected palatal regions, and an example of such an adaptation and its use in the investigation of coarticulation is provided in Gibbon, Hardcastle and Nicolaidis (1993). In this study, anterior and posterior COG

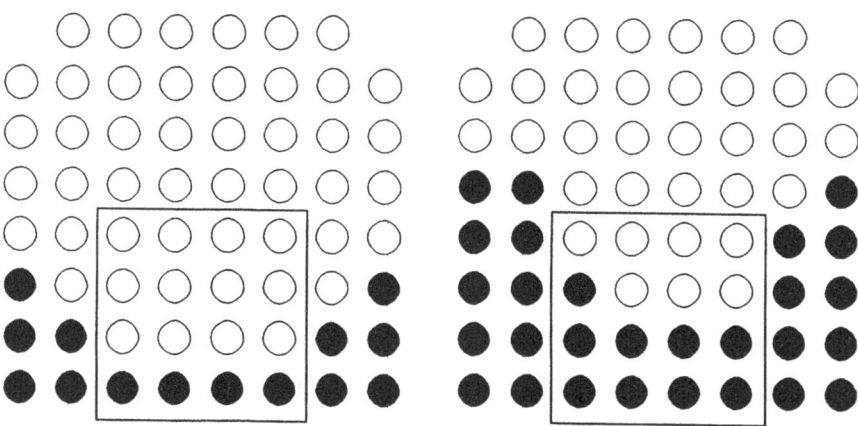

Figure 10.5   Individual EPG frames from [ɑkə] (left palatogram) and [ikɪ] (right palatogram) at the point of maximum constriction (frame 71 in Figure 10.4a and frame 157 in Figure 10.4b). Only the electrodes in the posterior midsagittal region (within the squares) were used to calculate posterior COGs in the Gibbon, Hardcastle and Nicolaidis (1993) study (see text for details). The following formula was used:

$$\text{posterior COG} = \frac{(0.5 \times R8) + (1.5 \times R7) + (2.5 \times R6) + (3.5 \times R5)}{R8 + R7 + R6 + R5}$$

(where R8 = the number of activated electrodes in row 8, and so on). Index values for these /VkV/ sequences are 0.5 for [ɑkə] and 1.17 for [ikɪ]. The higher posterior COG score for [ikɪ] reflects the more anterior placement for [k] in the close vowel environment.

indices were calculated by measuring electrodes contacted in the four mid-sagittal rows of electrodes in the four anterior rows and the four posterior rows respectively. The aim was to quantify lingual contact in different contexts, in this case alveolar /l/ and velar /k/ produced in singleton and /kl/ cluster contexts.

Figure 10.5 illustrates two EPG patterns from which the posterior COG index (as used in Gibbon, Hardcastle and Nicolaidis 1993) was calculated to quantify contextual variability in lingual contact at the EPG frame of maximum contact in VCV sequences (V = i, a, C = k). The posterior COG values (0.5 for [ɑkə], and 1.17 for [iki]) capture the different lingual placements that occur in these vowel contexts, i.e. the higher COG score for [iki] reflects the more anterior placement for [k] in the close vowel environment. Indices such as these provide valuable quantitative single measures which are amenable to more rigorous analyses than raw data observations.

Contact distribution indices

Anteriority, posteriority and centrality contact indices are proposed and described in detail for the Reading EPG system by Recasens *et al.* (1993) and Fontdevila, Pallarès and Recasens (1994). These indices quantify both the *distribution* and *degree* of tongue–palate contact across the palate. The anteriority and posteriority indices quantify changes along the sagittal axis of the palate and the centrality index along the coronal axis. For the calculation of the anteriority and posteriority indices the palate is divided into eight rows while for the centrality index the palate is divided into four columns (column one comprises lateral electrodes on both sides of the palate, and similarly for the central electrodes). The formulae used for the calculation of the indices are included in Fontdevila, Pallarès and Recasens (1994). The rationale for these indices is that the contribution of a single electrode in a row (or column for the centrality index) is always higher than the contribution of all the activated electrodes in previous rows (or columns). In the Recasens *et al.* (1993) study, the contact indices were calculated separately for the alveolar and palatal regions for the investigation of alveolar and palatal consonants in Catalan and Italian. The contact indices were used not only to examine vowel-to-consonant coarticulatory effects in the different tongue regions, but also to investigate interarticulator coordination between the tongue front and dorsum.

Coarticulation index

A coarticulation index (CI) was devised by Farnetani, Hardcastle and Marchal (1989) to quantify the coarticulatory effects of contiguous vowels on a particular phase of consonant production. Overall, the index measures differences in degree of electrode activation during the production of a segment in two different contextual environments. CIs calculated for symmetrical environments (for example /ata–iti/) at the consonantal mid-point show global effects of the vocalic environment on the consonant. CIs calculated for pairs of sequences such as /ata–ati/ or /ata–ita/ at the points of consonantal closure and release determine possible anticipatory and carryover coarticulatory effects respectively. For example, an anticipatory CI can be calculated for the sequences /ata–ati/ to quantify anticipatory effects of /i/ versus /a/ at the onset of closure for /t/. Similarly, a carryover CI can be calculated for the sequences /ata–ita/ to determine carryover effects of /i/ versus /a/ at the consonantal release. The calculation of the index is described in the caption to figure 10.6 and more fully

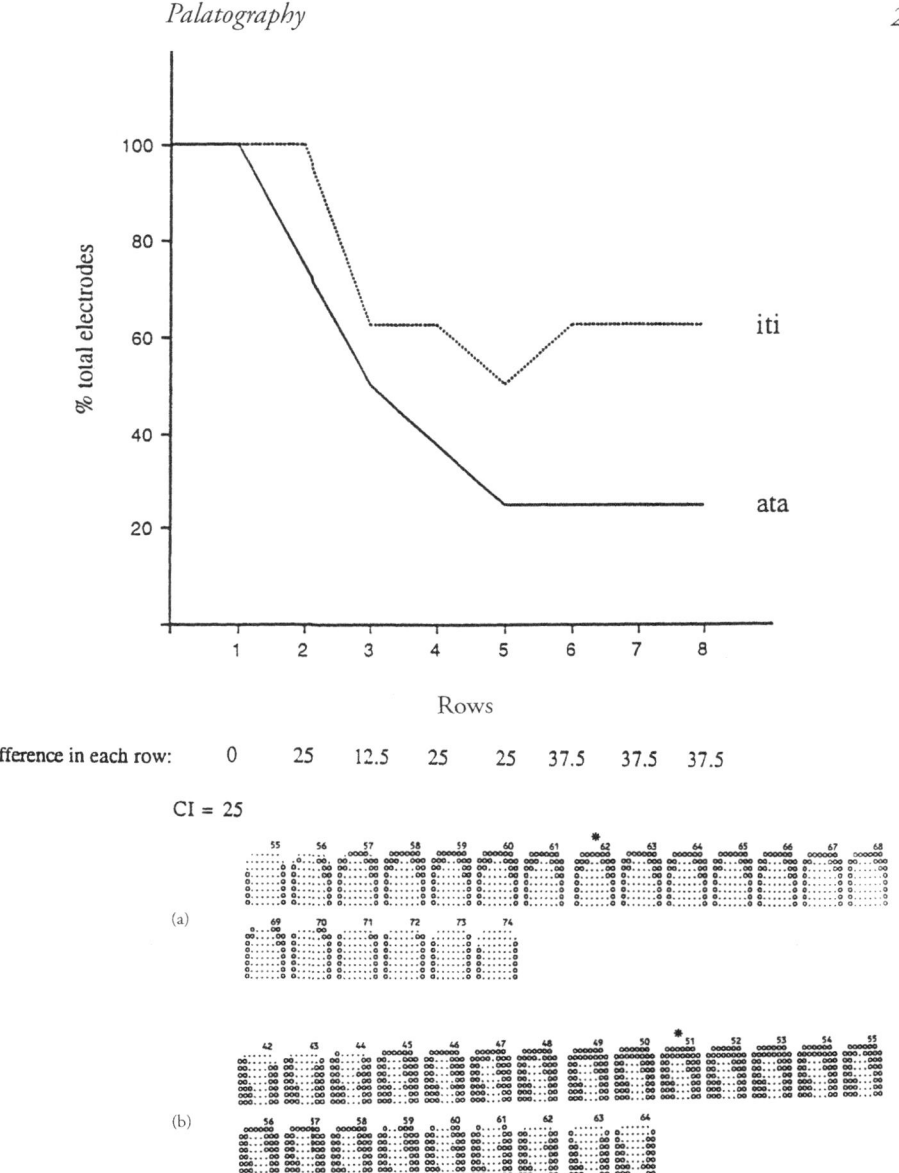

Figure 10.6   Calculation of the coarticulatory index (CI). Full EPG printouts of the sequences (a) /ata/ and (b) /iti/ are shown at the bottom of the figure. The frame at the temporal mid-point of each stop is marked with *. The graph above plots the total number of activated electrodes in each row. This is expressed as a percentage of the total possible contactable electrodes per row at the marked frame. The index is calculated by averaging the absolute value of the differences between the totals of each row (see numbers below each row).

in Farnetani (1990). The index can be calculated for different parts of the palate (e.g. front/back) when clear differences exist between the two regions.

Other indices

An articulatory reduction index was devised by Farnetani and Provaglio (1991) to measure the degree of electrode activation during a segment produced with different speech styles (e.g. isolated words versus connected speech). This measure may reflect a variation in the frequency of electrode activation or in the overall extent of the articulatory gesture on the palatal surface between the different speech styles.

An asymmetry index was proposed by Marchal and Espesser (1987) to express the asymmetry of contact pattern between the left and right sides of the palate (see also Farnetani 1988; Hardcastle, Gibbon and Jones 1991). The index can also be calculated for different regions of the palate (e.g. front/back).

An interesting phenomenon that may occur in VCV sequences (especially when the consonant involves an articulatory gesture which is relatively independent of the vowel, e.g. bilabial stops) is a change in electrode activation during stop closure that has been interpreted as lingual relaxation. A 'trough' index was devised by Engstrand (1989) to capture this phenomenon (see also Hardcastle, Gibbon and Nicolaidis 1991).

To quantify inter-utterance and/or contextual variability, two 'variability' indices based on EPG data have been proposed. The indices can measure gestural variability in selected tongue regions (for a description of the calculation of these indices, see Sudo, Kiritani and Sawashima 1983; Farnetani and Provaglio 1991).

Multi-channel recordings

The advantages of recording EPG simultaneously with other channels are becoming increasingly recognized. A multi-channel approach can provide additional information which allows for a more accurate understanding of the complex relationships that exist between articulatory gestures involved in speech production. An example of how multi-channel recordings can assist in the description of complex articulations is illustrated in figure 10.7, which shows simultaneous laryngograph, acoustic, EPG and oral airflow traces during production of an affricate /tʃ/ in the word 'starchy'. It is known that in certain accents of English affricates may be preceded in some phonetic contexts by a glottal stop and, in these cases, the approach phase of the oral stop as seen on the waveform can be masked.

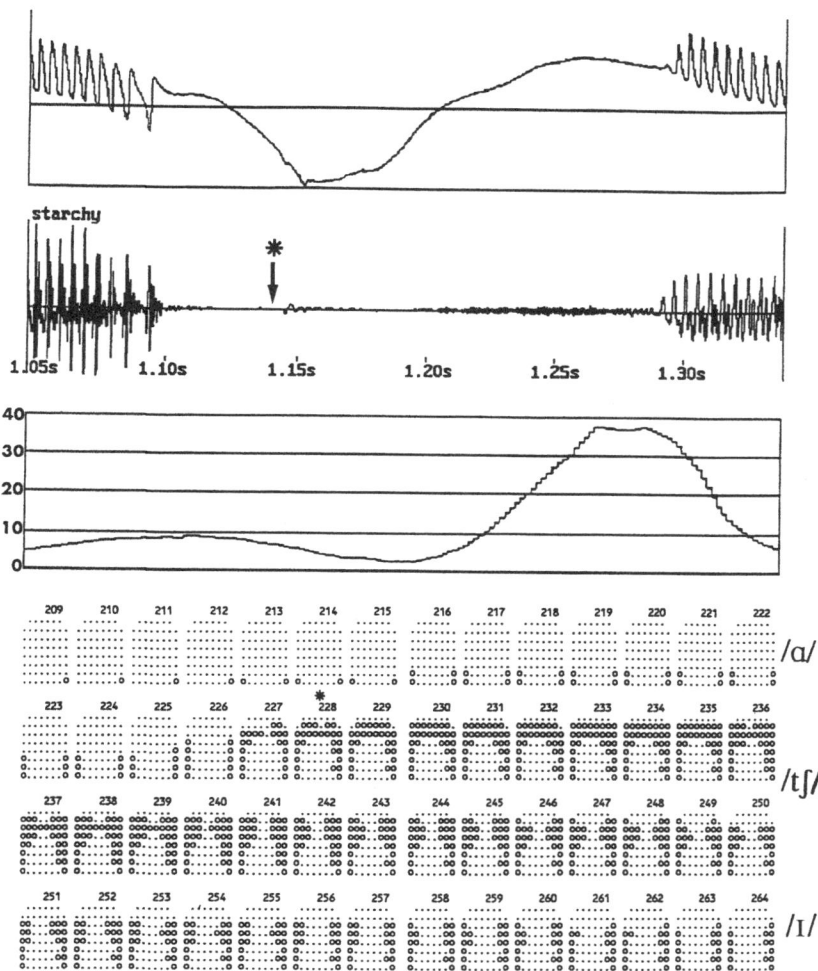

Figure 10.7   Multi-channel screen display of [ɑʔtʃɪ] in the word 'starchy' showing laryngograph trace (upper), acoustic waveform (middle) and the oral airflow trace (lower). Below the screen display is a full printout of the EPG patterns (sampled at 200 Hz, with frames occurring at 5 ms intervals). The total duration of the display is 28 ms (1.05 s–1.33 s on the acoustic trace, EPG frames 209–264). The asterisk marked on the acoustic waveform indicates the onset of complete closure for /t/, as shown by the EPG data (frame 228). Preglottalization occurs at around 1.10 s on the acoustic trace and this corresponds to EPG frame 219, where there is minimal contact present. The release of the stop component of the affricate (EPG frame 239) occurs at 1.20 s on the acoustic trace. A rapid rise in oral airflow coincides with the release of the stop component and continues to increase during the fricative component of the affricate.

In figure 10.7 a glottal stop occurs before the affricate in 'starchy' [ˈstɑʔtʃɪ]. From the EPG trace, complete closure for the alveolar gesture can be seen to occur at frame 228, and is marked on the waveform by *. Observation of the acoustic signal alone could not have revealed the precise timing of the approach and onset of closure phases of the stop component of the affricate. Likewise, observation of the EPG records alone would fail to identify the presence of preglottalization. For this purpose, the laryngograph trace is useful in revealing the presence of a characteristic 'kink' after the end of vocal fold vibration for the vowel, providing additional evidence of preglottalization. It is evident that simultaneous analysis of waveform, EPG and laryngographic traces can provide a more precise view of the timing relationship and coordination between the different motor systems.

Knowledge that EPG registers only tongue–palate contact emphasizes the need to incorporate complementary instrumental techniques within the experimental set-up. EPG cannot reveal which part of the tongue is touching the hard palate or its proximity to it. In order to gain a more accurate picture of the overall tongue shape and its positioning within the vocal tract, EPG needs to be combined with techniques such as electromagnetic transduction (Hoole, Nguyen-Trong and Hardcastle 1993) and ultrasound (Stone *et al.* 1992).

In addition, it has become increasingly recognized that it is important to take into account the anatomical dimensions of the speaker's hard palate when interpreting EPG data (Hardcastle *et al.* 1991; Jones and Hardcastle 1995). In all the systems, the relationship between the positioning of electrodes on the artificial palate and the EPG frames is unavoidably schematic. However, recent developments using a Reflex microscope linked to a personal computer (e.g. Speculand, Butcher and Stephens 1988) have enabled the precise calculation of XYZ coordinates for all the electrodes of the artificial palate. In another development, an enhanced EPG (eEPG) system uses digitized palate shape data to display the tongue–palate contact patterns in three dimensions (Chiu, Shadle and Carter 1995). These palate shapes are obtained using a colour-coded structured light digitization system.

The use of a combination of techniques, as described here, can provide essential three-dimensional data on palatal shape and relative tongue–palate proximity, making it possible in the future to deduce more precisely the shape and movement trajectories of the tongue from the EPG contact data alone, information that is central to the study of lingual coarticulation.

Acknowledgments

We acknowledge financial support from the European Economic Commission DGXIII under the auspices of ESPRIT II Basic Research Action (ACCOR Project 3279) and the British Medical Research Council (Project no. G8912970N). Thanks are due to Wilf Jones who designed the Reading EPG system and provided technical support.

11

Imaging techniques

MAUREEN STONE

Introduction

This chapter is concerned with how imaging systems can be used to answer the questions and address the issues pertinent to coarticulation. At first glance one might be sceptical about the role of systems which are static or limited to video frame rates in answering subtle coarticulatory questions about the interaction of articulators and phonemes in the rapid movements used for speech. On further consideration, however, there are many issues that can be explored via imaging techniques and some questions that can only be answered using such techniques.

The patterns of speech events are well captured by image sequences, like those created using X-ray and ultrasound. Image sequences display important features of articulatory behaviour, which are often difficult to obtain, such as the interaction of several articulators, pharyngeal behaviours, cross-sectional tongue movement and three-dimensional components of tongue behaviour. Point tracking systems have advantages over current imaging systems. Point tracking techniques have a much faster sampling rate than imaging systems and they measure the movement of actual tissue points. However, imaging techniques have advantages over point tracking measures. Imaging techniques provide true two-dimensional (2D) movement data, such as the movement of the entire tongue profile, rather than the one-dimensional movement of a single point or series of points. Images also indicate the true high point of the tongue, not the point of the highest marker. In addition, although point tracking measures provide better timing information, shape information is degraded for deformable articulators such as the lips, tongue and velum, since the experimenter must infer the shape contour between points. Furthermore, tracked midsagittal points provide no information on articulator behaviour in the cross-sectional plane.

Table 11.1 *Physiological features of the vocal tract that are readily observed, measured and analysed using imaging techniques.*

	CT	MRI	X-ray	Ultrasound*
Two-dimensional images	X	X	X	X
Multiple viewing planes	X	X	X	X
Static shape features				
Lengthwise VT shape	X	X	X	X
Crosswise VT shape	X	X		X
Multiple articulators	X	X		X
3D reconstruction	X	X		X
Time-varying movements				
Lengthwise movement			X	X
Crosswise movement			X	X
Pharyngeal movement			X	X

Notes:
*tongue features only

Imaging techniques

There are four imaging techniques most commonly used to image the vocal tract. They are X-ray, computed tomography (CT), magnetic resonance imaging (MRI) and ultrasound. This chapter will discuss each of these techniques and then consider coarticulatory issues that are best addressed by imaging techniques. Table 11.1 indicates the features discussed below with respect to each of the imaging techniques.

Lateral X-ray

X-ray is the most well known of the imaging systems and differs from the others in significant ways. In a lateral X-ray image, an X-ray beam is projected from one side of the head, passes through all the tissue of the head and is recorded on a plate on the other side. Similarly, an anterior/posterior (A/P) X-ray passes through the head from the front to the back. Often, soft tissue structures like the tongue are difficult to measure with X-rays because the jaw, palate and teeth obscure much of the tongue. A second problem with X-ray is that unless a contrast medium such as barium is used to mark the entire surface of the tongue, it is difficult to tell if the highest and most visible edge is the only edge or if the mid-line of the tongue is grooved relative to the edges. This is particularly problematic since the tongue is often grooved during speech. Finally, the potential hazards of exposure preclude the collection of large quantities of data with X-rays.

Imaging Techniques

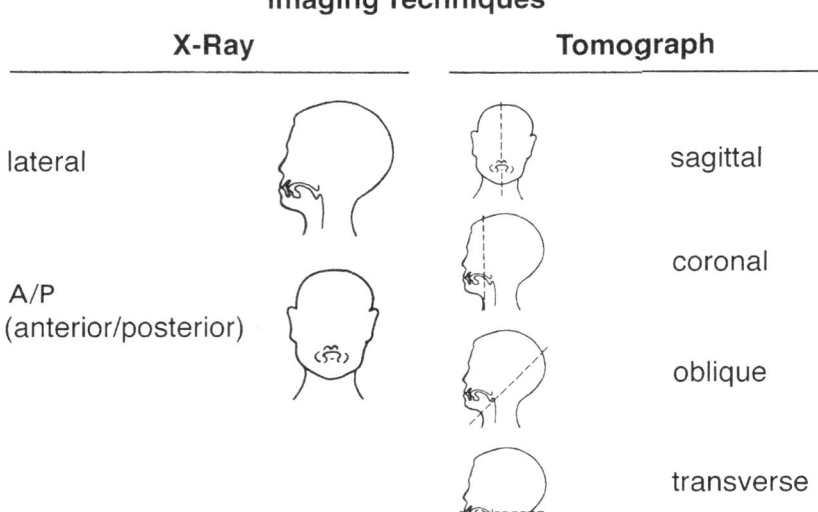

X-Ray	Tomograph

lateral

A/P
(anterior/posterior)

sagittal

coronal

oblique

transverse

Figure 11.1   Depiction of medical sections and terminology used to describe imaged data. Lateral and anterior/posterior X-rays give similar information to sagittal and coronal tomographs.

The other three techniques, CT, MRI and ultrasound, create images in a fundamentally different way. These techniques visually construct a tomograph, or slice of tissue, made by projecting a thin, flat beam through the tissue in a single plane. There are four tomographic planes of interest, shown in figure 11.1. They are sagittal, coronal, oblique, and transverse (axial). The lateral and A/P views seen on X-ray correspond most closely to the sagittal and coronal tomographic planes.

Computed tomography (CT)

The first tomographic technique is computed tomography (CT). CT uses X-rays to image thin slices (2 mm) of the body. Figure 11.2 depicts a CT scanner. The scanner rotates around the body taking multiple images, at different angles, of a single section of tissue. A computer then creates a composite, including any stuctures that were visible in some scans but obscured in others. Figure 11.3 shows a transverse CT of the oropharynx at rest. Bone appears bright white in the image. The jaw is seen at the left of the image and a vertebra at the right. The hyoid bone is horseshoe shaped, in the middle of the image. The air in the vocal tract appears black, and the epiglottis can be seen within the vocal tract. The tongue and other soft tissue are grey. CT can

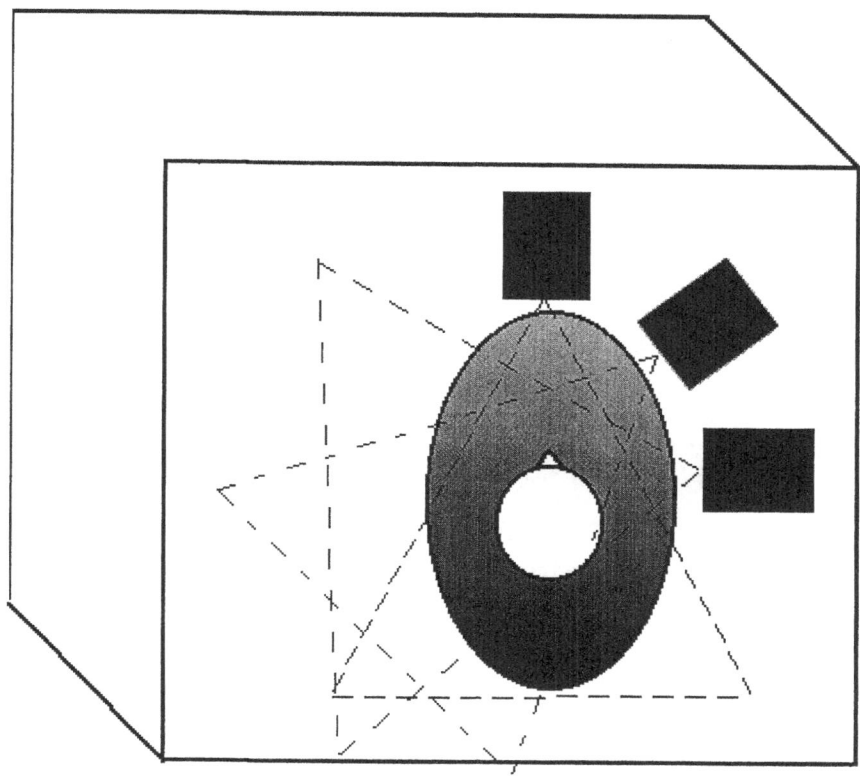

Figure 11.2   View of a subject's head (face up) in a CT scanner. Subject is lying supine. The CT takes a series of tomographic X-rays, in a single plane, which are reconstructed into one image.

image soft tissue more clearly than X-ray because it produces a composite X-ray. By digitally summing a series of scans, the composite section has sharper edges and more distinct tissue definition.

CT has three major limitations. First, CT scans take about two seconds per frame, too slow for real-time speech. Future technology may eliminate this problem. The second limitation is the radiation exposure. CT is an X-ray. Lastly, the scan images are limited to the transverse and oblique planes because the patient can only be tilted to about 45 degrees from horizontal.

Magnetic Resonance Imaging (MRI)

The second tomographic technique, Magnetic Resonance Imaging (MRI), uses a magnetic field and radio waves rather than X-rays to image a section of tissue. An MRI scanner consists of electromagnets that surround

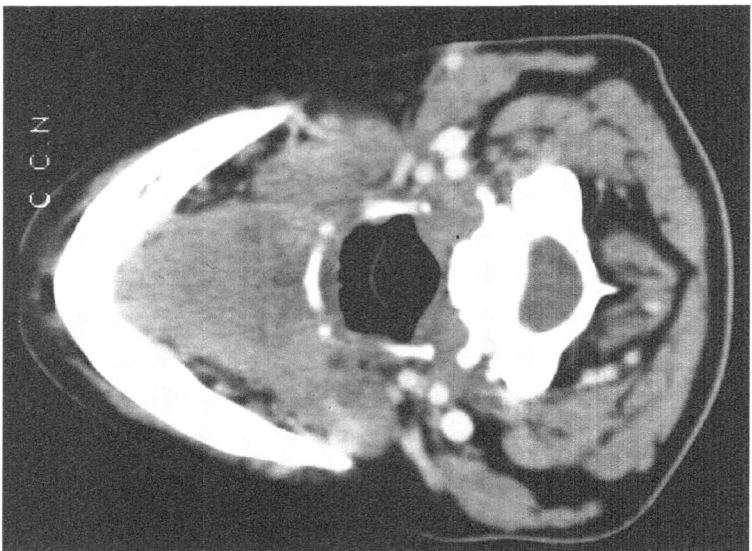

Figure 11.3   CT image of a transverse section of the oropharynx at rest.

the body and create a magnetic field. MRI scanning detects the presence of hydrogen protons, which occur in abundance in water and therefore in tissue. In figure 11.4, picture A represents a hydrogen proton spinning about an axis which is oriented randomly. B shows what happens when a magnetic field is introduced. The proton's axis aligns along the direction of the field's poles. Even when aligned, however, the proton wobbles, or precesses. In picture C a short-lived radio pulse, vibrating at the same frequency as the wobble, is introduced. This momentarily knocks the proton out of alignment. D shows the proton re-aligning, within milliseconds, to the magnetic field. As it re-aligns, the proton emits a weak radio signal of its own. These radio signals are then assembled as an image indicating hydrogen density, or water content, thus clearly differentiating between different types of tissue. Because the emitted signal is weak, repeated emissions are summed over time.

Figure 11.5 shows a sagittal MRI image of [ɑ] taken in the midsagittal plane. The subject held the [ɑ] for 45 seconds to make this image. The vocal tract appears black, as do the teeth, since neither contain water. The marrow in the palate, which is high in water content, and the fat surrounding the head, which is high in hydrogen, are bright white. Although the edges are not as crisp as on CT, they are quite clear and easily measurable. Most recently, fast MRI machines, such as echo planar imaging techniques, allow rapid imaging in a single plane (50–500 ms per image). However, the machine can acquire

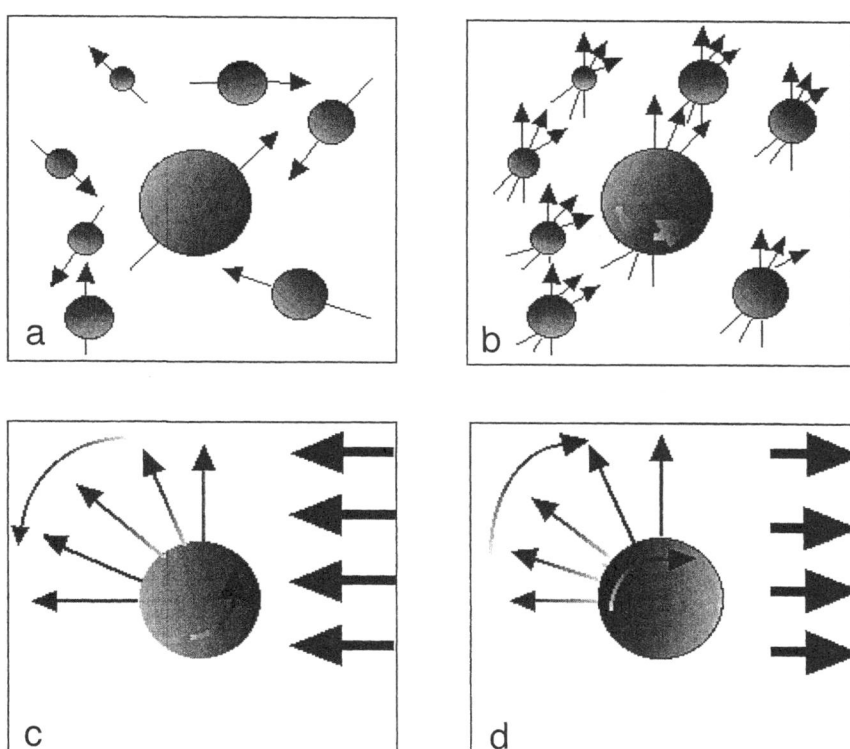

Figure 11.4   Artist's rendition of the effects of MRI scanning on hydrogen protons. a. Hydrogen protons have randomly oriented axes. b. They align to the MRI magnetic field, but with some precession. c. They are knocked out of alignment by a radio wave. d. They return to alignment emitting their own radio signal.

7–10 frames per second. Often, however, the images are composites summed over several repetitions, and the image quality is often poorer when using the short acquisition times.

One drawback of MRI is the width of the section: usually at least 5 mm wide. A tomographic scan compresses a three-dimensional space into two dimensions, like displaying a cylinder as a circle. Therefore, in a slice that is 5 mm wide, items that are 5 mm apart in the cross-sectional plane of the image will appear to be in the same plane. Thus the entire epiglottis may appear in one axial slice blurring the edges and misrepresenting the actual size and shape. A second drawback is that the teeth and bony palate appear black and are not distinguishable from the airspace. Thus, measurements of the tongue

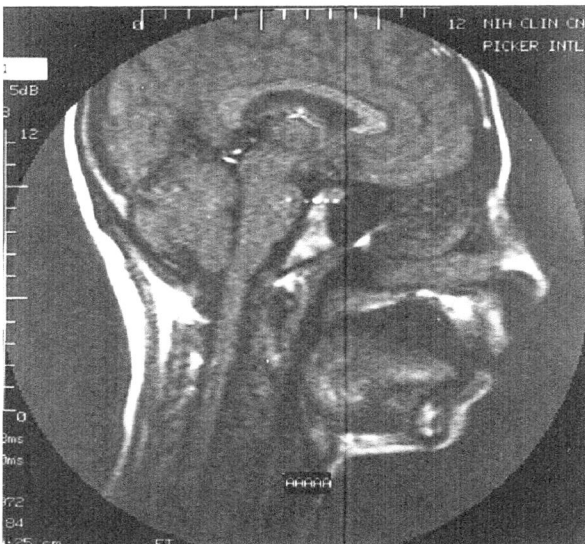

Figure 11.5   MRI image of a midsagittal section of the tongue during the production of [ɑ].

or airspace from an MRI cannot be completely accurate. A final possible drawback for both MRI and CT is that the subject must be lying down, which changes the location of gravity relative to the oral structures. There is no documentation to date on whether this is a problem.

The advantages of MRI and CT are the acquisition of unique and valuable images of the soft and hard tissue of the vocal tract with no obscuration. In addition, MRI technology is advancing rapidly, to allow higher sampling rates.

Ultrasound

The final imaging technique is ultrasound. Ultrasound produces an image by using the reflective properties of sound waves. A piezoelectric crystal stimulated by electric current emits an ultra-high-frequency sound wave. The sound wave travels through soft tissue and reflects back when it reaches an interface with tissue of a different density (like bone) or when it reaches air. In order to see a section of tissue, rather than a single point, multiple crystals sequentially emit sound waves and receive the reflected echoes. The echoes are processed by computer and displayed as a video image (cf. Hedrick, Hykes and Starchman 1995).

For speech research, ultrasound provides excellent studies of the tongue. The transducer is placed below the chin and the beam angled upward to pass through a 2 mm thick slice of the tongue. The sound reflects back from the

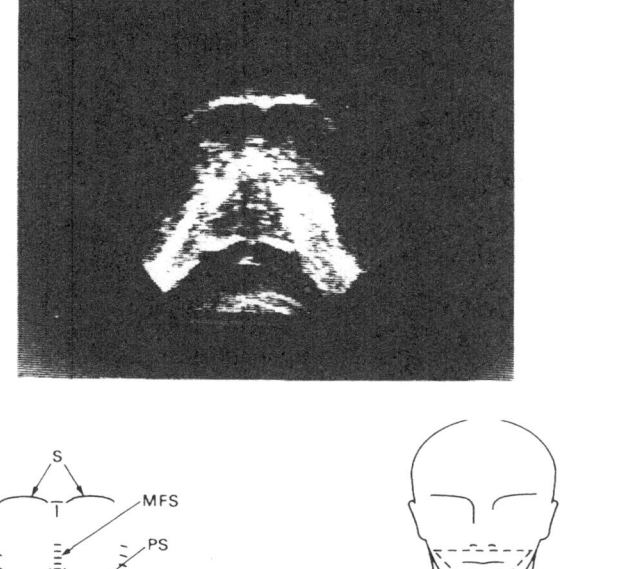

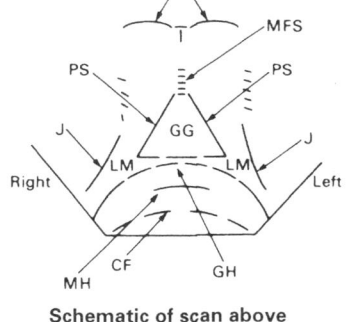

Schematic of scan above

Transducer placement

S, Tongue Surface; GG, Genioglossus;
GH, Geniohyoid; MH, Mylohyoid;
MFS, Median Fibrous Septum;
LM, Lateral Muscles; J, Jaw Inner Aspect;
PS, Paramedian Septum; CF, Cervical Fascia.

Figure 11.6   Ultrasound image of a coronal section of the tongue at rest, a schematic of the structures imaged, and a schematic showing the location and direction of the ultrasound beam (from Stone *et al.* 1988).

air at the surface of the tongue and from intermuscular interfaces within the tongue. Figure 11.6 depicts the coronal (cross-sectional) tongue. The bright white line at the surface of the tongue is the reflection caused by the sound hitting the air. The black area immediately below is the surface tongue mucosa. The interface between the air (white) and the mucosa (black) is the actual surface of the tongue.

Three-dimensional (3D) ultrasound is being developed, and is applicable to speech research. Two approaches are being used. In the first, a three-dimensional transducer collects sixty tissue slices, each one degree apart. The images are then spatially aligned to produce a 3D volume. These reconstructions are quite good (figure 11.7). The transducer takes

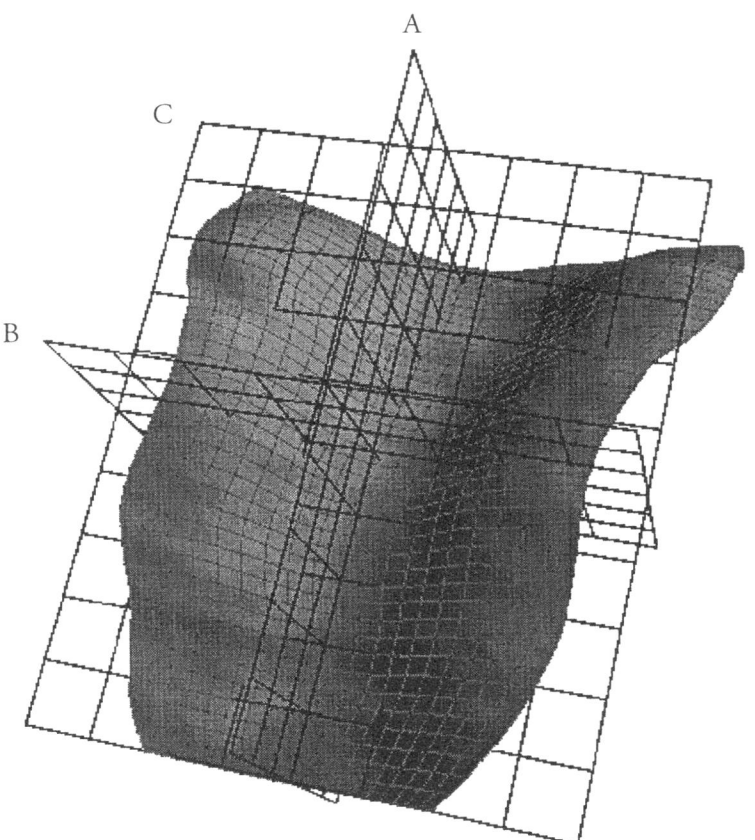

Figure 11.7   Three-dimensional tongue surface reconstruction of the sound [ʃ].

eight to ten seconds to collect all sixty slices, however, so this is not yet a real-time device. The second approach is a transducer holder that positions the transducer in a single plane for a short time, then moves it through a radial arc to several different locations allowing it to collect short-term time-varying data in each plane. The resulting images can be used to make 4D reconstructions, i.e. 3D volumes that move over time, when spatially and temporally aligned.

   The main disadvantage of ultrasound is the inability to see anything but the tongue. The air at the tongue's surface reflects the sound wave, therefore, the palate and posterior pharyngeal wall cannot be seen. The jaw and hyoid bone appear as shadows in the image and cannot be reliably measured. Finally, the tongue tip often is not imaged due to the air beneath it. Ultrasound, however, produces time–motion displays. Scan rate is between thirty and sixty

Table 11.2 *Coarticulatory issues well suited to exploration by imaging techniques.*

- linearity of pattern changes over time
- cross-correlation of interarticulator timing
- stability of movement patterns across repetitions
- left-to-right symmetry of articulator movement
- motor equivalent vocal tract shapes and movements
- coarticulatory effects in non-primary articulators
- articulatory overlap in adjacent and non-adjacent articulators
- fine-tuning existing models of the vocal tract and tongue
- developing new models of vocal tract geometry in motion
- gaining insight into articulator movement strategies, particularly for non-rigid articulators like the tongue and correlated articulators like the tongue and jaw
- visualization of 3D and 4D behaviour

---

scans per second, adequate to image vowels and most consonants in real time. In addition, the tongue surface is easily seen and measured. Moreover, the development of 3D ultrasound makes it the first instrument to provide almost complete 3D tongue-surface data.

Coarticulation

In recent years, theories of coarticulation have begun to merge with theories of speech motor control. This merger is entirely sensible since coarticulation is the result of the execution of speech motor programs. Coarticulation is the interaction of the current articulatory state and its movement to the next state, as determined by task and system constraints (cf. Jordan 1991). Often such theories focus on the timing of events (c.f. Kelso, Saltzman and Tuller 1986). One can, however, examine the patterns of events and changes in those patterns to reveal articulatory organization. Table 11.2 lists coarticulatory issues appropriate for examination using imaging techniques. Very few studies actually have used images, however, to consider coarticulatory effects in speech.

Applications of imaging techniques

One application of imaging techniques to coarticulatory questions is in understanding the relationship between state (position) and movement events. Three-dimensional vocal tract shapes can be reconstructed from 2D MRI, ultrasound or CT images. Time-varying images, such as X-ray and ultrasound, display the effects of starting and ending state on articulatory movement patterns. Several movement features of the CV transition would benefit from image analysis, for example, (i) linearity in the timing of pattern changes during the transition, (ii) regularity of the 2D and 3D movement patterns across repetitions, (iii) left-to-right and central-to-lateral uniformity of pattern change during the transition (cf. Stone, Faber and Cordaro 1991; Stone *et al.* 1992).

A second application of imaging techniques is in studies of motor equivalence. Imaging techniques are especially well suited to such studies, because they can view the vocal tract or tongue as a whole, and can expose difficult-to-observe parts of the pharynx and cross-sectional tongue. Increased completeness of vocal tract movement data will facilitate models of motor equivalence, and the 3D coordinate space used by the vocal tract. The effects of coarticulation on the non-primary articulators can be viewed and may be especially useful in understanding coarticulatory effects on vowels and sonorants for which the entire vocal tract shape is important. For example, Stone and Vatikiotis-Bateson (1995) used ultrasound to document tongue configuration modifications during /i/ that compensated for the lower versus higher jaw positons found in /l/ versus /s/ context.

A third application is in the examination of gestural organization or interarticulator timing. The degree of articulatory overlap in temporally adjacent sounds and its implications for how gestures are organized and how gestures combine ('gestural aggregation') has been seriously considered (Browman and Goldstein 1990a; Löfqvist 1990). Imaging techniques allow these concepts to be examined in terms of global movement patterns and provide more complete articulatory visualization at the point of maximum constriction. For example, an interesting question is whether *area* is the most important feature of the vocal tract constriction, or whether *shape* is important also. This was explored in Stone and Vatikiotis-Bateson's (1995) ultrasound, electropalatography and jaw tracking study, which found that constriction shapes were well described cross-sectionally using two features: shape and openness.

It is clear that different articulators and even different parts of the same articulator, such as the tongue or lips, do not reach maxima at the same time. Some structures do not reach a maximum at all in certain clustered sounds. Thus the notion of a target system configuration, a maximum articulatory position, a target, etc. is more theoretical than physiological. Imaging provides greater perspective in documenting physiological events. For example, does the continuous motion of the tongue during [ilɑ] indicate a lack of shape representation for the [l]? Ultrasound images indicate that this is not the case. Figure 11.8 presents a midsagittal view of the tongue saying [ilɑ]. The tongue profiles are 33 ms apart in time. The /l/ shape is sustained no longer than any of the other shapes intermediate between /i/ and /ɑ/. It is apparent, however,

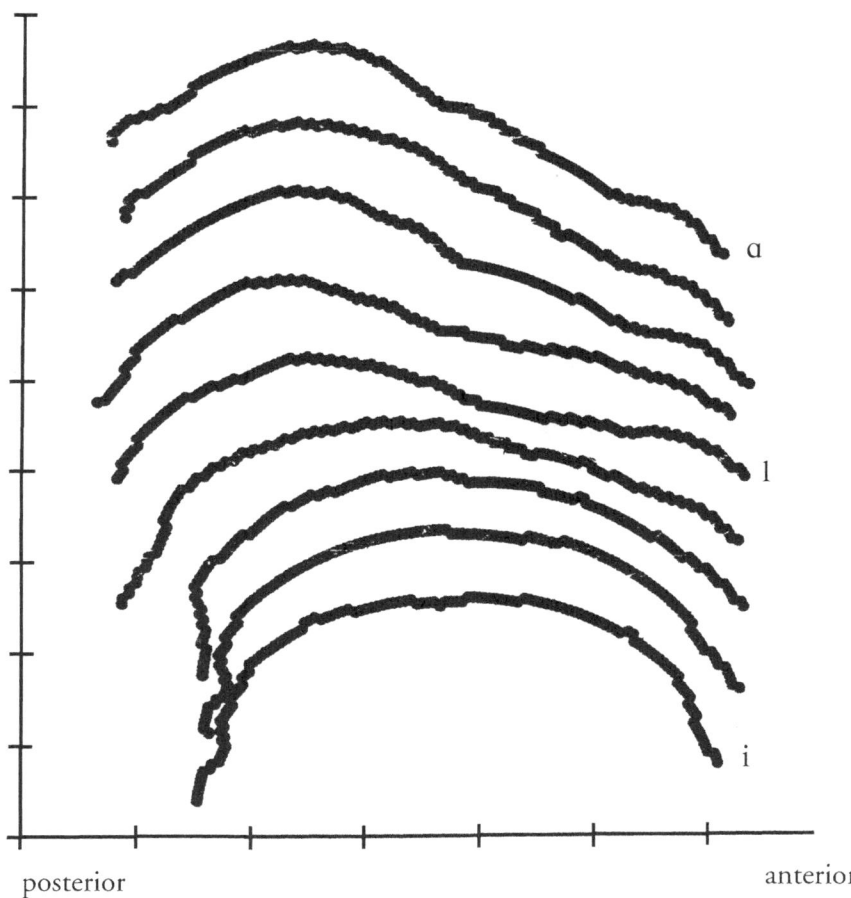

posterior   anterior

Figure 11.8   Sagittal tongue profiles of [ilɑ] measured from midsagittal ultrasound images.

that the /l/ shape is not merely a linear interpolation mid-way between the /i/ and /ɑ/. On the contrary, the /l/ shape has elevated anterior and posterior segments, with a depressed segment between. This shape is quite different from either the /i/ or the /ɑ/. Thus, the phoneme /l/ is represented as a unique shape in the [ila] movement, though not a steady-state target. Tracking two or three points on the tongue surface would not have revealed this so clearly.

A final application for imaging techniques is to gain insight into movement strategies. Two movement strategies are in need of exploration. The first is whether consonants and vowels use tongue–palate interaction in fundamentally different ways. This issue was explored in Stone and Lundberg (1994,

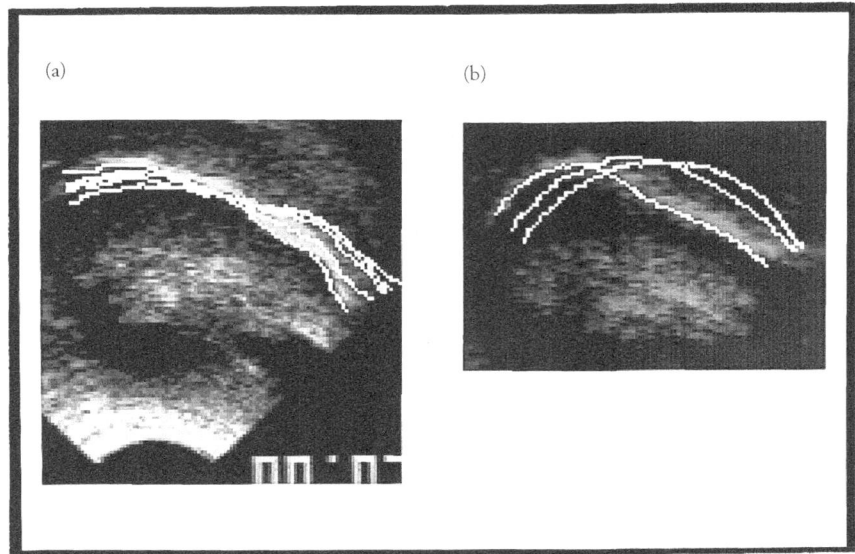

Figure 11.9   Two tongue movement strategies. (a) rotation (b) local displacement
(from Unser and Stone 1992).

1996). Those studies, using electropalatography and 3D ultrasound, found
only four categories of tongue shapes, which included both consonants and
vowels. This limited repertoire of shapes, however, was used differently by
consonants and vowels to create a wide variety of vocal tract shapes as well as
constrictions, obstructions and occlusions.

   The second movement strategy is the use of 'economical' tongue movement patterns, like stiffening and rotating, for executing difficult behaviours.
This question derives from observations of diadochokinetic repetitions of
[tʌtʌ...], [kʌkʌ...], and [tʌkʌtʌkʌ...]. During the first two utterances, an
observable tongue maximum and minimum appear during each syllable.
During repetitions of [tʌkʌ...], however, no minima appear. Instead the
tongue surface stiffens to become level, and rotates from the [t] to the [k], with
the [ʌ] being produced during the transition. That is, the tip elevates and the
dorsum lowers for [t]. The opposite occurs for [k]. There is neither a pause
nor a shape change between the two consonant positions that would suggest
a target for [ʌ]. It would appear that for this rapid, demanding task voicing is
produced during the C-to-C transition with no tongue shape specification.
Front to back tongue rotation also has been observed in CV transitions where
the high point of the tongue shifts from front to back, as in [tɑ] (cf. Stone,
Faber and Cordaro 1991). Figure 11.9 shows (a) rotation and (b) local dis-

placement used as movement strategies by the tongue. These strategies are easily visible because the ultrasound images provide an almost complete representation of the 2D tongue surface.

Summary

Four imaging techniques, X-ray, CT, MRI and ultrasound, are used to image vocal tract behaviour during speech. These techniques can be applied to the study of coarticulation in several ways. First, by providing 2D time-varying and 3D static images of the end states of speech movements in their entirety, or focused on key features such as the vocal tract constriction. Second, by imaging multiple articulators, or completely visualizing a single structure, imaging techniques provide information on gestural organization and motor equivalence. Finally, time-varying images allow in-depth exploration of movement strategies like tongue rotation, and consonant–vowel differences.

12

Electromagnetic articulography

PHILIP HOOLE and NOEL NGUYEN

Introduction

Electromagnetic articulography (EMMA[1]) belongs to the category of transduction device that provides data on the trajectories of articulator fleshpoints in a two-dimensional Cartesian space. It thus provides data comparable to that available from the well-established X-ray microbeam system (cf. Westbury 1994). This contribution reviews some of the methodological issues involved in employing EMMA for phonetic investigations, particularly for studies of coarticulation. On the face of it, EMMA is extremely well suited to the study of coarticulation since it allows a wide range of utterances to be recorded in a single session (sessions of thirty minutes or more being feasible). Moreover, since it provides kinematic data in readily analysable form it should help to remedy one of the most serious failings of instrumental studies of coarticulation to date, namely the small number of subjects per experiment. EMMA is able to monitor the movements on the midsagittal plane of most of the articulatory structures that have been the focus of coarticulatory studies, i.e. lips, jaw, tongue and velum,[2] but it is probably of most interest for the tongue, since for the lips and jaw other well-established techniques are readily available. Currently three main systems are available to individual laboratories: the MIT system (cf. Perkell *et al.* 1992), the AG100 system (Carstens Medizinelektronik, Göttingen, Germany) and the Movetrack system (Botronic, Hägersten, Sweden, cf. Branderud 1985). Various other implementations of the electromagnetic measurement principle have also been reported in the literature (e.g. Hixon 1971; Panagos and Strube 1987; Sonoda and Ogata 1992; Ogata and Sonoda 1994). For more detailed discussion of the issues raised here the reader is referred in particular to Perkell *et al.* (1992) as well as to Gracco (1995) and to the proceedings of a workshop on EMMA collected in FIPKM 31 (= Forschungsberichte des Instituts für Phonetik und Sprachliche Kommunikation, Munich).

The following topics will be covered: measurement principle and sources of error; environmental conditions and combination with other equipment; disturbances to the subjects' speech; safety. A number of issues that are not specific to EMMA but rather are common to fleshpoint tracking systems in general, will not be covered here. These include issues that can in fact be crucial to the interpretability of the data, such as correction for head movement and definition of anatomically based coordinate systems. In addition to the above sources an extremely valuable discussion of these issues is to be found in Westbury (1994). Examples of the analysis of issues relevant to various ramifications of the topic of coarticulation can be found in Hoole, Gfroerer and Tillmann (1990); Katz *et al.* (1990); Perkell (1990); Hoole, Nguyen-Trong and Hardcastle (1993); Kühnert (1993); Keating *et al.* (1994b); Harrington, Fletcher and Roberts (1995); Hoole and Kühnert (1995); Löfqvist and Gracco (1995); Mooshammer, Hoole and Kühnert (1995); Ní Chasaide and Fitzpatrick (1995); Recasens (1995); Romero (1996).

Measurement principle and sources of error

When an alternating magnetic field is generated by a transmitter coil the strength of the signal induced in a transducer (receiver coil) is approximately inversely proportional to the cube of the distance between transmitter and receiver. This basic configuration of a transmitter–receiver pair formed the foundation for the use of magnetometer systems in studies of respiratory kinematics (Hixon, Goldman and Mead 1973), in which the variable of interest is simply the distance between the transmitter and receiver. For studies of tongue movement more information is required, namely the coordinates of the fleshpoints in two-dimensional space. Under ideal conditions, two transmitters would suffice to determine these coordinates by triangulation. Particularly when monitoring tongue movements it is unfortunately the case that ideal conditions do not apply: specifically, the fleshpoint locations are only transduced accurately when the main axes of transmitter and receiver coils are parallel to each other. Misalignment of transmitter and receiver can result from rotation of the receiver coils about either of the two axes shown in figure 12.1 (following Perkell and Cohen 1986, these rotational movements will be referred to as 'twist' and 'tilt' or together as 'rotational misalignment'). When rotational misalignment occurs the effective surface area presented by the receiver coils to the magnetic field is reduced, and the induced signal declines proportional to the cosine of the angle of misalignment; the apparent distance between transmitter and receiver thus increases. Clearly rotational shifts (especially tilt) are to be expected with an organ such as the tongue which is highly deformable and which may be pressed against the vaulted shape of the hard palate.

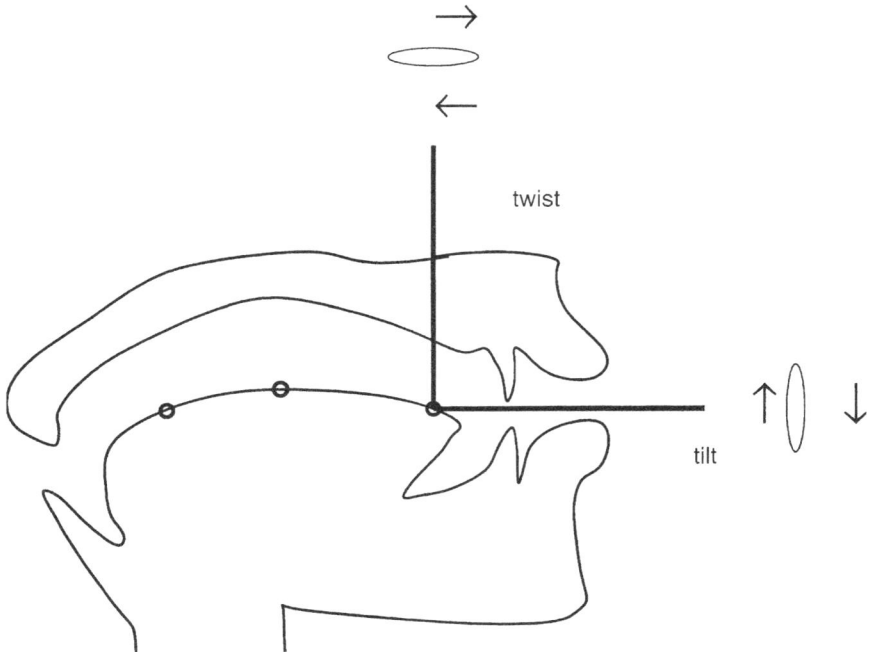

Figure 12.1   Rotational axes of magnetometer sensors that lead to a reduction in the induced signal for typical sensor locations on the tongue.

Since van der Giet (1977) pointed out this problem various solutions have been tried. In this chapter we will concentrate on the approach followed in the current MIT system[3] (Perkell *et al.* 1992) and in the commercially available AG100, both systems being based on a solution developed by a group in Göttingen (Höhne *et al.* 1987; Schönle *et al.* 1987; Schönle 1988; Schönle, Müller and Wenig 1989). The idea is essentially that the use of a third transmitter provides the additional information needed to determine and correct for the rotational misalignment. For the amount of misalignment likely to be encountered in speech, the problem can be considered resolved (see e.g. Perkell *et al.* 1992). There remains, however, the less tractable problem of errors caused by displacement of the transducers out of the plane on which the transmitters are located (usually the mid-line). Due to the curvature of the lines of magnetic flux, this will have an effect somewhat similar to rotational misalignment since the axis of the transducer is no longer parallel to the lines of flux (see figure 5 in Perkell *et al.* 1992; cf. also Gracco and Nye 1993). Published tests of both the MIT and the AG100 system agree in showing a sharp rise in measurement error when off-midline placement is combined with rotational misalignment (see e.g. Schönle, Müller and Wenig 1989; Perkell *et al.* 1992; Honda and Kaburagi 1993). For example, Honda and Kaburagi found for the AG100 system about 1.5 to 2 mm of error with 5 mm displacement from the mid-line and twenty degrees of twist, increasing to 4 mm of error with 10 mm of displacement and a further increase to 10 mm of error for 20 mm of displacement and twenty degrees of both twist and tilt. Perkell *et al.* (1992) summarized the results for the MIT system (which appears slightly less sensitive to this source of error than the AG100) as showing that the error should remain below 1 mm as long as displacement is less than 5 mm and misalignment less than twenty degrees.

Thus great care must be taken to place the transducers on the mid-line and measurements with large amounts of rotational misalignment may well need to be discarded.[4] (An additional consideration, compounding the off-mid-line problem, is that monitoring the angle of rotational misalignment to detect unreliable data is itself less reliable when the sensors are not mounted on the mid-line.) One must further be able to assume that the tongue does not show substantial lateral deviations during articulation, which may not be justified for some pathological populations. Complete resolution of these problems will only be achieved if a full 3–D system proves feasible (cf. Branderud, McAllister and Kassling 1993; Zierdt 1993). On condition, however, that appropriate precautions in experimental technique are taken (e.g. Perkell *et al.* 1992; Alfonso *et al.* 1993; Hoole 1993b) then the problems are clearly not an insuperable obstacle to acquiring valid data of the kind typically required in coarticulation experiments.

Having discussed the main problems we now summarize the accuracy to be expected from such systems. For the MIT system, which is the one most extensively tested to date, the accuracy approaches 0.5 mm over a range of measurement positions sufficient to capture the main speech articulators (Perkell *et al.* 1992). It was initially not possible to demonstrate this level of accuracy so convincingly for the AG100 (cf. Schönle, Müller and Wenig 1989; Tuller, Shao and Kelso 1990; Honda and Kaburagi 1993) but work by Hoole (1993b, 1996) suggests that this may be largely due to the fact that calibration hardware and software was originally much less sophisticated for the AG100 than for the MIT system. Finally, Nguyen and Marchal (1993) report a clearly acceptable level of accuracy for the Movetrack system, at least for non-misaligned conditions. Two further points must be made here, however.

Firstly, it is important to be clear about the kind of accuracy required in any given experiment (cf. Perkell *et al.* 1992: 3085–6). The accuracy referred to above can be designated 'absolute accuracy'. This kind of accuracy is relevant if one is interested in measuring the distance between, say the tongue and the hard palate. In coarticulatory studies one will often be more concerned with relative accuracy, in other words the accuracy in transducing *differences* in the position of a point on the tongue as a function of context. Relative accuracy will generally be better than absolute accuracy, if, as will often be the case, error vectors do not change much within the small portion of the measurement field to which a single fleshpoint is restricted (typically an area of no more than two by two centimetres). Relative accuracy may also still be quite good at large angles of rotational misalignment, as long as the misalignment stays fairly constant. If one is simply interested in timing as opposed to spatial measurements then the demands on accuracy are probably even less stringent (for example, the transillumination technique is known to give valid information on laryngeal timing, even though the signal cannot be calibrated, cf. chapter 15 in this volume).

The second point to make is that while there has been fairly extensive bench testing of magnetometer systems, there have been few direct attempts to validate performance during actual speech utterances (see Hoole 1993b, for an indirect assessment of the plausibility of EMMA data, based on comparison with EPG data). For monitoring the tongue, the most direct approach to date is to be found in work by Honda and Kaburagi (1993) comparing simultaneous ultrasound and EMMA (AG100) transduction of tongue configuration. The difference between the position of the tongue measured magnetically and ultrasonically averaged out at slightly over 1 mm. This is of the order of the estimated measurement error for the ultrasound and EMMA system and may be regarded as fairly satisfactory, particularly as Honda and Kaburagi used only a simple technique for calibrating the EMMA system. In addition, reconstruction of complete tongue contours from the four EMMA transducers on the tongue also gave satisfactory results. Recently, Hertrich and Ackermann (1997) found very close agreement between the results from a passive optical system and simultaneously acquired data from the AG100 when monitoring movement of upper and lower lip.

Environmental conditions and combinations with other equipment

As discussed by Gracco and Nye (1993) the user needs to pay careful attention to any sources of electromagnetic interference (e.g. computer screens) whenever a new installation of a magnetometer system is carried out. Our own experience suggests that a stable ambient temperature and generous warm-up time are advisable.

The question of environmental conditions leads on to the issue of what other instrumental procedures can be combined with EMMA without resulting in unacceptable levels of mutual electromagnetic interference. Both Schönle (1988: 23, using a forerunner of the AG100) and Perkell *et al.* (1992, using the older MIT two-transmitter system) report no problems in combining EMMA and EMG. The AG100 has been successfully combined with ultrasound (Honda and Kaburagi, see above) and with EPG (Hoole 1993b; Rouco and Recasens 1996), though the latter authors do note that EMMA sensors can cause some (probably) recoverable 'excavation' of EPG patterns on the mid-line. Informal tests in our laboratory suggest no major interference between the optoelectronic SELSPOT system and the AG100; however, Kaburagi (personal communication) has noted interference between the AG100 and a different optoelectronic device (Hamamatsu Photonics); similarly the OPTOTRAK system is reported to cause interference in the MIT EMMA system (Vatikiotis-Bateson, personal communication). The AG100 interferes massively with the laryngograph signal at the transmitter frequencies, but appropriate filtering of the laryngograph signal would probably eliminate this problem.

This indicates that many useful combinations are feasible. However, since the different EMMA systems operate at different frequencies and power levels, unproblematic combinations with one EMMA system may not prove so with another one.

Interference with subjects' articulation

The situation here can be considered comparable to the X-ray microbeam system since the EMMA sensors are roughly the same size (i.e. about 3 to 4 mm square and 2 to 3 mm high) as the microbeam pellets. The latter have not generally been considered an undue source of disturbance. The authors' own experience (see also Perkell *et al.* 1992: 3081) suggests that subjects feel irritated if a transducer on the tongue is placed closer than about 1 cm to the tongue tip (it is also important to run lead wires out of the side of the mouth, rather than over the tongue tip). Thus for details of tongue tip articulation EMMA may need supplementing by techniques such as EPG (cf. Hoole 1993b). A simultaneous combination of EMMA and EPG did, however, result in distortion of fricative articulation in one subject reported on in Hoole, Nguyen-Trong and Hardcastle (1993). There remains a need for comparative acoustic analysis of speech sounds produced with and without EMMA transducers in place, especially for sounds such as fricatives.

Safety

The possibility of harmful effects from long-term exposure to electromagnetic radiation is a matter of ongoing public concern. The

International Radiation Protection Association has published (1990, see also Bernhardt 1988) a set of guidelines on exposure to magnetic fields. However, it is important to note that in the absence of conclusive evidence of long-term effects, the exposure limits set out therein were related to magnetic field strengths known to cause *immediate* biological effects. The basic criterion used was the current density occurring naturally in the human body. This is of the order of 10 mA/m^2. Magnetic fields inducing current densities of this order correspond to the exposure level at which demonstrable biological effects start occurring. At current densities of the order of 100 above this criterion level acute danger to health can be expected (e.g. cardiac malfunction). The magnetic flux density expected to induce the criterion current density of 10 mA/m^2 is 5 mT (milliTeslar). The IRPA recommendation (for 50/60Hz fields) is that occupational exposure at this level is permissible for up to two hours per day. The limit for continuous occupational exposure is set at 0.5 mT and the limit for continuous exposure of the general public is set at 0.1 mT. By way of comparison, average household levels have been estimated to be in the range up to 1 µT, though some household appliances (e.g. hair-dryers) can generate substantially stronger fields (up to 1 mT). It should be reiterated that the above limits refer to immediate biological effects. If adverse effects of long-term exposure to weak magnetic fields are demonstrated, then a substantial downward revision of these limits may be required.

For users of EMMA systems one problem is that there is little research targeted specifically at the frequency ranges at which these devices operate. As discussed by Perkell *et al.* (1992) the most relevant source of epidemiological information is probably from studies of long-term exposure to computer terminals, since one of the main frequency components in the latter, namely the horizontal line frequency, is comparable to the frequencies found in EMMA systems. Perkell *et al.* give the field strength to which the subject is exposed in the three-transmitter MIT system as 0.163 µT and have found this to be comparable to a typical computer terminal. Field strengths of this order have also been reported for Movetrack. No measurements of field strengths in the AG100 have been published but they are clearly higher than in the MIT system and have been estimated (A. Zierdt, personal communication) to be of the order of 10 µT. Recent measurements made by M. Hasegawa-Johnson at UCLA indicate that a slightly higher figure may be more realistic. These findings are available as an internet document (http://pc241.icsl.ucla.edu/emma/report-nomu.html) which includes an excellent discussion of the relevant biophysical background. Currently there are no grounds for disquiet but it is probably advisable to avoid pregnant subjects and wearers of pace-makers (Bernhardt 1988: 23) and to remain alert to further epidemiological findings in this area.

Illustration of coarticulatory effects

Finally, an illustration of the kind of coarticulatory effects that can be observed with a typical magnetometer experimental set-up is given in figure 12.2. This shows the influence of symmetric flanking consonants on tongue configuration for the two vowels /eː/ and /ɛ/.[5] Note, for example, that the areas of the ellipses enclosing all data points for a given fleshpoint are generally larger for the short vowel /ɛ / (figure 12.2, bottom) than for the long vowel /eː/ (figure 12.2, top). This is probably a straightforward effect of the shorter vowel overlapping more with the flanking consonants, and thus showing stronger contextual influences. A more interesting contextual effect which is common to both vowels (and which to our knowledge has not previously been pointed out in the literature) is that fleshpoints on the anterior part of the tongue (refer especially to the front three sensors in figure 12.2) may well be located more *posteriorly* in /t/-context than in /k/-context, even though we customarily think of /t/ as being articulated further forward than /k/. The explanation may be that the tongue body has to retract somewhat to give the tongue tip room to elevate for the alveolar articulation of /t/.

Thus, use of the magnetometer helps to make it clear that there can still be much to learn about the organization of even very simple sound sequences recorded, as here, within what is undoubtedly one of the commonest paradigms for examining coarticulatory effects.

Notes

1 We will use the abbreviation introduced by Perkell *et al.* (1992) for the Massachusetts Institute of Technology system. The second m stands for 'midsagittal'.

2 Application of the transducers to the velum may require sutures (see Engelke and Schönle 1991) rather than surgical glue.

3 An alternative approach followed in an earlier MIT system was to use two transmitters and a more complicated bi-axial receiver (Perkell and Cohen 1986; Perkell *et al.* 1992).

4 We have been assuming here that correction for rotational misalignment is essential for transducing tongue movements accurately. In fact, not much information is actually available on how much a transducer on the tongue changes its alignment during actual speech utterances. Hoole (1993b) has found a typical standard deviation of about three degrees in the course of an utterance for transducers on the tongue. Assuming a corresponding range of about +/− 2.5 standard deviations (i.e. fifteen degrees) this agrees well with Branderud, McAllister and Kassling

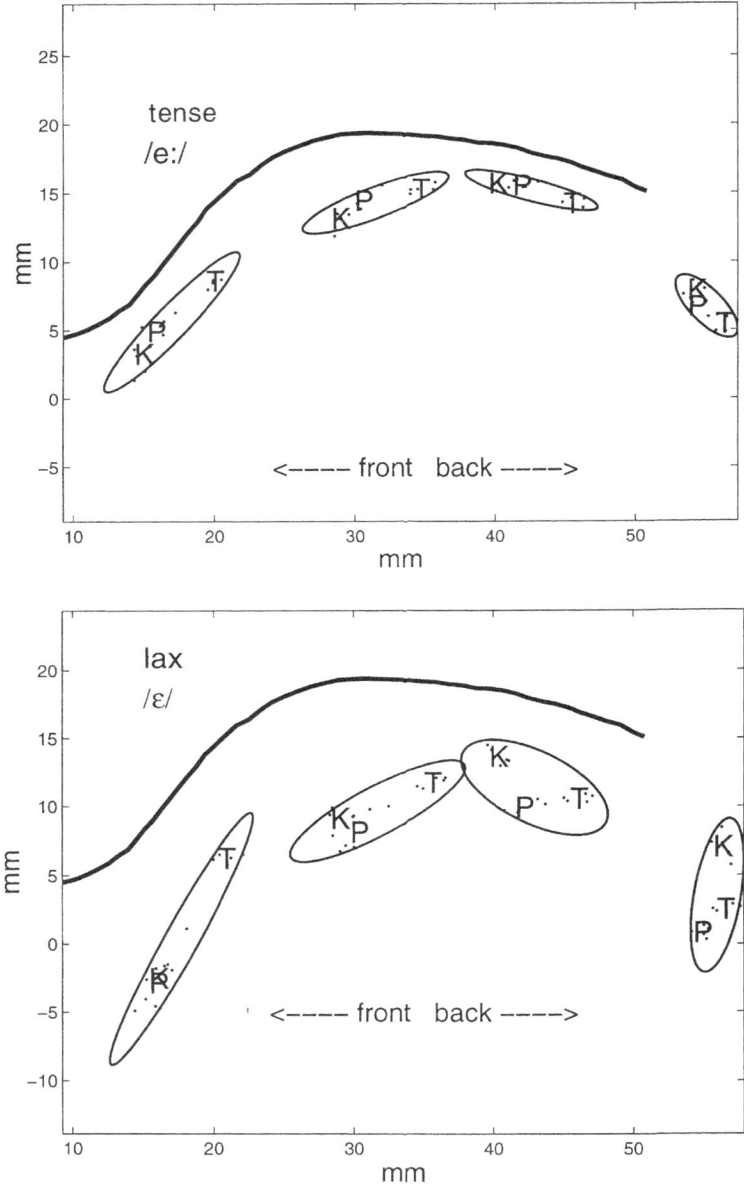

Figure 12.2   Positions of four fleshpoints on the tongue for the German tense–lax vowel pair /eː/ (top) and /ɛ/ (bottom) in the three consonantal contexts /p/, /t/ and /k/ (averaged over approximately five tokens per consonant). Ellipses enclose two-sigma areas of variation over all tokens and contexts at each fleshpoint. The contour of the hard palate is also shown

(1993) who have estimated that the tilt angle for a set of Swedish vowels covers a range of about fifteen degrees in both static and dynamic conditions. Branderud, McAllister and Kassling (1993) discuss the conditions under which it might be possible to assume that the two-transmitter Movetrack system (i.e. without compensation for rotational alignment) also gives an accurate picture of lingual articulation.

5 See Hoole and Kühnert (1995) for further discussion of patterns of contextual (coarticulatory) and token-to-token variability in the realization of the German vowel system.

13

Electromyography

WILLIAM J. HARDCASTLE

Introduction

Most of the techniques discussed in these chapters are designed to record, directly or indirectly, movements of the various respiratory, laryngeal or supralaryngeal (articulatory) structures involved in the production of speech. However, there is considerable interest also amongst speech scientists in the underlying neuromuscular control mechanisms that make such movements possible, the patterns of contraction and relaxation in the various muscles and muscle groups and the electrical discharges that accompany such contractions. It is these changes in electrical activity within muscles which the technique of electromyography (EMG) aims to record. Although the simple detection of electrical changes in muscles as they increase in tension is a relatively straightforward process, the interpretation of the records of such changes in terms of the functions of particular muscles and the resultant movements of speech organs is extremely complex and far from straightforward. This brief outline of EMG techniques discusses the various components of the EMG system (the types of electrodes, amplification, recording apparatus), signal processing techniques used in data reduction, the type of research that can be carried out with the technique into aspects of both normal and pathological speech and the general problems associated with the use of EMG for speech research purposes. Before discussing the technique itself, however, it is useful to outline the main neuromuscular features of muscle activity as background for interpreting the electromyogram.

Traditionally, the main functional unit of muscle activity is called the motor unit which consists of a single motoneuron and the group of muscle fibres which it innervates. The motoneuron consists of a cell body and a long process called the axon the branches of which terminate at each muscle fibre within a muscle at a specialized junction called a motor end-plate.

When the motoneuron is activated by the higher centres of the brain, neural impulses in the form of tiny electrical charges travel along the axon and impinge on all the end-plates roughly simultaneously, there releasing a chemical substance called acetycholine. The resultant chemical change has the effect of depolarizing the muscle fibre or more precisely, it changes the muscle fibre membrane from a resting potential of −70 mV to a positive 20 mV. For more details of the complex electrochemical changes at the neuromuscular juncture see MacLean (1980) and Basmajian and De Luca (1985). After a delay of about 1 ms from the arrival of the neural impulse, the depolarization spreads along the muscle fibre in both directions at velocities up to 4 m per second and may last for as long as 9 ms. This is the so-called 'action potential' and it generates an electromagnetic field in the vicinity of the activated muscle fibre. An electrode placed in the vicinity of this electromagnetic field will detect a potential or voltage change (with respect to ground). In the technique of EMG usually two electrodes are used and the aim is to record the difference in electrical potential between these electrodes. If they are placed in close proximity within a muscle, such that the two electrodes are in parallel to the muscle fibres that make up a whole muscle, a recorded discharge will represent a number of single muscle fibre action potentials.

The shape and amplitude of the discharge will be dependent on a number of factors including: the position of the electrode in relation to the geometry of the muscle fibres; properties of the muscle and other tissue; characteristics of the detecting electrode and its associated instrumentation (e.g. filtering properties).

The action potential causes a mechanical change in the muscle fibre (called a 'twitch') and the result of this is for the muscle to shorten in length sometimes by as much as 57%. It is changes in length such as this in the thousands of muscle fibres that make up any given muscle that are the basis for most movements of the speech organs. In normal muscle contraction, the neural impulses arrive sufficiently fast (e.g. at frequencies of 50 Hz but some may be very much higher, e.g. 280 Hz, MacNeilage, Sussman and Powers 1977) so that each individual twitch merges into the next thus creating a smoothing effect (called tetanus).

Muscle fibres of motor units tend to be randomly distributed throughout a sub-section of normal muscle and to intermingle with fibres belonging to different motor units. Thus the output from an EMG electrode may not represent the unique firing from a single motor unit but a complex pattern with components from a number of different motor units even some belonging to different muscles. This is particularly likely in the case of some of the speech muscles such as the intrinsic tongue muscles which are characterized by a great deal of interdigitation of fibres from adjacent muscles. Another complicating factor in interpreting EMG traces is that the motor units themselves are differently distributed throughout the muscle; in some parts of the muscle they may be considerably denser than at others. Because they also differ in the size of the cell body, the diameter of the axon and the properties of the muscle fibres, they have different thresholds to excitation; some will fire earlier than others and in some the electrical potential lasts longer. Maintaining an orderly recruitment of motor units throughout the muscle is one of the ways in which a smooth graded contraction of the muscle can take place, rather than an abrupt on–off mechanical effect which would result if all motor units in a muscle fired simultaneously.

Increased tension in a muscle may be brought about by three main mechanisms: (i) by increasing the firing frequency in the motor units themselves; (ii) by activating increasing numbers of motor units throughout the muscle (the principle of 'recruitment') and (iii) by synchronous firing of different motor units (occurring in extremely strong contractions or in fatigue in normal muscle resulting in augmented recorded potential, duration and amplitude (Herberts 1969; Hirano 1981). It has been suggested that gross control of muscle may be exercised by motor unit recruitment and fine control by firing frequency (Abbs and Watkin 1976). Also small muscles may rely on firing rate and larger muscles predominantly on recruitment (Basmajian and De Luca 1985: 167). These different mechanisms by which muscle tension can develop are of considerable importance in the interpretation of electromyograms as each may be reflected in patterns of EMG activity.

Increased tension in a muscle can have a variety of mechanical effects depending on a whole complex of factors. These include the relatively constant inherent characteristics of the muscle itself (e.g. the muscle architecture, arrangement of fibres, etc., and mechanical properties of the tissues) as well as the changing external conditions that prevail at any given time (e.g. temperature, metabolic rate changes, length of the muscle fibres, firing history of particular fibres, etc.; see full discussion in Blair and Muller 1987, for the periorial system). External conditions affecting muscles will be changing constantly in activities such as speech. For example, if one end of a muscle is fixed, increased tension in the muscle will result in shortening which moves the origin of the muscle towards its insertion. If, however, external resistance is applied to one end of the muscle acting in the opposite direction, depending on the magnitude of the external force, the movement of the muscle may be restricted. If the external resistance is equal to the force developed in the muscle no movement will take place (isometric tension). Anisometric tension will develop in the muscle if the external resistance is greater or smaller than the muscle force.

Comprehensive models of the transference of bioelectric to mechanical energy are not yet available for the cranial nerve muscle system, although such models are desirable if we are to interpret EMG patterns in a maximally meaningful way.

When interpreting tension changes in muscles in terms of movements of speech organs we need to consider more than the mechanical constraints mentioned above; we need to take account also of the variety of functions a given tension change can fulfil depending on the external forces operating on a muscle at any given time, and the desired effect the movement is to have. In achieving a desired speech movement, a number of different muscles may be involved, each contributing in some way to the overall target movement. The functional names given to these muscles are usually prime movers (or agonists), antagonists, fixators and synergists. Agonist muscles are primarily responsible for achieving the movement of an organ in a prescribed direction. Antagonists may be inhibited from activity during contraction of the prime-mover or they may actively contract to oppose the movement thus contributing to a balanced, controlled movement. Fixator muscles provide a stable fixed base from which other muscles can contract. Synergists may contract to assist the prime-mover in effecting a particular movement.

The problems facing the experimenter in interpreting an EMG pattern in terms of muscle activity are therefore considerable. It is extremely difficult to attribute a particular EMG output to a function in a given muscle and even more difficult to infer movement of a speech organ from such an output. Ideally the EMG recording should be accompanied by some direct monitoring of the speech organ or organs under investigation and the recorded electrical activity should be interpreted in the light of the movement data and within a framework of biomechanical constraints operating in the system.

The beginnings of a comprehensive biomechanical framework for physiological research on human perioral muscles has already been offered recently in the literature (see e.g. Abbs and Eilenberg 1976; Blair and Smith 1986; Blair and Muller 1987; Folkins *et al.* 1988; Wohlert and Goffman 1994) and there is an urgent need to extend this comprehensive approach to other speech organs.

The technique of electromyography

EMG is commonly used in physiology, particularly in the diagnosis of a wide range of pathological neuromuscular conditions. For speech purposes, probably the first well known EMG work was by Stetson and Hudgens (1930) but many researchers since have recognized the potential of the technique for gaining greater insight into the complex control mechanisms used in the speech production process (see reviews in Fromkin and Ladefoged 1966; Gay and Harris 1971; Abbs and Watkin 1976; Hirano 1981; Baken 1987). In general, unlike physiologists, speech researchers are not so interested in the characteristics of single motor units, although these are important for identifying pathological conditions, for example vocal fold pathologies (see Hirano 1981). They are interested more in the timing of EMG activity in relation to movements of particular speech organs and the relationship between EMG patterns and specific speech sounds or prosodic effects. Typical questions are, for example: which muscles contribute to a particular speech movement (but note the difficulties as mentioned above); when does electrical activity in a muscle begin and cease in relation to a speech gesture; what is the time interval between onset of EMG activity and peak amplitude of the signal during a speech gesture; does the electrical activity undergo relative changes with corresponding changes in movement patterns? These questions are very relevant to the instrumental study of coarticulation and the technique has been widely used for the investigation of this phenomenon (see e.g. Mansell 1973; Gay 1981; Sussman and Westbury 1981; Lubker and Gay 1982; Gracco 1988; Boyce 1990; Honda, Kusakawa and Kakita 1992).

EMG electrodes

A crucial part of the EMG system is the electrode which detects electrical potentials in active muscle fibres. The size and type of available electrode varies considerably and the choice will depend largely on the purpose of the investigation (for fuller descriptions of electrodes and their characteristics, see Geddes 1972; Basmajian and De Luca 1985).

There are three main types of electrodes in current use: needle electrodes, hooked-wire, and surface electrodes. Most speech research involves the use of either hooked-wire or surface types.

Hooked-wire electrodes are fine wires usually of platinum–iridium alloy (diameter in the region of 0.002 in) inserted into the body of the muscle by means of a hypodermic needle, following local anaesthetic. Small hooks in the end of the wires retain the position in the muscle. For a detailed description of the preparation and insertion of hooked wire electrodes see Basmajian and Stecko (1962) and Hirose (1971). Folkins *et al.* (1988) use two separate needles for insertion to ensure electrodes are 4 mm apart. This distance they have found most suitable for monitoring action potentials from the perioral musculature. At the end of the study the hooked wire can be removed with a firm steady pull on the wires.

Most of the speech muscles have been investigated with hooked-wire electrodes, including relatively inaccessible muscles such as the velopharyngeal muscles (e.g. Bell-Berti 1976; Kuehn and Moon 1994), the laryngeal muscles (e.g. Hirose 1977; Hirano 1981; Hoole in chapter 15 of this volume) and the tongue muscles (e.g. Bole 1965; Baer, Alfonso and Honda 1988). The periorial muscles, particularly the orbicularis oris muscle of the lips, have also been extensively studied (see e.g. Leanderson, Persson and Öhman 1971; Gay and Hirose 1973; Abbs and Eilenberg 1976; Kennedy and Abbs 1979; Blair and Muller 1987; Folkins *et al.* 1988). One of the major problems associated with hooked-wire electrodes, as with all systems of EMG is the problem of where to place the electrodes to ensure the particular muscle under investigation is in fact being recorded. Most of the muscles used in speech particularly those in the velopharyngeal and laryngeal region are relatively inaccessible and lie deep within the speech organs themselves. The investigator must rely on current knowledge concerning the detailed anatomy of the region and his/her own intuition and experience in placing the electrode. Various quite detailed verification procedures have been devised for different speech structures such as the lips (Kennedy and Abbs 1979; O'Dwyer *et al.* 1981; Smith *et al.* 1985), the larynx (Hirose 1971; Hirano 1981) and the soft palate (Bell-Berti 1973). The usual procedure is to insert the electrodes into the region where the investigator thinks the target muscle is located then confirm the placement by having the subject carry out some activity thought to consistently involve contraction of the target muscles (see Shipp, Fishman and Morrisey 1970). For example, verification of placement in the cricothyroid muscle would occur if a steadily rising EMG pattern accompanies a rise in pitch (Hirano and Ohala 1969). One of the main problems, however, with the verification procedures is the lack of detailed anatomical descriptions of the speech musculature and the lack of suitably comprehensive models of the sorts of biomechanical constraints operating on the systems under investigation. In referring to the labial musculature, Folkins *et al.* (1988) in fact claim that the need to relate activity to traditionally defined muscles may not be as important as knowing the functional constraints on activity in different parts of the speech producing systems. The problems with verification make it even more important to monitor movement patterns of the organs along with the EMG signals.

There are a number of disadvantages associated with the use of hooked-wire electrodes:

- although discomfort is minor, subjects nevertheless usually are aware of the presence of the electrodes and this may affect the naturalness of their speech;
- specialist knowledge is needed for the insertion procedure, for example, an intensive and detailed knowledge of the anatomy of the

region for accurate placement, avoidance of blood vessels etc. The need for specialist medical personnel makes the technique less suitable for the average speech research laboratory;

- there are difficulties in verifying placement of the electrodes and possible biasing of the results due to the specific verification procedure adopted (see above);
- although the positions of the electrodes in the muscle are relatively fixed some migration may take place, particularly during rapid, strong contractions. Basmajian and De Luca (1985: 34) suggest such migration is particularly likely during the first few contractions of a muscle after insertion. They advise contracting and relaxing the muscle six times before any measurements are made to stabilize the electrodes. But changes in position are still possible in the course of a recording session and such changes may affect the amplitude of the detected signal by as much as 75%. Possible minor shifts in position, also, make it extremely difficult to relate the recorded signal to individual motor units.

Hooked-wire electrodes can record signals from individual motor units identified as spikes in the pattern. Gross muscle activity represented by signals from a large number of motor units can be detected by another type of electrode – surface electrodes. Surface electrodes are thus useful when an indication of the response of the muscle as a whole is required (Cooper 1965). There are many different types of surface electrodes but three types are most commonly used for speech research purposes (see Blair and Smith 1986; Baken 1987):

- commercially available types in the shape of small silver cups (e.g. outside diameter 4 mm): a hole in the top allows the insertion of electrode jelly which comes in contact with the skin. They adhere to the skin with special adhesive paper or are cemented on with adhesive;
- suction type developed by Haskins Laboratories (Harris *et al.* 1964) specially for use in the oral region on structures such as the tongue which pose considerable problems of adhesion. They are made from hollow silver jewellery beads connected to a vacuum manifold. The suction keeps them in place and they have been used on many structures including the tongue, posterior pharyngeal wall, anterior and posterior faucal pillars, anterior and posterior palate;
- paint-on-type (Allen, Lubker and Harrison 1972) primarily for use on the facial muscles. They are made from a mixture of 10 g of silver powder suspended in 10 g of Duco cement thinned with a few millilitres of

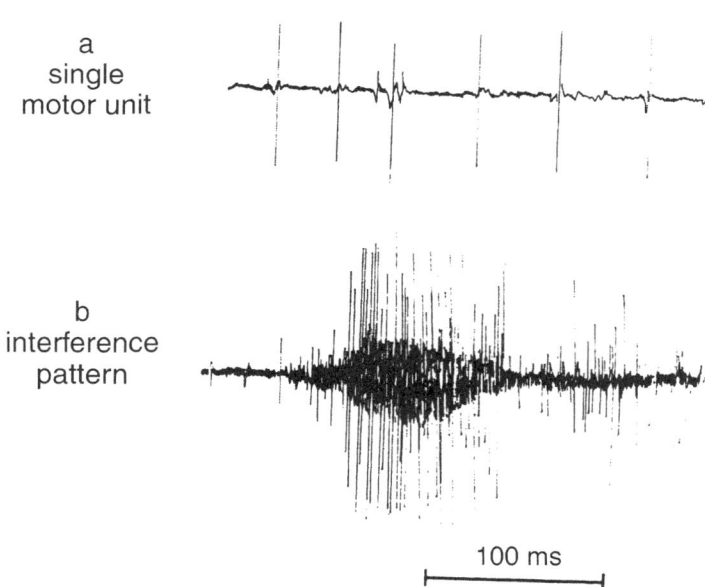

a
single
motor unit

b
interference
pattern

100 ms

Figure 13.1 Two records of electrical activity recorded with a hooked-wire electrode from the mentalis muscle:
a firing of a single motor unit during minimal voluntary contraction
b interference pattern recorded during production of the utterance [æpæ] (from Abbs and Watkin 1976: 45).

acetone to form a paste. The mixture is painted in small daubs on the skin and a fine 38–40 gauge wire sandwiched between two layers of the paste. In general their performance is not as good as cups (Basmajian and De Luca 1985) but they are far less obtrusive and thus offer some advantages for speech research purposes.

With most types of surface electrodes it is advisable to reduce the electrical insulation between the electrode and the skin by (a) continuing pressure of contact (e.g. by using a strip of surgical tape), (b) by using a saline electrode jelly and (c) by removing the dead surface layer of skin and any protective oils by light abrasion (e.g. with an eraser) prior to electrode placement.

Because of their relatively large area, surface electrodes are suitable for recording responses from a relatively large number of motor units in a muscle and from muscles immediately below the electrodes. This response from a number of motor units is usually called an 'interference' pattern and it is extremely difficult to identify single motor unit responses in such a pattern (see figure 13.1). As the muscle tension increases, as mentioned above, more and more motor units are recruited and this increasing recruitment is reflected in the interference pattern by an overall increase in the amplitude of the response. EMG recordings from surface electrodes are thus useful when the response from a substantial part of a muscle is required. Often such a response can be more indicative of the activity of the muscle as a whole than the response of a single motor unit in a particular muscle.

There are a number of advantages of surface electrodes over hooked-wire and needle electrodes:

- they are easy to apply and need no specialist knowledge in their application;
- they are painless and non-invasive and are therefore quite suitable for children who normally will not tolerate needles;
- they are normally not so susceptible to interference from radio, power lines, etc., so there is no need for special shielding (see below).

Extensive research has been carried out by phoneticians using surface electrodes to record responses from a range of speech organs, primarily the lips (Wohlert and Goffman 1994), the soft palate (e.g. Lubker 1968) and the tongue (e.g. MacNeilage 1963). However, there are considerable limitations in using surface electrodes in EMG (Eblen 1963; Basmajian and De Luca 1985). These are:

- the pick-up is very widespread and it is extremely difficult to interpret the response pattern in terms of specific activity in a given muscle. However, as Wohlert and Goffman (1994) point out, it may be more productive to describe the aggregate activity of motor units in a given area, for example, in the perioral region, than attempting to describe the activity of a single muscle;
- the technique is restricted to the investigation of superficial muscles only such as the orbicularis oris, superior longitudinal muscle of the tongue, etc., and is quite unsuitable for investigating deeper placed muscles e.g. intrinsic laryngeal muscles;
- there are practical difficulties in attaching the electrodes onto moist intra oral surfaces. Special adhesives are necessary (see Allen, Lubker and Turner 1973) or special instrumentation to provide suction (see the above mentioned Haskins technique, Harris *et al.* 1964);
- the impedance may vary considerably during an experiment giving variable results when amplified and displayed.

Basmajian (1973: 508) summarizes the disadvantages thus: 'We must condemn the exclusive use of surface electrodes to study fine movements, deep muscles, the presence or absence of activity in various postures and in short, in any circumstances where precision is desirable.' For many purposes in speech research such precision is not required: the aim frequently being to record simply the time-course of EMG discharge and relative amplitude of response related to movement of a particular speech organ. Surface electrodes are also very useful for biofeedback studies in modifying muscle tension in patients with neuromuscular disorders (see e.g. Daniel and Guitar 1978; Stemple *et al.* 1980; Andrews, Warner and Stewart 1986).

Amplification

The signals from EMG electrodes are extremely small (typically ranging from 100 μV to about 2 mV) so high amplification is needed to display and record them on conventional laboratory equipment. The amplification system used should also have broad band widths appropriate to the type of electrodes used (Basmajian and De Luca 1985).

The small wires used in hooked-wire electrodes present a potential problem; they act like miniature antennae and pick up any stray electromagnetic radiation, for example from mains power lines in the building. The shorter the lead the better, so generally a low gain preamplifier (e.g. with gains to 40 dB, noise levels 5 mV RMS) is positioned as close as possible to the electrodes (less than 10 cm) and increases the power of the electrical potentials before conducting them to the main amplifier. The amplifier is a differential amplifier with relatively high common mode rejection ratio (ideally greater than 100 dB, Basmajian and De Luca, 1985).

Another requirement of the amplifier is that its input impedance be high (100 times higher than the electrode impedance). The electrode impedance will depend on the type, being higher for hooked-wire than for surface or needle electrodes. Higher impedance means a greater influence of radiated energy from mains electrical power lines so some recommend that the area should be shielded (McLeod 1973).

Signal processing

For most purposes in speech research some signal processing of the EMG needs to be carried out. The EMG signal is a noisy signal with disturbances coming from a variety of sources including mains hum, background physiological noise (e.g. 'tissue' noise, Hayes 1960), fluctuations in the physiological properties of the tissue, microphony (i.e. EMG electrodes acting as a transducer picking up periodic vibrations accompanying voicing), movement artefacts resulting in spikes in the signal due to jerky movements of the electrodes, electrode surfaces touching, etc. Most of this noise can be filtered out using a band-pass filter (Kewley-Port 1977 high pass filters at 80 Hz, Folkins *et al.* 1988 high pass at 30 Hz). Rischel and Hutters (1980) compared different electrodes and experimented with different filter settings. They warn against generalized statements about useful frequency range of EMG signals as this will depend on the muscle type and type of activity taking place. There may be important differences between the small, fast-acting cranial muscles used in speech production and the slower moving limb muscles widely investigated by physiologists. One difference might be a preponderance of higher frequency energy in the smaller muscles, which may be due to small motor units, shorter duration of motor unit potentials and other features. Also the type of electrode is relevant; surface electrodes pick up from a more diffuse area and are a greater distance from motor units than needle or hooked-wire so there may be more low-frequency emphasis. Hooked-wire electrodes may result in relatively high amounts of high frequency energy.

Rischel and Hutters (1980) found for most subjects, signals from some intrinsic laryngeal muscles showed most useful EMG energy in the region above 100 Hz. Spurious spikes tended to occur in the 100–150 Hz range and microphony could be easily removed by HP filtering 100–250 Hz. Some mains interference can be removed by HP filtering with cut off somewhere between 50–200 Hz but the best way to deal with mains 'hum' is to avoid it by proper shielding, grounding and recording.

For speech research most investigators recommend rectifying and smoothing the EMG signal. Usually full wave rectification is used (i.e. all signals are made positive) and the low pass filter time constant used for smoothing the rectified signal depends somewhat on the muscle and the particular type of experimental task (Abbs and Watkin 1976). In general, the time constant should be relatively long compared to the duration of each spike and the time interval between spikes, but short in relation to the number of times per second the muscle activity changes during production of a speech sound (Fromkin and Ladefoged 1966: 230). Figure 13.2 illustrates the smoothing effect on the signal of applying different time constants to the rectified EMG pattern.

Another type of data reduction procedure used in speech research is the computerised multiple token averaging described in detail by Kewley-Port (1977). The procedure involves multiple repetitions (usually about twenty) of the same token and the EMG data from specified muscles are temporally aligned to some reference point chosen by the system user, e.g. the release of a stop (Fromkin and Ladefoged 1966). This averaging procedure has the advantage of cancelling out random spurious aspects of the muscle activity signal seen often in single repetitions, so that those elements of the signal that are consistently repeated are emphasized (Abbs and Watkin 1976).

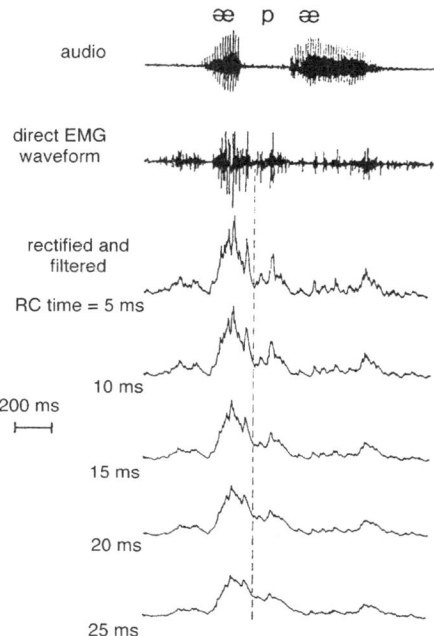

Figure 13.2   Illustration of the smoothing effect of different time constants on the rectified EMG pattern (from Abbs and Watkin 1976: 53).

Measurements

The onset of EMG activity in relation to speech movements is of particular interest to speech researchers and this is perhaps the most widely used measure. Typical delays of between 60–100 ms have been measured between muscle activation and movement (see e.g. Boyce 1988; Honda *et al.* 1995). It should not be assumed however as indicated above that EMG activity generated by a particular muscle implies movement of its associated structure (Lubker and Gay 1982). The muscle may be functioning as agonist, antagonist or fixator. If a number of muscles are recorded then the temporal sequence of response during a particular speech activity can be investigated. Honda, Kusakawa and Kakita (1992) used EMG waveforms from a number of different tongue and lip muscles to construct an 'articulatory score' meant to represent the time-course of motor commands to particular muscles during an utterance (see figure 13.3).

Another important measure is time to peak EMG amplitude. This has been found to be a relevant measure in studies of the coordination of multiple articulation (e.g. lip and jaw movement, Gracco 1988).

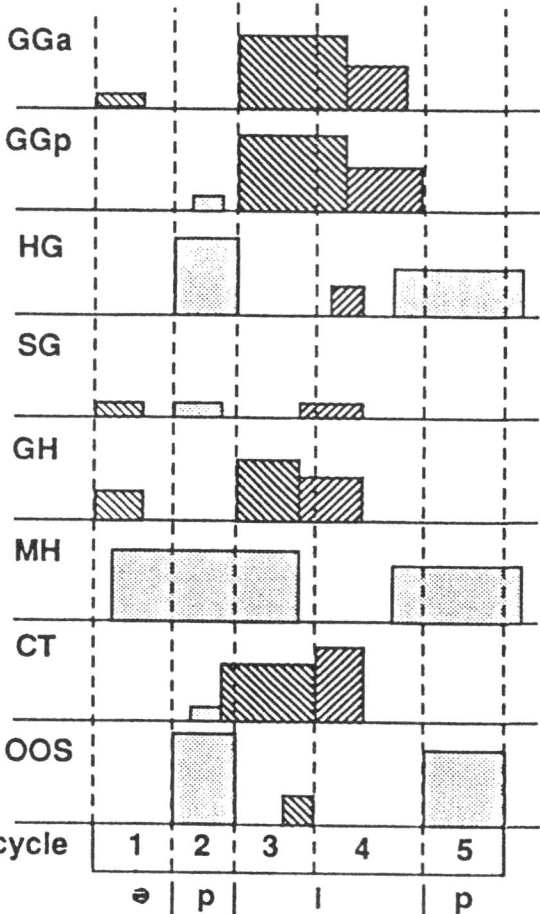

Figure 13.3   A 'motor score' showing schematized results of EMG signals from various different muscles during production of the utterance /əpip/. (GGa = anterior genioglossus; GGp = posterior genioglossus; HG = hypoglossus; SG = styloglossus; GH = geniohyoid; MH = mylohyoid; CT = cricothyroid, OOS = superior orbicularis oris) (from Honda, Kusakawa and Kakita 1992).

Limitations of EMG

EMG is an important technique in speech research as it remains the only way of directly monitoring activity in particular muscles. Indeed much of our current knowledge concerning the physiology of speech production comes from detailed and carefully controlled investigations using this technique. Increasingly, as was mentioned above, the most useful approach is a multi-channel one, where

EMG is used in conjunction with other instrumental techniques such as specialized movement transducers, fibre optic endoscopy, magnetometers, ultrasonics and others which monitor, relatively directly, the movements of the organ or organs under investigation. As we explore the relationship between movement patterns and EMG responses from a number of different muscles thought to contribute to such movements, we will be in a better position to formulate the type of comprehensive models of speech production that are urgently needed. The confident interpretation of EMG patterns also awaits much more detailed models of the inherent constraints that operate on the speech mechanisms – the mechanical properties of the systems – details of elasticity, mass, inertia, etc., as well as the neuromuscular control mechanisms, and the implications of such constraints for the dynamics of speech organ activity during speech production. An important start has already been made in this direction with a number of detailed studies on the lip and jaw mechanisms (see e.g. Abbs and Eilenberg 1976; Kennedy and Abbs 1979; Blair and Muller 1987; Folkins *et al.* 1988). These investigations combine EMG with lip and jaw transduction and the results are interpreted in terms of known mechanical features of the system. Such an approach can be extremely important for interpreting the electromyogram. Notwithstanding the problems of methodology and interpretation indicated above the technique remains a useful one for investigating speech physiology. EMG studies have increased our understanding of the underlying mechanisms of speech production, the contributions of various muscles to articulatory activity and timing relationships between EMG activity and actual movements.

14

Transducers for investigating velopharyngeal function

MICHEL CHAFCOULOFF

Introduction

In phonetic and clinical research, the study of velopharyngeal function has received considerable attention during the past decades and in both domains numerous instrumental techniques have been used either singly or in combination. The techniques employed for collecting physiological, acoustical and aerodynamic data about speech sounds have been described by Abbs and Watkin (1976) in phonetic research and by Baken (1998) in clinical research. The most complete survey of the instrumental techniques used for the investigation of nasalization and velopharyngeal function has been published by Krakow and Huffman (1993) with critical comments on their respective advantages and limitations.

As a result of intensive work carried out by means of these devices, valuable information on nasal sounds has been obtained. However, because of factors such as invasiveness, discomfort, limitations or expense, these techniques have proved useful in one specific domain of research, but not necessarily in others.

In the following sections, two types of instrumental techniques will be distinguished:

- the first type concerns indirect observation techniques such as aerometry, electromyography and acoustics;
- the second type concerns direct observation techniques such as radiography, endoscopy, photodetection, mechanical devices and more recent techniques such as ultrasound, magnetic resonance imaging and electromagnetic articulometry.

Indirect observation techniques

Aerometry

To gain insight into the aerodynamics associated with nasalization (Warren, Dalston and Mayo 1993), various devices have been designed for measuring oral and nasal airflow. Among these devices, electro-aerometers or warm-wire anemometers fitted to nasal masks or arranged in front of the nostrils are well-known instruments among phoneticians and clinicians (for physical bases and construction see Baken 1998). However, it should be noted that in the study of nasal coarticulatory effects, relatively few researchers have used these devices. Farnetani (1986a) has used the Frokjaer-Jensen anemometer simultaneously with an electropalatograph to examine the coordination of velar and lingual movements in the production of /n/ in Italian. She found that carryover velar coarticulation had a greater temporal extent than anticipatory coarticulation and that the timing of the velar opening/closing gestures was essentially context-dependent. However, because of several limitations, e.g. transducer sensitivity, dead volume from the mask, airflow leaks, low-frequency response, difficulty of calibration, etc., the reliability of these devices has remained questionable and consequently large amounts of data have not been collected.

Among aerometric instruments, the pneumotachograph has been most popular among clinicians and phoneticians. Briefly described, it consists of a flow meter and a differential pressure transducer. As air flows into the flow meter, a pressure drop is recorded by the transducer and converted into an electrical voltage. It requires the use of a facial mask to channel separately both oral and nasal airflows (for a detailed description of instrumentation see Lubker 1970; Warren 1976; Teston 1984; Baken 1998).

In clinical research, it has proved a most suitable tool for the needs of speech therapists to assess the amount of nasal leakage in the speech of individuals with cleft palates or similar maxillofacial defects. For a review of speech therapy for the rehabilitation of patients with velopharyngeal incompetence, see Dickson and Maue-Dickson (1980).

In phonetic research, the pneumotachograph has been used routinely to measure a number of respiratory parameters associated with speech, e.g. volume velocity of supraglottal airflow, and has been used for estimating volume displacements, area of constrictions, etc. Concerning variations in velopharyngeal orifice as a function of changes in transglottal airflow, Warren (1967) has used the pneumotachographic technique to show the existence of a relationship between orifice area and intraoral pressure at different rates. Warren and Devereux (1966) have found that the critical area of the velopharyngeal orifice should be approximately 20 mm^2 for inducing the perception of a nasal voice quality. Emanuel and Counihan (1970) have provided information about the timing of the coupling of the oral and nasal cavities and Lotz, Shaugnessy and Netsell (1981) have used a pneumotachograph to measure velopharyngeal resistance to airflow during the production of a sustained nasal consonant.

As far as the study of nasal coarticulatory effects is concerned, the pneumotachographic technique has been used either singly or in combination with other techniques. From the measurement of nasal airflow patterns, Benguerel (1975) reported a case of right to left coarticulation effect in French. He showed that for both nasal consonants and nasalized vowels, the velar opening gestures starts well ahead of the nasal sound itself, and that the closing gesture of the velum is faster than the opening gesture. Similar results were found by Clarke and Mackiewicz-Krassowska (1977) who used a divided mask to show the presence of nasal air pressure in vowels preceding nasal consonants. In combination with other techniques, Lubker and Moll (1965) used cineradiography simultaneously with airflow measurements. Lastly, Ali, Daniloff and Hammarberg (1979) used a combination of spectrographic and nasal airflow patterns to show the presence of intrusive stops in nasal–fricative clusters in English.

Estimation of velopharyngeal function from measurement of airflow has been employed by many investigators (see review in Warren 1996). However, it is difficult to make inferences concerning velar opening from a signal which (directly or indirectly) records nasal airflow. A number of factors can influence the amplitude of the signal including oral airflow resistance, and the action of the glottis and respiratory systems.

Electromyography

Electromyography (EMG) was used in the sixties for investigating velopharyngeal function. However, due to the surface electrodes employed in the earlier experiments, few reliable results were obtained concerning the particular activity of any muscle (Harris, Schvey and Lysaught 1962). With hooked-wire electrodes, the participation of specific muscles (e.g. levator palatini) in velar movement patterns was established with greater accuracy (for a review of EMG work, see Bell-Berti 1980 and chapter 13 in this volume).

It has been reported that the palatopharyngeal muscle has a greater activity level for /a/ than for /i, u/ (Fritzell 1969) and that the levator palatini EMG patterns were consistently correlated with changes in velar positions (Bell-Berti 1973; Ushijima and Hirose 1974). However, investigators disagreed concerning the role of the palatoglossus muscle which was found to be involved in tongue-dorsum elevation. In this respect, the data of Benguerel *et al.* (1977a) were not consistent with those collected by Bell-Berti (1976).

In order to determine how changes in muscular activity were related to structural movements, EMG was used simultaneously with cineradiography by Lubker (1968) who reported a correlation between the activity of the levator palatini and the velum raising movement. Using the same combined technique, Fritzell (1969) found a relation between the activity of the palatoglossus muscle and velum lowering. Moreover, it was found that this muscle was also involved in the production of velar consonants /k, g, ŋ/. Later, endoscopy was used in combination with EMG to demonstrate that an increase in EMG potentials corresponded to changes in velar height (Bell-Berti and Hirose 1975). For a fuller account of electromyography and the limitations of the technique see chapter 13 in this volume).

Acoustics
    Because of the intricate and complex relationship between the vocal system and the nasal sub-system, the acoustical description of nasal sounds has caused serious problems to researchers. Actually, one should differentiate between the type of instrumentation used in phonetic research and that used in clinical research.

In acoustic phonetics, the introduction of the spectrographic method has been decisive in contributing to knowledge of the main correlates associated with nasality. Through the analysis of spectral patterns, Delattre (1954) in French and Hattori, Yamamoto and Fujimura (1958) in Japanese have identified some of the spectral features of nasalization for vowels (e.g. additional nasal formant at 250 Hz, decreased intensity of F1, anti-formant between 500 and 1000 Hz, emergence of additional components in the upper F-pattern).

As the spectrographic method was limited in locating pole-zero pairs, Fujimura (1961a) used a spectrum-matching strategy for the analysis of nasalized vowels. Moreover, he showed that within the murmur of the nasal consonant, acoustic zeros varied as a function of vowel context and place of articulation (Fujimura 1962).

Fujimura and Lindqvist (1971) used sweep-frequency measurements for obtaining data on the transfer function of nasals and nasalized vowels. The same experimental set-up was used by Lindqvist-Gauffin and Sundberg (1976) for the estimation of the transfer function of the nasal tract.

To investigate correlations between the acoustic and articulatory aspects of nasality i.e. to determine to what degree the envelope spectrum of a vowel is affected by changes in the velopharyngeal port opening, articulatory synthesis was a most powerful method. By varying the cross sectional area of a section of a nasal tract added to an electrical analogue of the vocal tract, Fant (1960) and House and Stevens (1956) found that vowel nasalization was characterized by several attributes: a decrease of overall amplitude, an increase of bandwidth coupled with a frequency shift of F1, the presence of pole-zero pairs at different frequencies according to vowel quality etc.

After hardware synthesizers, articulatory modelling was used. Guérin and Mrayati (1977) showed that some attributes of nasality, among others the reduced amplitude of F1, were correlated not only with velum lowering, but also with compensatory adjustments of the pharyngeal cavity. In simulation experiments, Maeda (1982) examined the role of the nasal cavity in the production of nasal vowels. He found that a pair of spectral peaks at 250 Hz and 1000 Hz were strong perceptual correlates of nasalization (Maeda 1984). The same author has reported that a flattening of the spectrum in the F1–F2 region could also be considered as an attribute of vowel nasalization (Maeda 1993).

In clinical research, several instrumental techniques have been used for the measurement of nasal sound pressure level. The simplest device is a microphone positioned in front of the nose, or a probe microphone inserted in the nares of the subject. Otherwise, an accelerometer can be employed to detect nasal vibrations of the soft tissues of the nose, the output signal providing a feedback for the assessment of nasality in the speech of deaf children (Stevens, Kalikow and Willemain 1975). Given that variation in the nasal amplitude signal may be partly due to the speaker's vocal intensity, another system based on accelerometry was proposed by Horii (1983) for calculating a nasal-to-voice amplitude ratio. At this point, it should be noted that these devices are essentially used as evaluative tools for detecting nasality and/or hypernasality and seldom, if ever, as research tools of acoustic analysis.

The nasometer, whose technical principle is similar to that of the TONAR system (Fletcher 1970), has enjoyed a wider use than the devices reviewed previously. Its basic principle rests on a separation of the oral and nasal signals by means of two microphones positioned on each side of a dividing plate. The output signal is computed as the amplitude nasal/oral ratio (nasalance) in a varying range of the speech frequency spectrum. Although the main problem with such speech-training aids is the difficulty of obtaining significant correlation scores between objective quantitative measurements of nasalization and subjective perceived nasality, the nasometer has been used as a diagnostic tool for the clinical treatment of hearing impaired speakers and those with velopharyngeal incompetence (Dalston, Warren and Dalston 1993).

In phonetic studies, the nasometer has been employed to determine the temporal extent of nasal anticipatory coarticulation in comparison to carry-over coarticulation (Flege 1988). By means of the Nasometer 6200 marketed by Kay Elemetrics, Rochet and Rochet (1991) compared nasal assimilation patterns across English and French. They report greater anticipatory effects in the former language, but carryover effects were found to prevail in the latter.

As a conclusion, it should be pointed out that, because of several factors, i.e. interdependence of the vocal and nasal cavities, anatomical differences across speakers, velar opening differences across vowels, it has been highly problematic to find consistent acoustic information that would signal nasalization reliably at different points of the speech signal. Taking into account the fact that the search for invariant features of nasalization turned out to be fruitless (Curtiss 1968) and as the interpretation of acoustic data was a difficult task, researchers have generally relied on the examination of physiological data to investigate how and to what extent nasal sounds would coarticulate with other speech segments.

Direct observation techniques
Radiography

Among the imaging techniques, radiography has been a most efficient tool for providing useful information on the articulatory structures of the speech mechanism. (For a fuller description see chapter 12 in this volume.)

In the early 1940s, radiology was used for providing shapes of the vocal tract and positions of articulators during the production of speech sounds. From the examination of static X-ray lateral views, Harrington (1944) reported significant differences in velar elevation across vowels. Later, dynamic information about the movement patterns of the velopharynx was obtained by means of cineradiography and cinefluorography. Dickson (1961) observed that the velum was completely closed during the production of high vowels in a plosive context, but not in a nasal consonant context. From the analysis of vowels uttered in context, Moll (1962) confirmed previous findings that velar elevation varied as a function of vowel height. Kent and Moll (1969) provided measures of velar height and velopharyngeal aperture together with measures of other articulators' movements, i.e. jaw, lips, tongue. Moll and Daniloff (1971) showed that nasal anticipatory coarticulation may extend as far as the initial consonant in a CVV sequence.

However, it must be acknowledged that the radiographic method suffered from serious drawbacks: radiation risk due to a prolonged exposure to X-rays, poor visualization of soft tissues in contrast to the bony structures, tediousness of a frame-by-frame analysis. To further reduce the X-ray risk and at the same time make the analysis easier, new imaging techniques were developed for obtaining complementary physiological data.

Videofluorography, which gradually replaced cinefluorography, was employed for a multiple viewing of the velopharyngeal region, i.e. lateral, frontal and submentovertical views (for an historical review of clinical work, see Dickson and Maue-Dickson 1980). Later, this technique was combined with endoscopy for observing lateral pharyngeal wall motion (Croft, Shprintzen and Rakoff 1981).

As mentioned above, one of the main drawbacks of the radiographic method was the difficulty of drawing precise contours of the soft tissues. To circumvent these problems of graphic analysis, Kent, Carney and Severeid (1974) used the fleshpoint tracking technique. It is based on the use of metal pellets which are attached to the articulators, e.g. tongue, lips, jaw, velum, for viewing their displacements on a vertical–horizontal axis. Although it was difficult to fix the pellet on the velum due to its extreme mobility and sensitivity, they reported evidence of velum–tongue coordination movements, i.e. the closing gesture of the velum started prior to the tongue alveolar contact in the production of the consonant /n/. A computer controlled X-ray microbeam system was developed by Kiritani, Itoh and Fujimura (1975) for obtaining data on velum movement patterns by reference to other articulators. In a specific study on the velum, Vaissière (1988) has found that the height and timing gestures of this articulator are influenced by suprasegmental factors such as stress patterns and speech rate. In part because of its high cost, this research technique which presents considerable advantages of relative safety and efficiency has not been much used so far.

Endoscopy

In the study of velopharyngeal function, endoscopy which consists of inserting a flexible fibreoptic endoscope through the nasal passage was employed in Japan in the early seventies for viewing the raising and lowering gestures of the velum (see also discussion in chapter 15, section A of this volume). By means of this technique, the relationship between velar elevation and vowel height, previously established through cineradiography, i.e. the velum is higher in a close-vowel context than in an open-vowel context, was confirmed by Ushijima and Sawashima (1972) and later by Bell-Berti *et al.* (1979).

Although there was general agreement concerning vowels, different conclusions were drawn on consonants. Ushijima and Sawashima (1972) could not find any specific dependence on velum height on duration and context, but Bell-Berti and Hirose (1975) reported that in similar vocalic environments, the velum was higher for /b/ than for /p/, which reflected oral cavity differences for these stop articulations. In French, Benguerel *et al.* (1977a) found that the velum was highest at the release of voiceless plosives and during the fricative noise portion of voiceless fricatives.

However, due to several limitations including the optical lens and viewing angle which may introduce distortions and the lack of clear-cut contours between velum and lateral pharyngeal walls, endoscopy did not prove an adequate investigation technique for collecting quantitative data about velopharyngeal port or velum elevation. Consequently, other techniques were introduced for the observation of velar movements.

Photodetection

The principle of photodetection is based on the use of a light source and a light detector inserted through a catheter in the nasal and pharyngeal cavities. The amount of light varies as a function of the opening of the velopharyngeal port, thus providing a proportional analogue voltage.

The first photoelectric device, the nasograph designed by Ohala (1971) had the peculiarity of having the light source and photocell located respectively above and below the velopharyngeal port. Among many studies of the latter author on the general topic of nasalization, it was used in an experiment to demonstrate the presence of spontaneous nasalization in non-nasal environments, and particularly in a glottal and pharyngeal consonantal context (Ohala 1975).

The velograph was developed to measure the degree of velar elevation (Kuenzel 1977). It differed from the previous device in that it was positioned on the nasal floor, and the phototransistor was close to the light source in the nasal cavity. By this technique, it was reported that the velum was highest for voiceless stops, and that its raising motion was longer for these sounds than for their voiced cognates (Kuenzel 1979).

However, these photoelectric devices had two serious drawbacks. One concerned their calibration, as there was no strict linear relation between the amount of light reflected and the velar port area or velar height. The other one concerned the frequent shifts in the position of the catheter in running speech.

Nevertheless, in spite of these shortcomings and partly to compensate for them, the photoelectric technique was used in combination with other techniques such as cineradiography (Zimmerman *et al.* 1987), endoscopy (Karnell, Linville and Edwards 1988) and nasometry (Dalston 1989). A method of measuring the velic port area with reference to the luminous component of the video signal was proposed by Hoole (1989). This procedure, which was designed for the processing of endoscopic or photoelectric images, looks promising and extensive data about velic movement patterns are expected.

Mechanical devices

As it had been previously observed by means of cineradiography that velar position varied even in the case of a complete closure, a mechanical device, the velotrace, was designed to monitor vertical changes in the position of the velum (Horiguchi and Bell-Berti 1987). It consists of an internal lever which rested on the upper surface of the velum, together with a connecting push-rod and an external lever whose corresponding angular displacements reflected the vertical movements of the velum. The system involves an optoel-ectronic position sensor which tracks the movements of the external lever using infrared diodes. The audio speech signal is recorded simultaneously. By comparing velotrace data to radiographic or endoscopic data, it was reported that the analogue signal accurately reflected the fast-varying movements of the velum even in entirely oral speech.

This technique has been used in studies aimed at assessing the theoretical relevance of some speech production models, and in particular the coproduc-tion model (Bell-Berti and Krakow 1991). The latter authors have shown that non-segmental influences such as syllable position, sentence duration, stress and speaking rate may affect velic movements (Krakow 1993). Moreover, it was demonstrated recently that there exists an interactive coordination between oral (upper lip and jaw) and nasal (velum) articulators (Kollia, Gracco and Harris 1994). In addition to its use in normal speech, this device may have applications in the domain of speech pathology for the investiga-tion of speech defects. However, one should not underestimate its invasive nature, and data should be interpreted with caution since potential distur-bances cannot be discounted *a priori.*

Recent techniques
Ultrasound

By comparison with other physiological or acoustical recording tech-niques, the ultrasound scanning technique is relatively new as it was first intro-duced in the late 1960s (see chapter 11 in this volume for a fuller description of this technique). Originally employed in clinical studies for laryngeal exam-ination, ultrasound was used for studying lateral pharyngeal wall motion through the pulse–echo technique (Kelsey, Woodhouse and Minifie 1969). However, because the ultrasound beam did not penetrate the mandible, its one limitation was that the system could not track the lateral wall motion of the nasopharynx.

Using the pulse-through transmission technique, Zagzebski (1975) and Skolnick, Shprintzen and McCall (1975) have combined naso-pharyngoscopy and ultrasound to examine lateral pharyngeal motion at two levels in the vocal tract. A correlation was found between velic height and displacement of the lateral pharyngeal walls. This finding was consistent with previous cineradio-graphic observations (Bjork 1961) and confirmed the view that the velopharyn-geal mechanism functioned as a sphincter (Skolnick, McCall and Barnes 1973).

However, it must be acknowledged that in its present state, the ultrasonic technique, mainly because of the different transmissive properties of the tissues traversed by the ultrasound signal, has been of limited use in speech research and has not been applied to the tracking movements of the velum.

Magnetic resonance imagery

As cineradiography and videofluorographic devices have been progressively ruled out because of radiation risks, researchers have been encouraged to use other methods for transducing movements of supraglottal articulators. Magnetic resonance imagery (MRI) presents the advantage of non-ionising radiation. It produces high-quality images similar to computed tomography in three-dimensional planes, i.e. axial, coronal, midsagittal (see chapter 11 in this volume). Although this technique has its limitations (see Baer *et al.* 1991), valuable information on vocal tract shapes and dimensions of sustained vowels has been obtained. One of the drawbacks of MRI is that the subject must be in a supine position and although gravity effects on articulatory movements are reported to be minimal, MRI is not in its present stage of development adequate for tracking these movements in continuous speech. Nevertheless, new equipment is being tested and fast progress is being made for improving previous systems (Stone and Davis 1995).

Electromagnetic articulometry (EMMA)

As discussed in chapter 13 in this volume, EMMA has been mainly used to investigate lower lip and jaw movements but it is in theory possible to attach a transmitter coil to the soft palate. One of the problems is that relatively few subjects can tolerate this because of the sensitivity of the soft palate.

So far, there has been a single attempt to track velum movements in the speech of normal and apraxic subjects (Katz *et al.* 1990; cited in Krakow and Huffman 1993: 25).

Conclusion

One of the main conclusions of this brief review of tranducers for investigating velopharyngeal function is that there is no single ideal instrument for directly tracking movement of the velum. For coarticulation studies the best solution is probably to use a combination of techniques (e.g. pressure/flow linked to photoelectronic methods) to obtain a more complete representation of the function of this important organ during speech production.

15

Techniques for investigating laryngeal articulation

Section A: PHILIP HOOLE

Section B: CHRISTER GOBL and AILBHE NÍ CHASAIDE

Introduction

In this discussion we will deal with techniques which permit investigation of two rather different aspects of laryngeal behaviour. Philip Hoole deals with the articulatory aspect in Section A and this specifically concerns those laryngeal adjustments of abduction and adduction involved in the production of voiceless segments, and which can conveniently be referred to by the term 'devoicing gesture'. This section will accordingly look mainly at techniques for assessing the kinematics of this gesture.

Christer Gobl and Ailbhe Ní Chasaide deal with the second aspect which concerns the detailed acoustic analysis of phonation itself. A number of studies in recent years have highlighted the fact that even during what would be termed modal phonation there is considerable modulation of the voice source as a function of the prosodic and segmental content of utterances. Of particular interest here are exploratory studies which indicate that the phonatory quality of a voiced segment may be affected by laryngeal adjustments associated with an adjacent voiceless consonant, and which suggest that there may be striking cross-language differences. These phonatory variations may yield valuable insights into the nature and timing of laryngeal gestures associated with these segments. Section B of this chapter provides a brief outline of the techniques that may be used to analyse the voice source, concentrating especially on those used to obtain the data presented in chapter 5.

Section A: Investigation of the devoicing gesture: Philip Hoole

It can be assumed that the immediate aim of any investigation of devoicing is to obtain measurements of the amplitude, form and timing of the abductory–adductory cycle, either directly in terms of the time-course of the separation of the vocal processes of the arytenoid cartilages, or indirectly through the resulting transillumination signal, or through the underlying electromyographic activity. Other indirect techniques for investigating aspects of laryngeal activity, notably electrolaryngography, are not discussed in detail here. The reader is referred to recent accounts such as Abberton and Fourcin (1997). As discussed further in chapter 5 the wider aim of such analyses is to gain further insight firstly into the nature of laryngeal–oral coordination in different categories of consonants and secondly into the blending processes occurring in clusters of voiceless sounds. We will discuss how the data for such analyses can be acquired most effectively using a combination of fibreoptics and transillumination, and will also look more briefly at EMG and pulse-echo ultrasound. The emphasis on the first technique is motivated by the fact that it is probably the one most accessible to laboratories involved in coarticulation research. The reader is referred to Löfqvist (1990) for very convenient illustrations of some typical voiceless sequences since transillumination and EMG signals are shown in parallel.

Fibreoptic endoscopy, transillumination, and their combination
In 1968 Sawashima and Hirose presented an endofibrescope that for the first time made it possible to routinely investigate laryngeal activity in running speech. For a description of fibrescope construction see Sawashima and Ushijima (1971). For a representative early study examining the voiced and voiceless consonants of English see Sawashima *et al.* (1970).

One of the main problems in analysing laryngeal films (*ceteris paribus*, this also applies to transillumination) is caused by the fact that the distance between objective lens (i.e. distal end of the fibrescope) and the glottis is not constant and not known. Differences in this distance can be caused, of course, by vertical movements of the larynx but also by the influence of velar movement on endoscope position. These influences must be minimized by careful choice of the speech material since methods that have been proposed to control for the varying distance between endoscope and glottis, such as radiographic monitoring (Kiritani 1971) or stereoscopic procedures (Sawashima and Miyazaki 1974; Fujimura, Baer and Niimi 1979; Yoshioka 1984), are unlikely to prove suitable for routine use, at least in coarticulatory studies. Thus most investigations must currently content themselves with relative rather than absolute measurements of glottal opening. Assuming suitable phonetic material is employed the stability actually achieved in a particular recording must essentially be judged by the experienced investigator.

One reason why a combination of fibrescopy and transillumination is attractive is that at standard video or cine frame-rates the temporal resolution of an endoscopic film is rather low, particularly if it is desired to locate the offset and onset of voicing in the devoicing gesture (cf. Hirose and Niimi, 1987).

One of the main attempts to circumvent the above limitation involves the use of specialized digital video equipment (Honda *et al.* 1987; Kiritani, Imagawa and Hirose 1992). CCD (charge coupled device) cameras allow trade-offs between spatial and temporal resolution, so an adequate frame-rate is certainly achievable. Use of image-processing to extract parameters such as glottal area or distance between the vocal processes should be feasible. However, in view of the fact that such algorithms tend to be computationally expensive and that some compromises with regard to spatial resolution have to be made it seems that at the present time this represents essentially a rather roundabout way of arriving at something that is not very different from a straightforward transillumination signal, at least as far as the gross characteristics of the devoicing gesture are concerned. Nonetheless, for the investigation of the way in which patterns of vocal fold vibration are modified at transitions between vowels and consonants the technique already appears to offer much promise (it should also be ideally suited to investigating irregular or asymmetric phonatory phenomena such as creak or diplophonia). With further technological advances more routine application of this technique should become possible.

The transillumination technique initially developed independently of fibreoptic endoscopy. It essentially involves a light source and a phototransducer located on opposite sides of the glottis; the amount of light passing through the glottis, and accordingly the output voltage of the phototransducer amplifier, is modulated by the changes in the size of the glottal aperture occurring during speech and respiration. Over the years various different arrangements of these two basic components have been tried out (see e.g. Sonesson 1960; Malécot and Peebles 1965; Ohala 1966; Frøkjær-Jensen 1967; Lisker *et al.* 1969), mainly regarding whether the light source is applied externally to the neck below the glottis, and with the phototransducer in the pharynx, or vice versa. See Hutters (1976) for a valuable overview of methodological issues.[1]

Once fibreoptic endoscopy started to become widespread in phonetic research, it was natural to employ an arrangement with the fibrescope functioning as light source in the pharynx and with the transducer applied externally to the neck[2] (Löfqvist and Yoshioka 1980b). The great advantage of this approach is, of course, that the endoscopic view allows the stability of the positioning of the light-source in the pharynx to be monitored, at least qualitatively.

There are essentially two positions in which the transducer can be applied to the neck, either between the cricoid and thyroid cartilage, or below the cricoid cartilage. Following Frøkjær-Jensen, Ludvigsen and Rischel (1971) we can assume that devoicing mainly involves modulation of the width of the posterior glottis, while in phonation the main modulation of the width occurs at more anterior locations. It appears (and is anatomically plausible) that the lower transducer position weights the posterior devoicing activity more strongly, while the upper position weights phonatory activity more strongly.[3] Accordingly, the sub-cricoid position is preferable for studies of devoicing; in particular, a more stable (albeit sometimes rather weak) signal is obtained since in the upper position the signal can be strongly influenced by changes in laryngeal height and orientation, related, for example, to the intonation pattern of the utterance. Thus, Löfqvist and Yoshioka found a good correlation between the amplitude of the transillumination signal and the glottal width as measured from a fibreoptic cine film, but only when the lower transducer postion was used.[4]

In our own implementation (Hoole, Schröter-Morasch and Ziegler 1997), we became convinced that it is essential to record the whole experimental session on videotape (cf. Hirose 1986) since if a permanent record of the endoscopic view is not available it is very easy for the human observer to overlook brief retractions of the tongue root or epiglottis that have a massive influence on the transillumination signal. Explicit synchronization of the video and transillumination signals is also very important.[5] In order to further facilitate the recognition of such artefacts, it seemed to us that one obvious approach would be to record from *two* phototransistors simultaneously, one between cricoid and thyroid, and one below the cricoid cartilage. Based on the above discussion of transducer positioning one can expect that the reduction in light intensity caused by shadowing will in general either be greater at the upper transducer position or will at least start earlier there. In other words, when the two signals diverge, a departure from ideal recording conditions may have occurred.[6]

In figure 15.1 typical traces obtained with the twin transducer system are displayed for the German sentence 'Lies "die Schiffe" bitte' ('Read "the ships" please'). The sentence contains the voiceless sounds /s/, /ʃ/, /f/ and /t/. Each of these sounds is associated with a peak in the amplitude of the transillumination signals. Main stress in this sentence fell on the first syllable of 'Schiffe' and it will be observed that much the largest amplitude of the devoicing gesture in this utterance is associated with the fricative /ʃ/ at the onset of this syllable, peak glottal opening occurring at about the temporal mid-point of the fricative. Vocal fold vibration is visible in the transillumination signal as a high-frequency modulation overlaid on the gross abductory and adductory movements. As is to be expected from the above discussion, this phonatory activity is a more salient feature of the signal

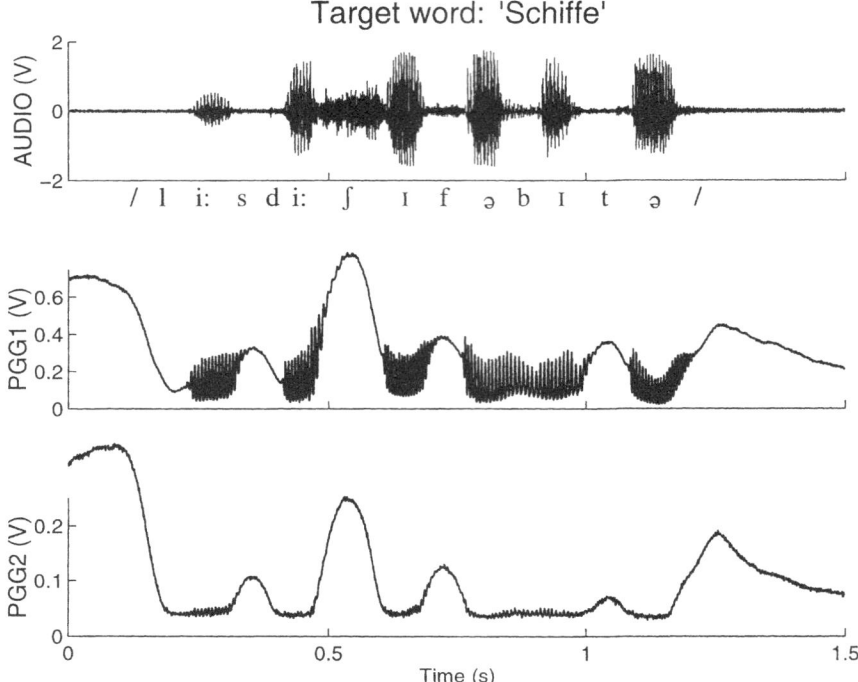

Figure 15.1   Example of two-channel transillumination signal for a German sentence ('Lies die Schiffe bitte') containing several voiceless sounds. The trace labelled PGG 1 (middle panel) is derived from a phototransistor applied externally to the neck between thryroid and cricoid cartilages. For PGG 2 (bottom panel) the phototransistor was located below the cricoid cartilage.

labelled PGG1, which corresponds to the transducer position between thyroid and cricoid cartilages. A consistent feature of voiceless fricatives that can be easily followed here (especially for the stressed /ʃ/) is the hysteresis effect by which vocal fold vibration dies out rather gradually during glottal abduction for the fricative but does not recommence for the following vowel until the glottis is almost completely adducted again.

Normally, as here, the relative amplitude of glottal abduction for the different voiceless sounds in the sentence is the same at both transducer positions, the two traces proceeding essentially in parallel. If, however, this is not the case, (for example, if abduction for /ʃ/ were to appear greater than for /f/ in the PGG2 trace but smaller in the PGG1 trace) then this is an indication that recourse should be had to the video film to check for shadowing of the glottis etc.

Electromyography of the larynx

Laryngeal EMG has clearly contributed much to our understanding of articulatory functions of the larynx. See for example the work of Hirose (1975) in clarifying the status of the posterior cricoarytenoid (PCA) as a speech muscle, and in establishing the typical reciprocal pattern of activity of PCA and INT (interarytenoid) in the devoicing gesture (Sawashima and Hirose 1983). The specific role with respect to the devoicing gesture of the other intrinsic muscles LCA (lateral cricoarytenoid), VOC (vocalis) and CT (cricothyroid) appears to require further clarification (e.g. Hirose and Ushijima 1978).

The use of laryngeal EMG for articulatory investigations received its major stimulus from the development of hooked-wire electrodes (Basmajian and Stecko 1962) since, in contrast to the concentric needle electrodes more common in clinical investigations, these electrodes allow the subject freedom of movement and cause little discomfort once the insertion (by means of hypodermic needle) has been completed (Hirano and Ohala 1969; Shipp, Fishman and Morrisey 1970; chapter 13 this volume). The path of electrode insertion as further developed by Hirose (1971; summaries also in Hirose 1979 and Hirano 1981) involves a percutaneous approach for CT, LCA and VOC and a peroral approach for PCA and INT. Further details of electrode construction, insertion and verification are to be found in the cited articles, as well as in Harris (1981) and Honda (1983).

The obvious drawback to the technique, unanimously alluded to by the above authors, is the amount of practice required, including for example electrode insertions on cadaveric material. Hirano and Ohala also point out that the insertion of hooked-wire electrodes probably requires more skill than needle electrodes. A final consideration is the extent to which topical anaesthesia of the laryngeal mucosa and premedication of the subject (Shipp, Fishman and Morrisey 1970; Hirose and Gay 1972) is necessary and compatible with the aims of a specific experiment.

Pulse-echo ultrasound

The ultrasound technique has provided much useful kinematic data on several articulatory systems (e.g. Keller and Ostry 1983; Munhall, Ostry and Parush 1985; chapter 11 this volume). Munhall and Ostry (1985) report on its application to laryngeal kinematics. Briefly, the procedure is designed to measure the distance between an ultrasound transducer applied laterally to the thyroid cartilage and the moving vocal fold, sample rates of 1 kHz or more being possible. A potential advantage of the ultrasound technique is that, in contrast to transillumination, absolute values for the excursion of the vocal fold can be achieved. However, this may only be an apparent advantage because it is never possible to indicate precisely which point (or rather small area) on the vocal fold forms the basis of the measurement at any given moment or in any given session. Perhaps the main drawback currently with this interesting technique is that there are relatively few published investigations, so that little is known about possible sources of error; there are no studies of which we are aware which compare the technique with parallel recordings made with an alternative procedure such as fibreoptics (but see Hamlet 1981 for extensive discussion of the utility of ultrasound in the analysis of phonation).

Section B: Techniques for analysing the voice source:
Christer Gobl and Ailbhe Ní Chasaide
Introduction
With methods of analysis that yield detailed voice source measurements, a small but growing body of data is emerging on the dynamic variation of the voice source as a function of non-linguistic and linguistic factors. It is of course well documented that the mode of phonation of a segment or syllable may serve a linguistically contrastive function (see for example Ladefoged 1983). Perhaps less well known is the extent of voice source modulation that occurs in utterances, considered to be spoken with normal modal voice, as a function of their segmental and prosodic content (Fant 1980; Gobl 1985; 1988; Gobl and Ní Chasaide 1988; Löfqvist and McGowan 1988; Pierrehumbert 1989; Ní Chasaide and Gobl 1993). Of particular interest to investigations of coarticulation is the finding that the mode of phonation during a voiced segment (vowel) may be influenced by the consonantal context, particularly by voiceless consonants. These findings are illustrated and discussed in chapter 5 section B.

In the remainder of this chapter we describe the techniques that may be used for the acoustic analysis of phonation and we attempt to evaluate the strengths and weaknesses of different approaches. As most experimental studies of the human voice source have involved inverse filtering of one kind or another, this method will be dealt with in detail later. There is a fairly wide range of inverse filtering techniques available, ranging from fully automatic implementations to ones that permit very detailed manual fine-tuning of individual source pulses. Other techniques which have been used for obtaining the voice source signal are also described. The following sub-section details a technique whereby the source signal can be quantified: it involves parameterization of the glottal waveform using a model of differentiated glottal flow. Then some of the voice source parameters that are likely to be most important acoustically and

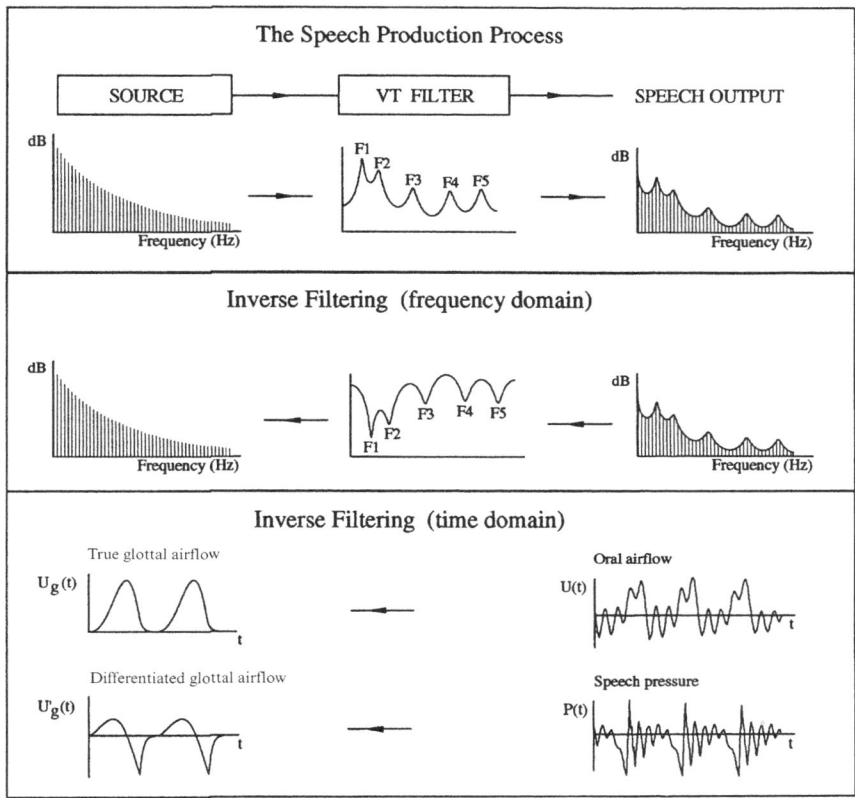

Figure 15.2 Simplified schematic representation illustrating the principle of inverse filtering.

perceptually are described. Finally, some of the ways in which inferences concerning the glottal source can be gleaned from the speech pressure waveform are detailed. The reader should note that the illustrations of source data in chapter 5 section B were derived using a manual interactive technique of inverse filtering and of LF-model matching. Source measurements are presented there in terms of the source parameters described in this chapter.

Inverse filtering

The vocal mechanism can, in very simple terms, be represented by a model of a source and a filter (see figure 15.2). The vibrations of the vocal folds provide the source for voiced speech and the voice source is defined as the airflow through the glottis during voicing. The acoustic spectrum of the sound generated by the source is characterized by harmonics whose amplitude decreases with increasing frequency. This is generally modelled by a spectral slope of − 6 dB per octave. The filter comprises the supraglottal cavities: oral, pharyngeal and nasal. Depending on the particular configuration adopted by the supraglottal tract at any instant in time, this filter will be characterized by resonances (or formants) with specific frequencies and bandwidths. The formants shape the source spectrum so that the speech output is determined by the source and filter characteristics together. This account is oversimplified in a number of respects. First of all, it omits from discussion the radiation effects at the lips. Furthermore, it clearly does not fully cover speech segments such as fricatives which involve an alternative or additional source.

The basic principle

Inverse filtering is essentially an attempt to implement a reversal of the normal speech production process. If the speech signal is fed through a filter which is the diametric opposite of the true filter, we will in principle derive the source in its pre-filtered form. The signal which is filtered is typically the speech pressure waveform. However, the oral airflow signal can also be filtered (see later). The middle panel of figure 15.2 illustrates the effects of inverse filtering in the frequency domain (in terms of the signal's frequency components). The third portion of the figure illustrates the same effects in the time domain (in terms of the glottal airflow). When the vocal tract resonances have been removed one is left with the true glottal flow. The radiation effect at the lips is approximately the equivalent of a + 6 dB per octave pre-emphasis. If the inverse filter does not cancel this effect, the output will be the differentiated glottal flow. Note that the differentiated flow is the equivalent of a representation of the rate of change in the true glottal flow. In many implementations the former signal is preferred. The additional pre-emphasis of the source signal can be useful in permitting better definition of higher frequency ranges. Furthermore, the differentiated glottal flow allows a more accurate estimate of some of the perceptually important source features.

Filter structure

The structure of the inverse filter can be described in terms of complex–conjugate zeros and poles which cancel out the poles and zeros respectively of the estimated vocal tract transfer function. If the differentiated glottal flow is desired, this structure is sufficient. If the true glottal flow is desired a real pole must be added to the inverse filter at zero frequency, thus effectively cancelling the radiation effect at the lips, which is approximately equivalent to a real zero at zero frequency.

Very often the vocal tract is approximated by an all pole model for all sounds, not only the vowels. The vocal tract inverse filter can then be represented by zeros only. Although the cancelling then becomes less accurate for sounds that comprise zeros, the advantages are obvious. Most importantly, the filter approximation is hugely simplified. The formants (poles) are typically easy to identify, whereas it is often very difficult to estimate or even detect the zeros with certainty.

The number of zeros needed for the inverse filter depends on the vocal tract length and on the bandwidth of the signal which is determined by the sampling frequency. For a typical male with a vocal tract length of 17.5 cm, the average spacing between formants is 1000 Hz. Thus, for a sampling rate of 20 kHz, the inverse filter should in principle have 10 anti-resonances.

Implementations of the inverse filter

One of the major difficulties with inverse filtering is of course that of finding the correct transfer function of the supraglottal system. Any error in the parameters of the inverse filter will more or less distort the glottal pulse. The pulse shape is very sensitive to erroneous settings of the frequencies and bandwidths of the first formant, especially when F1 is low. Minor errors in the higher formants have little effect on the main pulse shape and its corresponding frequency spectrum (Gobl 1988).

Numerous methods for estimating formant frequencies and bandwidths have been suggested in the literature. Early implementations tended to be hardware-based. Most current systems are software-based and may operate in a fully automatic way or, alternatively, may allow the user to manually fine-tune the inverse filter in an interactive way, on a pulse-by-pulse basis if necessary.

Hardware implementations   Inverse filters have been implemented in a variety of hardware and software systems. In the early pioneering studies of the voice source, analogue anti-resonance circuits were used and these were manually tuned to cancel out the formant pattern. The analogue methods would now be considered outdated, lacking as they do the flexibility that computer analysis of the voice source offers. However, the results of much of the earlier work are still valid: note that major voice source work by Fant (1979, 1980, 1981, 1982a, 1982b) was carried out with analogue equipment. Furthermore, hardware inverse filters, whether analogue or digital, can still be very useful when real time inverse filtering is required. If there is no need to be able to vary the articulation, this method of inverse filtering is very effective. This may be the case, for instance, when the general vocal behaviour is of main interest, as in the analysis of certain types of voice disorders. Also, for voice training, the immediate feedback offered by real-time hardware systems can be useful.

Automatic software implementations   Automatic methods of inverse filtering are typically based on linear predictive coding (LPC) analysis of the speech signal (see for example Rabiner and Schafer 1978, and references therein). There are two different formulations of LPC which are used particularly often in speech analysis: the autocorrelation and the covariance method. The advantage of the covariance method is that it can be used for pitch synchronous 'closed phase' analysis, as the filter estimate can be carried out using a very short time window, corresponding to the closed period of one single pulse. Closed phase covariance LPC is generally considered to yield a better filter estimate than autocorrelation LPC, which requires several pitch periods in order to obtain a reliable result and thus arrives at an estimate based on samples pertaining to the open and closed phases of several pulses. In this interval, the losses vary as a function of the time-varying glottal impedance. Furthermore, the vocal tract transfer function might also undergo change. Both factors may cause results to be less accurate.

To sum up, the closed phase covariance analysis is likely to be the more appropriate technique. We should point out, however, that it is not a trivial matter to obtain a reliable estimate of the closed phase directly from the speech signal, something which is very important for accurate closed phase analysis. Often, an additional simultaneous glottographic recording is carried out to facilitate the estimation of the closed phase (see below).

The linear prediction model of speech is an all pole model (AR – autoregressive – model) and spectra including zeros are thus approximated by an all pole filter. Experiments with pole/zero modelling (ARMA – autoregressive moving average – modelling) of speech have been carried out (e.g. Fujisaki and Ljungqvist 1987; Boves and de Veth 1989). However, at present these methods are not very widespread and very little data using them have been published.

One of the major problems with linear predictive analysis is that it assumes the excitation source to have a flat spectrum, i.e. an impulse train for voiced sounds and white noise for voiceless sounds. In order to overcome these problems, modified formulations of the linear predictive analysis have been presented (Hedelin 1984, 1986; Ljungqvist and Fujisaki 1985b, Fujisaki and Ljungqvist 1987). The modification is obtained by changing the basic LPC equation so that it includes coefficients that correspond to the voice source. Minimizing the squared error leads to a different set of equations that includes estimation of voice source parameters as well as vocal tract parameters.

Although automatic methods may work reasonably well for certain types of simple uncomplicated signals (e.g. a steady state vowel for a speaker with an efficient mode of phonation), they perform rather badly on more complex materials. For example, they deal rather less well with the types of transitions found in natural running speech, where the vocal tract is undergoing rapid change. They also are likely to perform less well when the mode of phonation is non-modal, and even with transitions from voice to voicelessness.

Interactive software implementations   More accurate source data can be obtained if an interactive facility is incorporated, permitting the experimenter to assess the validity of the inverse filter on a pulse-by-pulse basis, manipulating the frequencies and bandwidths to yield the optimal settings. How this process works is illustrated in figure 15.3. This figure shows two stages in the analysis of a single glottal period. A cursor in the uppermost window marks the glottal period being analysed. The next three windows show: (a) an expanded version of the speech waveform, centred on the period under analysis; (b) the differentiated wave, output of an inverse filter where the formants are effectively cancelled and (c) the differentiated wave, output of a less accurate inverse filter which has failed to cancel F1. The lowest window shows the spectra corresponding to all three waveforms. In (A) all the formants can be seen; in (B) one can see that all the fomant peaks have been eliminated to yield the differentiated waveform of (b), whereas in (C) we still have a clear F1 peak, just as we can see the ringing of F1 in the waveform of (c). The crosses in the lowest window indicate the individual formants, which determine the inverse filter. With the mouse each of these can be moved to effect changes in the frequency (horizontal dimension) or bandwidth (vertical dimension) of the formant. In fine-tuning the values the user is guided by both the time and frequency information.

Figure 15.3 is taken from a software system developed at Trinity College, Dublin (see Ní Chasaide, Gobl and Monahan 1992). Similar software is the INA program developed at KTH, Stockholm. A further program which allows interactive inverse filtering without the possibility of frequency domain matching is described by Hunt, Bridle and Holmes (1978).

A comparison of interactive and automatic methods   The main advantage of the interactive methods over automatic ones is the greater control of the estimation of the inverse filter. The experimenter can assess the validity of the inverse filter on a pulse-by-pulse basis. The speech knowledge of the experimenter can be exploited to avoid the unreasonable filter settings that often occur with automatic methods. This last point could also be turned on its head as an argument against manual interactive methods. Automatic methods may produce errors, but they have the advantage of always keeping to the same strategy for estimating the inverse filter. Different users of manual methods

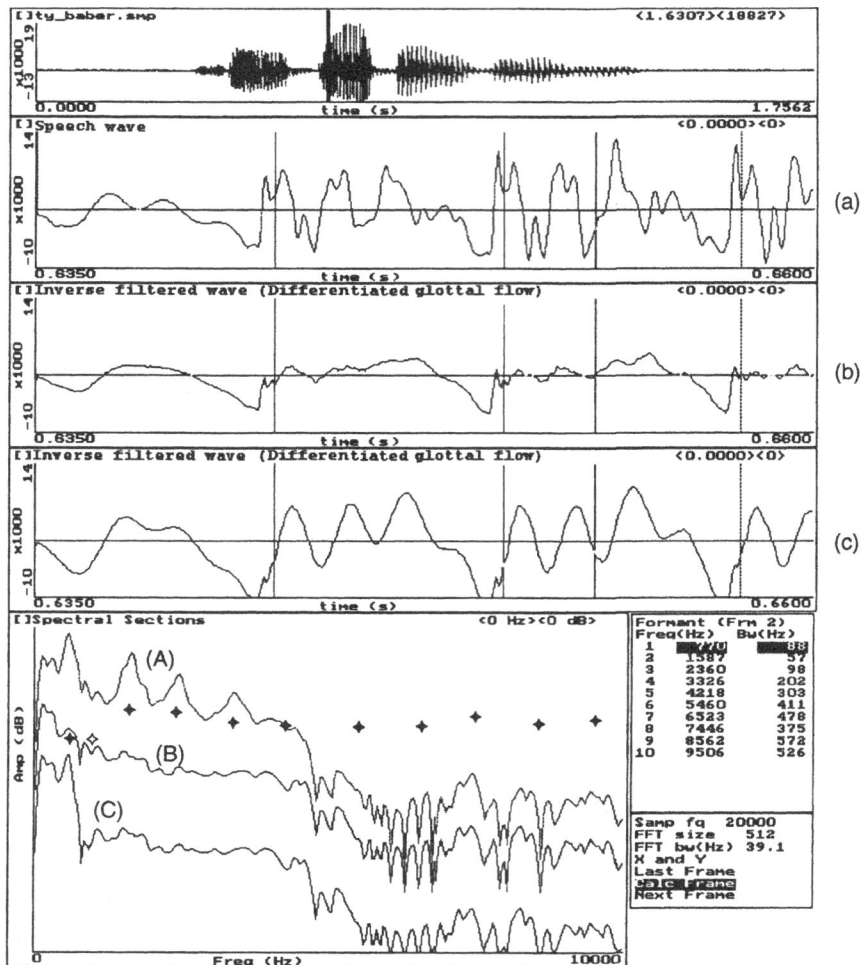

Figure 15.3   Modified screen display of an interactive inverse filtering program.

may adopt different strategies and therefore arrive at different results: even one and the same user might change strategy over time. This is likely to be more of a potential than an actual drawback: different users can generally be trained to be very consistent with each other and with themselves. This has been confirmed by the authors as well as by Hunt (1987).

A major advantage of using an automatic method is of course the reduction in analysis time needed. Even with programs like INA which help the user by providing a first filter estimate, the analysis of long utterances becomes extremely time-consuming. If the corpus is large and many speakers need to be analysed, the only reasonable option is to use an automatic method.

A problem with inverse filtering, both manual and automatic is the circular strategy that is necessary for estimating the inverse filter parameters. In order to carry out the analysis, one has to make certain assumptions concerning what the source function looks like. In the time domain, the criterion typically used is maximum flatness in the closed phase of the glottal cycle, as there can be no flow during the closed phased. This criterion only holds, of course, if complete closure is obtained during the glottal cycle. Recent studies have indicated that very many speakers have some glottal leakage during the so-called closed phase (see Holmberg, Hillman and Perkell 1988 and Södersten 1994). In the frequency domain, the main criterion is typically to obtain as even a source spectrum slope as possible, by cancelling out formant peaks and anti-resonances. Recent modelling of source-filter interaction has shown that many peaks and dips could originate from interaction effects rather than from the supraglottal transfer function (see the illustration of interaction ripple in figure 15.4). These 'problems' make inverse filtering a more difficult task. However, we feel that as the general knowledge increases, concerning the vocal tract and voice source functions as well as the interaction between the two, this will lead to better estimates of the inverse filter and thus to a better description of the voice source. These problems can in principle be overcome by using a direct method of estimating the glottal airflow (described in a later section).

Requirements on recording equipment

All the techniques discussed above assume high fidelity speech recordings, particularly in terms of preserving a phase linear response at very low frequencies. To achieve this the microphones and amplifiers need to be of very high quality. Furthermore, the recording would either have to be done on an FM tape recorder, digital tape recorder or straight onto computer. (Ways of compensating for phase distortion when using 'ordinary' audio equipment have been suggested in Holmes (1975), Hunt (1978), Ljungqvist and Fujisaki (1985c) and Hedelin (1986). Finally, the recording room should be anechoic or close to being anechoic.

Inverse filtering using an airflow mask

Glottal flow may also be estimated from an oral airflow recording carried out using a special airflow mask with a built-in differential pressure transducer. One advantage of estimating the glottal flow from the oral airflow signal is that the absolute glottal airflow level can be obtained, which is not

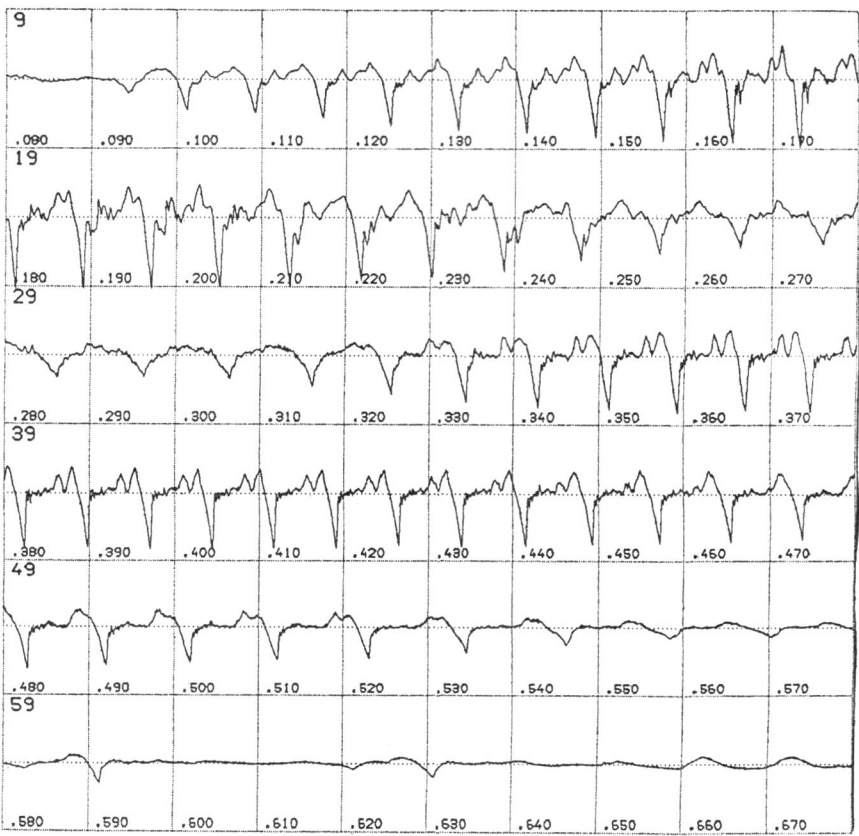

Figure 15.4   The inverse filter output (differential glottal flow) of the Swedish utterance /aˈjøː/. Note the source–filter interaction ripple in the glottal open phase (particularly in frames 34–47) and the frequently non-flat 'closed' phase

possible when the speech pressure waveform is used. Furthermore, an anechoic recording environment is not necessary when an airflow mask is used for recording the oral airflow. Note, however, that the quality of the recorder needs to be equally high, or even higher, as the recording has to be linear down to DC if absolute airflow levels are required. The vocal tract filter is eliminated in a similar fashion to that described above. Since the signal from the airflow mask is the oral airflow and not the pressure waveform, the signal obtained after inverse filtering is the true glottal flow. If the differentiated glottal flow is wanted, a first order differentiator (a real zero at zero frequency) has to be added to the inverse filter.

Two major drawbacks with the method of using an airflow mask are (i) the distortion introduced by the mask and (ii) its limited frequency response. Even the circumferentially vented pneumotachograph mask by Rothenberg (1973) which was specially developed for extended linear frequency response, has an upper frequency limitation of about 1–1.5 kHz.

To sum up, the method of using an airflow mask is most useful for estimating gross glottal airflow characteristics, general glottal behaviour and (particularly in combination with other methods) for studying the correlation between laryngeal control and voice source parameters. Its disadvantages, however, make it unsuitable for detailed spectral analysis of the voice source. Whenever such detailed voice source data are necessary (as for, for example, high fidelity synthesis purposes and speech recognition systems using source information), voice source estimation made from the speech pressure waveform still remains the only real option.

Inverse filtering in combination with glottography

In order to improve inverse filter estimation, additional glottographic recordings may be carried out simultaneously with the speech pressure (or oral airflow) recording. The most common use of an extra channel would be for estimating the closed phase in order to do automatic, pitch synchronous inverse filtering. By including a simultaneous recording of the vocal fold contact area as produced by a laryngograph, or of glottal area by means of photoelectric glottography, fairly accurate identification of the closed (or flat) portion of the glottal cycle can be obtained. This portion of the cycle is then used as the time window when using the covariance method of LPC (cf. Chan and Brookes 1989).

The advantage of including an additional recording is, as already stated, the possibility of achieving a more accurate voice source signal. In the case of introducing an intrusive method, the disadvantage might be that the equipment could interfere with the subject's normal behaviour. Also, it leads to a more complicated recording procedure compared to the otherwise very simple and straightforward microphone recording.

Other methods for obtaining glottal flow
The Sondhi Tube

The method described by Sondhi (1975) and used (in a slightly modified version) by Monsen and Engebretson (1977) utilizes a long metal tube into which the subject phonates (see figure 15.5). This tube then acts as a pseudo-infinite termination of the vocal tract. A microphone inside the tube picks up a signal that should in theory be the equivalent of the glottal airflow. The reason why this signal should approximate the volume velocity at the

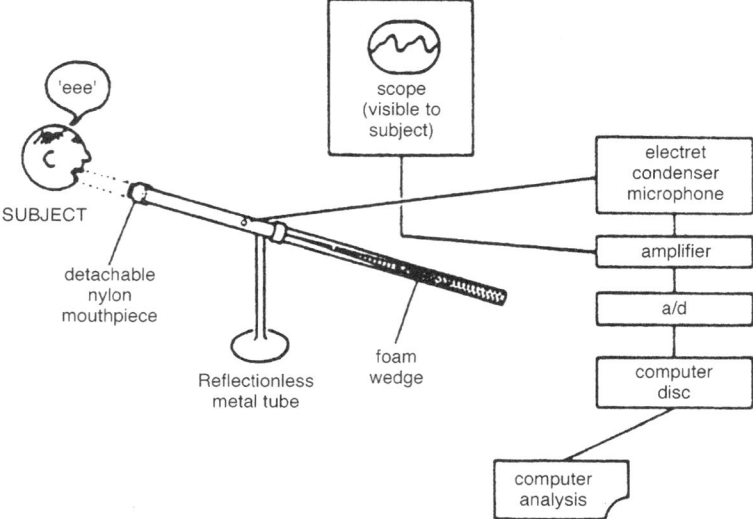

Figure 15.5   Schematic diagram of the experimental set-up using the Sondhi tube (after Monsen and Engebretson 1977).

glottis is that the reflectionless termination of the tube causes a considerable reduction of the vocal tract resonances.

In Monsen and Engebretson's application the steel tube was 1.8 metres long with an inside diameter of 2.2 cm. A conical wedge inside the tube provided the reflectionless termination. Although Sondhi (1975) used fibreglass material for the wedge, Monsen and Engebretson (1977) used polyurethane foam, which they found more efficient as an acoustic termination of the tube and easier and safer to handle. The length of the wedge is approximately 90 cm and is therefore effective for wave lengths of less than about 3.5 metres, i.e. for frequencies greater than about 90 Hz. The resonant frequencies of the tube (which is roughly ten times longer than a typical male vocal tract) would be roughly $50n$ Hz, where n is all positive odd numbers. All resonances but the lowest are damped by the terminating wedge.

The main advantage with this method is that no inverse filtering is necessary and thus no *a priori* assumptions have to be made concerning the voice source. Furthermore, as with the method using a mask, no special recording room is needed. The method also provides a wide frequency range. The phase response, however, is not linear at low frequencies and will cause distortion of the glottal pulse shape unless a phase compensation filter is included. The method is also very attractive in that it allows for analysis of the glottal waveform in real time.

The method of using the Sondhi tube has one severe disadvantage: in principle the method only works with phonation of a neutral vowel. Therefore, this method is not a useful tool for analysing dynamic aspects of the voice source in natural speech. Furthermore, phonating into a long tube is quite an unnatural task and the auditory feedback is distorted. Both factors might interfere with the subject's normal behaviour.

To sum up, the Sondhi tube can be useful for measuring source characteristics such as differences in overall voice source characteristics between speakers, phonatory settings, correlations between f_0 and the voice source, etc. Unfortunately, however, the method does not lend itself to analysis of the dynamic contextual variation of the voice source within utterances, which is of paramount importance to linguists.

Glottal waveform estimation using miniature pressure transducers

Glottal airflow estimates can be obtained from pressure measurements in the trachea and the pharynx. Accurate measurement of subglottal pressure has traditionally been difficult to obtain. A useful approximation for many purposes is oesophageal pressure, which has frequently been measured by means of a tiny inflatable balloon placed in the oesophagus, directly behind and beneath the vocal folds (see Ladefoged 1967b). Direct tracheal puncture is a technique which yields more reliable results. It has not been extensively used however, probably because of the potential medical risk factor and the unpleasantness for the subject. Direct subglottal measurements have also been obtained by means of a hollow catheter introduced through the glottis into the trachea. In this technique, as in the others mentioned, the pressure variations are conducted via narrow tubes to the external transducer, with the consequence that the frequency resolution is greatly impoverished. Edmonds, Lilly and Hardy (1971) have suggested that the frequency range for these methods tends to have an upper limit of about 300 Hz.

This particular difficulty has been overcome with the introduction of miniature semiconductor strain-gauge pressure transducers, with an excellent frequency response of up to 20 kHz. With this type of transducer, Cranen and Boves (1985) estimate that pressure can be measured with a resolution of 0.65 mm H_2O (see however below). These transducers (developed originally for medical applications such as heart catheterization) may be attached to a thin catheter and introduced into the trachea through the glottis in such a way that the catheter lies in the posterior commissure of the vocal folds. This technique has been demonstrated and some preliminary results have been presented by Kitzing and Löfqvist (1975) and Cranen and Boves (1985).

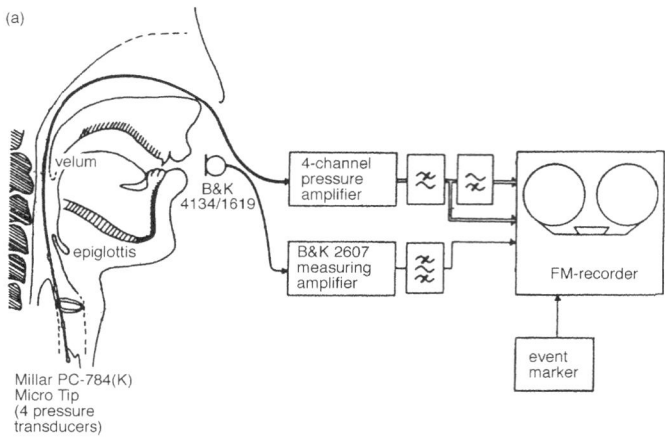

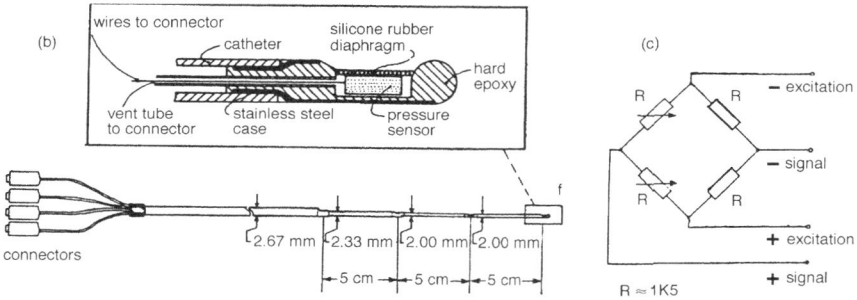

Figure 15.6   (a) schematic diagram of the experimental set-up using miniature pressure transducers (b) Dimensions of the Millar catheter [type: PC-784(K)] with its four pressure transducers (c) Electrical diagram of the transducer (after Cranen and Boves 1985).

In the latter study, by attaching multiple transducers to a single catheter, subglottal and supraglottal pressures were recorded at two locations 5 cm apart in both the trachea and the pharynx (see figure 15.6). From this an estimation of glottal flow can be made. Integrating the difference signal of the two pressure transducers in either cavity with respect to time yields a signal which is roughly proportional to the particle velocity. Particle velocity can in turn be considered as a scaled version of glottal airflow (volume velocity) with the cross sectional area of the tube as a scaling factor.

This technique has undeniable attractions. Firstly, it provides an estimation of glottal flow which does not depend on inverse filtering with its associated assumptions discussed above. Secondly, as sub- and supra- (and thereby) transglottal pressures are directly measured, it offers interesting opportunities for correlating these with the more derived measures such as particle velocity and glottal flow.

One major limitation with this technique is, however, that even though the transducer has an excellent frequency response, the formula for approximating the airflow is only valid for frequencies below 1500 Hz.

Other problems with this method concern the practicalities of calibrating and recording. A major difficulty arises out of the fact that the pressure transducers are extremely sensitive to temperature variation, due to the semiconductor material from which they are made. As described by Cranen and Boves, a change from room to body temperature can occasion an error of approximately 20% of the full scale over which variations are found in speech. Furthermore, the sensor outputs behave unpredictably when exposed to a sudden temperature change. For these reasons, very careful calibration must be carried out with the transducers in place. The procedure suggested by the above authors demands considerable sophistication of the subject (the ability, for example, of maintaining a constant pressure and an open glottis for a few seconds while blowing into a U-tube manometer). Care must be taken to avoid sudden or deep inhalations, which would cause temperature-induced measurement errors. Artefacts may also arise due to mechanical excitation of the sensors should they touch the vocal tract. All this must be borne in mind when analysing results.

Furthermore, conducting an actual recording is not without its problems. Local anaesthetic is needed and insertion must be made under medical supervision. Introducing the catheter through the vocal folds can involve considerable discomfort to the subject (personal experience). For some subjects, gagging reflexes may make insertion impossible. It is not clear whether and to what extent the intrusive catheter, the associated discomfort and the local anaesthetic may interfere with the subject's normal phonation.

For all these reasons, this technique in its present state of development does not seem all that well suited to large-scale studies, but rather to carefully controlled experiments on limited subjects and materials, perhaps as a supplement to broader studies involving other techniques.

Quantifying voice source characteristics: model matching

The methods discussed so far generate a glottal flow signal, which serves as the raw data for our analyses. An illustration of the differentiated glottal flow is shown in figure 15.4. As a next step one must quantify and interpret the salient characteristics of the source signal. Certain studies have employed a direct approach, measuring (as far as one can from visual displays of the glottal waveform) the kinds of parameters that are outlined below (see for example Huffman 1987a; Holmberg, Hillman and Perkell 1988). Another approach involves matching a model of source flow to the actual source signal so that the main characteristics are (hopefully) captured and then using the modelled signal to quantify these. This approach has been used in a number of recent descriptive studies (e.g. Gobl 1988; Pierrehumbert 1989; Karlsson 1990, 1992; Gobl and Ní Chasaide 1992; Kane and Ní Chasaide 1992) as well as in the generation of the source data detailed in chapter 5. As a measuring tool it can be particularly useful for quantifying certain source parameters such as the return phase (explained later) which, though perceptually important, are difficult to measure directly from the glottal waveform. This modelled signal can also be directly implemented in synthesis, an obvious attraction to the many researchers for whom this is the main application of the analysis.

There are many models of the true and differentiated glottal flow that could in principle be used for the matching procedure and a number of them are reviewed in Ananthapadmanabha (1984) and Ljungqvist and Fujisaki (1985a). A model which has gained particular popularity in recent years and which was used in the above mentioned descriptive studies is the LF-model of differentiated flow, illustrated in figure 15.7 and described in Fant, Liljencrants and Lin (1985).

In current implementations, the matching is carried out in the time domain. As in the case of inverse filtering, the process can be fully automatic or can involve an interactive methodology, where the experimenter fine-tunes the match for individual glottal pulses. The latter methodology was used to derive the source measurements illustrated in chapter 5 and figure 15.8 illustrates the screen display which guides the experimenter in the matching process. The top window in this figure shows the speech waveform with a cursor marking the glottal pulse currently being analysed. The middle window shows the inverse filtered wave (differentiated flow) centred on the pulse being currently matched. Superimposed on this pulse one can also see a matched model pulse (thick dark line). The shape of the matched model pulse is determined by the location of five vertical cursors which denote critical time points and a single horizontal cursor which denotes the negative amplitude of the main excitation. With the mouse, the user can change these time and amplitude cursors, thereby altering the shape of the model pulse. The object of the exercise is to approximate as closely as possible the underlying inverse filtered wave in its important dimensions. The spectrum of the inverse filtered pulse is shown in the lowest window and superimposed on it is the spectrum of the model pulse (thick black line). As with the fine-tuning of the inverse filter, the

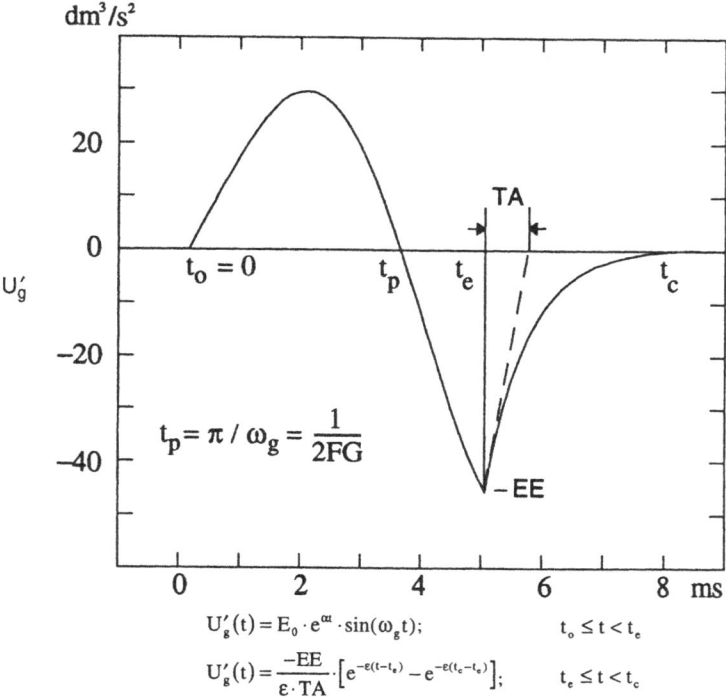

Figure 15.7 The LF model; a four-parameter model of differentiated glottal flow.

user is guided by the time domain information (middle window) and the frequency domain information (lowest window) to achieve the best possible match for the modelled pulse.

Automatic programs for model matching also exist. They are typically based on algorithms for minimizing the squared difference between the samples of the model and the glottal waveform. Examples of automatic matching programs are to be found in Ananthapadmanabha (1984) and in Chan and Brookes (1989). The advantages and disadvantages of the interactive, manual approach as compared to the automatic are similar to those discussed for inverse filtering. The main advantage of the automatic approach is, of course, the vastly reduced analysis time needed. As for the inverse filtering, if the corpus is large and many speakers need to be analysed, the only reasonable option is to use an automatic method. It has the advantage of always keeping to the same strategy for estimating the voice source parameters. The major disadvantage concerns the accuracy of the match. A much higher degree

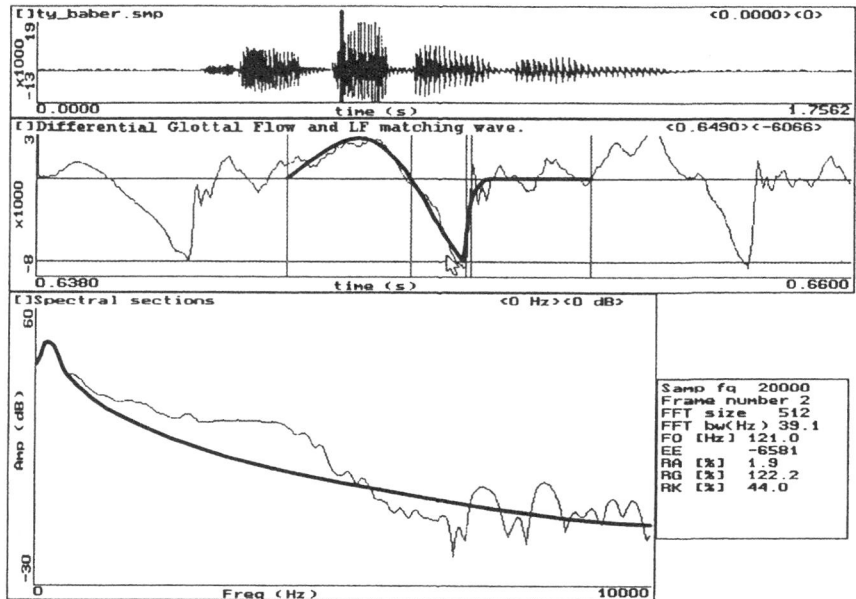

Figure 15.8   Screen display of an interactive model matching program.

of accuracy can be achieved using the manual interactive approach which gives the user control over the details of the matching.

A quite different approach to the parameter estimation of the voice source has been suggested in Fant (1988) and in Fant and Lin (1988). Relations between the time and the frequency domain are presented as well as formulae for calculating time domain parameter values from the amplitudes of the voice source spectrum. These time domain parameter values can be used to control the generation of most of the time domain parametric models described above. One advantage of this approach is that the model matching is done to achieve the best spectral resemblance. As it is probably more important perceptually to have the correct spectral characteristics than the correct details of the waveform fit, this method may turn out to be more desirable for some applications. Furthermore, as spectral properties are used for calculating the parameter values, it is no longer necessary to obtain low-frequency phase linear recordings in order to arrive at reliable estimates. The drawback with this approach is of course the lack of control over the matching in the time domain. The optimal match in the frequency domain does not necessarily generate the truest match in the time domain.

Important voice source parameters

An important measure of the source would be its spectral slope characteristics. This may be a difficult measure to obtain, as demonstrated in attempts by Jackson *et al.* (1985) to fit a single regression line to source spectra.

In effect, source data are typically presented in terms of time domain parameters. In this section a brief outline is provided of some of the main ones, thought to be acoustically and perceptually important and which are known to capture salient characteristics of the glottal flow pulse. By and large, they can also be correlated with aspects of the vibratory pattern of the vocal folds. The time domain (true and differentiated glottal flow) and frequency domain correlates of certain parameters are illustrated in figure 15.9. A fuller account of these and other parameters is to be found in Gobl and Ní Chasaide (1988). The reader should note that these parameters are used in the illustrations of source data in chapter 5.

EE, the excitation strength, is the negative amplitude at the time point of maximum discontinuity of the differentiated flow. It corresponds to the maximum slope of the falling branch of the glottal pulse, which typically precedes full closure (figure 15.9a). At the production level it is determined by the speed of closure of the vocal folds and the volume velocity of air through them. At the acoustic level it corresponds to the overall intensity of the signal (figure 15.9b).

RA is a measure of the residual flow (or dynamic leakage) from excitation to complete closure, or maximum closure if there is a DC leakage (figure 15.9a). At the production level RA relates to the sharpness of the glottal closure, i.e. to whether the vocal folds make contact in an instantaneous way or in a more gradual fashion along their entire length and depth. RA is an important determinant of the spectral slope of the signal (figure 15.9b). In terms of the LF model, the effect of the return phase on the voice-source spectrum is approximately that of a first order low-pass filter. The cut-off of this filter is determined by $FA = 1/2\pi TA$.

RK is a measure of the skew or symmetry of the glottal flow pulse. It expresses the relationship between the times of the rising and falling branches of the glottal pulse. The larger the RK value, the more symmetrical the pulse shape. At the acoustic level, RK mainly affects the lower part of the source spectrum, so that a high RK corresponds to a boosting of the lower harmonics.

OQ is frequently called the open quotient, and it expresses the relation between the open portion of the glottal pulse to the total pulse duration. It mainly controls the amplitude of the lower components in the source spectrum (see figure 15.9b).

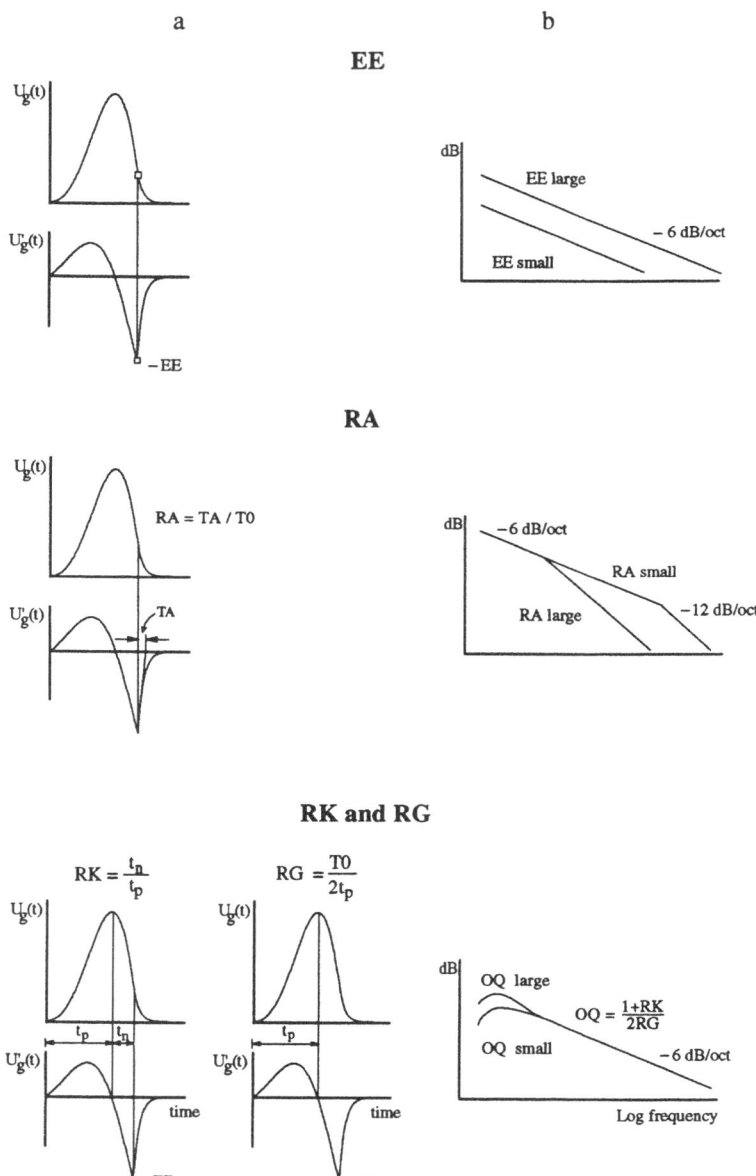

Figure 15.9   The voice source parameters EE, RA, RK and RG, in terms of (a) the true and differentiated glottal flow, and (b) the effect of a change in a parameter's value on the acoustic spectrum.

Measurements of the speech output signal
Spectral measurements
The spectral characteristics of the voice source are inevitably reflected in the speech output signal, and therefore, measurements of spectral levels of the latter yield valuable insights into the former. Where specialized analysis software and/or the ideal recording conditions are not available, these measurements may be the only option. A number of linguistic descriptive studies (see below) have shown them to be very useful for comparing speech tokens where the mode of phonation is contrasted (e.g. segments involving breathy voice as compared to modal voice).

Spectral measurements of the speech waveform generally take the form of a comparison of the spectral levels of F0 and some higher point in the spectrum. The level of F0 is a useful basis for comparison as it tends on the whole to remain relatively stable (see further discussion on this point in chapter 5). A particularly popular measure has been a comparison between it and the second harmonic ($H_1 - H_2$, as used, for example, in Fischer-Jørgensen 1967; Bickley 1982; Maddieson and Ladefoged 1985). Another measure frequently used is a comparison of the amplitude levels of F1 and the fundamental (L1 – L0), as, for example, in Gobl and Ní Chasaide 1992; Kirk, Ladefoged and Ladefoged 1984 (see also illustrations in chapter 5).

Caution is required with this type of measurement, as the slope characteristics of the source spectrum is only one of the determinants of spectral levels in the speech output. The frequency of a formant will affect its level: thus the (L1 – L0) measure would be entirely inappropriate if one were comparing, say, two vowels of a different quality. Formant levels are also affected by the degree of damping present, which depends on a combination of glottal and supraglottal factors. The comparison of H1 and H2 levels is highly sensitive to any change in the frequency of F0 or F1. The lower the frequency of F1 (and the higher the frequency of F0) the greater the likelihood of H1 (or H2) being boosted, simply due to their proximity to F1. For these reasons, spectral measurements of this type require an understanding of potential artefacts and a careful selection of speech materials to take account of them.

Estimates of time domain source parameters
In a descriptive study Gobl (1988) reported a striking correlation between the excitation strength of the source signal and the amplitude of the speech pressure waveform at the time-point of the excitation. A tendency for covariation of source parameters was also observed. The return phase, RA, is often negatively correlated with the excitation strength, EE. One also

often finds a positive correlation between RA and RK. For some similar observations, see Fant (1993) and Pierrehumbert (1989). In recent work Fant *et al.* (1994) and Fant and Liljencrants (1994) have elaborated proposals for estimating time domain source parameters directly from the speech pressure waveform. The starting-point of these estimates would be: (i) the measurement of the negative amplitude of the speech waveform (because of its correspondence to the source excitation, EE); (ii) an approximation of Up: by integrating the speech waveform one can obtain an approximate estimate of the AC component of the glottal pulse. It also calls for (iii) an estimate of a critical frequency for F0 below which EE and F0 exhibit a positive correlation and above which this correlation turns negative.

This last approach is still at the experimental stage and one can expect fuller elaborations and refinements in the future. By definition, it yields approximations rather than actual source measurements and considerable research will be required comparing estimated and direct measurements to establish where these calculations do and do not perform. Insofar as they permit source estimates to be carried out easily and rapidly on the speech waveform and insofar as low-frequency phase linear recordings are not required, these developments undoubtedly offer exciting prospects for the future.

Notes

1 One aspect of Hutter's work that deserves to be more widely followed is a procedure to determine the relationship between change in output voltage of the PGG (photoglottograph) amplifier for defined changes in light-intensity.

2 In contrast to custom-designed equipment such as the Frøkjær-Jensen photoelectroglottograph, the stability of standard endoscopic light-sources should not be taken for granted. Appreciable ripple at the first few harmonics of the mains frequency can be troublesome. Use of a DC power source may be advisable.

3 cf. Baer, Löfqvist and McGarr (1983) for this conception of the transillumination signal as the weighted sum of the glottal width at a series of points along its length.

4 It should not be overlooked, however, that the correlation is not based on two completely independent measurement methods; it will be probably be the case, for example, that changes in the distance between larynx and fibrescope will have a similar effect on the analysis of both the cine film and the transillumination signal (e.g. smaller image, lower signal amplitude).

5 We have found the following solution very convenient: a commercially available video timer (FOR-A VTG33) was modified according to a technique developed by N.R. Petersen at the phonetics lab of Copenhagen University. In addition to its normal function, which is to insert date and time into the video signal with a resolution of 1 cs, pulses for the one-second intervals were led out in a form which allowed them to be recorded on one track of an instrumentation recorder that was also used to record the photoglottographic and audio signals. Alternatively,

if the measurement signals are recorded online by computer, a straightforward solution would be to remote-control the video-timer using a digital i/o port, with the computer resetting and starting the timer at the start of each measurement sequence.

6 This double transduction may also increase the utility of transillumination for studies of phonation, since vibratory parameters may differ along the front-back dimension of the glottis (Baer, Löfqvist and McGarr 1983).

16

Acoustic analysis

DANIEL RECASENS

Acoustic analysis techniques

Techniques for acoustic analysis are more easily available than techniques for articulatory analysis which explains why the former have been used more extensively than the latter in studies on coarticulation. Criteria for data analysis on spectrograms and on acoustic waveforms were early established; nowadays the availability of fast and powerful acoustic analysis techniques allows processing large amounts of data which helps to improve our knowledge of the factors inducing variability in the acoustic signal. An increase in the explanatory power of the coarticulatory effects may be achieved through synchronous acoustic and articulatory measures; moreover inferences about articulatory mechanisms may be drawn from acoustic data on coarticulatory effects using general principles of acoustic theory of speech production (keeping in mind that articulatory–acoustic relationships may be non-linear).

Traditionally formant frequency information for vowels, laterals, rhotics, glides and nasals has been obtained from broad-band spectrograms at the centre of formants or from narrow-band spectral section peaks; narrow-band spectral sections have been mostly used to gather frequency information at the noise period for fricatives, affricates and stop bursts. Formant detection on spectrograms may be problematic when formant bands are too weak, two formants come close together (e.g. F2 and F3 for /i/) or F1 has a very low frequency (e.g. in the case of /i/).

Nowadays formant frequency trajectories are usually tracked using the all-pole model LPC (Linear Prediction Coding). LPC parameters vary depending on the event being measured; a review of acoustic studies from the literature reveals that LPC is usually performed with a 10–30 Hamming window, in 5–10 ms steps and with a number of coefficients which increases with the number of formants (e.g. ten to fourteen for oral vowels, fourteen to eighteen for nasal consonants and nasalized vowels). FFT (Fast Fourier Transform) spectral sections with the same parameters may also be used for the analysis of formant frequencies keeping in mind that the presence of glottal harmonic structure may mask vocal tract resonances (e.g. at the F1 region for high vowels). Information about the location of spectral zeros (for laterals, nasals, fricatives and stop bursts) can be achieved from FFT sections or using a pole-zero matching technique of a vocal tract transfer function with a transducer positioned on the neck above the larynx (Fujimura and Lindqvist 1971).

Segmentation and the estimation of segmental durations may be carried out on waveforms and on spectrograms (Klatt 1974; Ohde and Sharf 1975; Bladon and Al-Bamerni 1976). Fundamental frequency data are obtained on digitized waveforms using computerized tracking procedures based on time domain approach algorithms; traditionally F_0 has been calculated measuring the central frequency of selected high harmonics on narrow band spectrograms and dividing it by the order number of the respective harmonic (Lehiste and Peterson 1961; Umeda 1981). LPC and FFT are suitable methods for analyzing relative formant amplitude levels; average sound pressure levels have been measured on VU meter readings (Lehiste and Peterson 1959).

Segmentation

The selection of acoustic events for the analysis of coarticulatory effects involving adjacent phonetic segments depends on segmentation criteria:

- different criteria have been proposed for determining the acoustic boundaries of vowel segments from inspection of spectrographic displays (Peterson and Lehiste 1960; Espy-Wilson 1992) or acoustic waveforms (Luce and Luce 1985; McGowan and Nittrouer 1988): at F1 onset or at the onset of periodicity after a stop, and at those events or at frication noise offset after a fricative; at the abrupt cessation of formant energy before a stop and at the onset of high frequency energy noise before a fricative; at energy changes and formant discontinuities in the adjacency of a nasal consonant, and after /l/ and /r/ (with the help of F3 information for the two latter consonants); at a steady F_0 minimum before final /l/ and /r/ (with the help of F3 information); at the onset of a positive F2 trajectory in the context of /w/ and at a F3 frequency minimum with adjacent /j/. In some instances vowel segmentation may be harder than usual, e.g. it may be difficult to determine the offset of a vowel when voicing continues after closure onset for a following stop;

- several temporal events have been chosen as indicative of the transition's starting point at an acoustic stable portion during the vowel: the frame where the frequency change for each formant after an oral stop falls to less than 10 Hz per 5 ms frame, or where the formant back-tracks to the same value within four frames (Kewley-Port 1982); the first point where the formant frequency (F1) after an oral stop is greater than 80% of the frequency change (van Summers 1987); the point at which transition offset after /w/ increases by no more than 5 Hz in each of three subsequent pitch periods (Mack and Blumstein 1983); the point in time where the first derivative of a given formant equals zero (Lindblom 1963b); the minimum or maximum formant frequency turning point (Krull 1989). Problems in determining the boundaries of the formant transitions may be encountered for vowels uttered at fast speech rates, for vowels involving articulatory movement throughout (as in the case of rounded vowels) or for sequences exhibiting long range transitions (as in the case of the sequence /təp/);

- several acoustic events for consonants can be identified quite easily: closure onset, at the temporal point where vowel formant energy ceases to occur (Fischer-Jørgensen 1979; Zue 1980) or at a drop in waveform amplitude postvocalically or after a stop burst in consonantal sequences (Luce and Luce 1985; Docherty 1992); closure offset, at the onset of a release burst; onset/offset of a fricative noise, at amplitude discontinuities in intervocalic position or in fricative sequences (Docherty 1992); consonantal voicing, from the presence of pitch pulses on acoustic waveforms and of a voicing bar on spectrographic displays. Nasals, liquids and glides are signalled by a complex array of cues on the waveform (e.g. changes in shape and amplitude) and on spectrograms (e.g. spectral discontinuities and a decrease in formant intensity level) (Espy-Wilson 1992; Båvegård *et al.* 1993). Segmentation may be harder than usual in the absence of important acoustic cues such as the release burst or the silent closure in the case of stops produced with an incomplete closure, and the high intensity noise for fricatives produced with an open frication channel; moreover, linguopalatal contact data reveal that closure onset for nasals and laterals does not always coincide with the actual articulatory closure onset and that primary articulatory attributes of velarized /l/ may occur after voicing offset (Goldstein 1994);

- tonal contours have been identified at different events for the analysis of tone coarticulation, i.e. at the first F_0 value after voiceless stops or at the onset of an abrupt F_0 increase after voiced stops, at a change in F_0 direction or tonal turning point, and at the last F_0 value preceding formant energy offset or the direction of F_0 movement towards the following tone (Shen 1990; Gandour, Potisuk and Dechongkit 1994). Other measures include tonal height and tonal slope (Xu 1994).

Coarticulation involving adjacent phonetic segments
This section reviews methods applied in the literature for studying coarticulatory effects between adjacent segments at the acoustic level.

Formant transitions
Formant transitions, i.e. formant trajectories generated by articulatory movement, have been measured in order to investigate V-to-C coarticulation or else contextual invariance for stop consonants. Several events have been analysed:

- formant transition endpoints. As illustrated in figure 16.1 (top), formant frequency values at vowel onset in a CV sequence may be represented as a function of both consonant and vowel in F2 x F3 plots; figure 16.1 (bottom) also gives frequency ranges showing the degree of coarticulatory variability for the formant data in the upper graphs. The figure shows more variability for velars versus labials and alveolars and for voiced versus voiceless stops, and little or no overlap between consonantal categories when all data points are taken into account;
- formant transitions proper, which may be reproduced by means of straight line approximations (Kewley-Port 1982) or by parabolic curves (Stevens, House and Paul 1966). Data on CV transitions trajectories in figure 16.2 show that the direction, the frequency extent and the duration of the transitions at vowel onset vary with the vowel and the consonant; it is also worth noticing that F2 for some CV combinations, i.e. /ga/ and /du/, shows no appreciable vowel steady state portion. Broad and Fertig (1970) have proposed a linear model for eleven equidistant vowel points in /CɪC/ sequences according to which F1 and F2 trajectories can be modelled as the superposition of the initial and final transitions thus capturing the fact that the consonantal influence decreases with temporal distance. A later improvement of the model (Broad and Clermont 1987) includes additional components, i.e. pre-consonantal similarity (formant contours are shaped differently depending on the

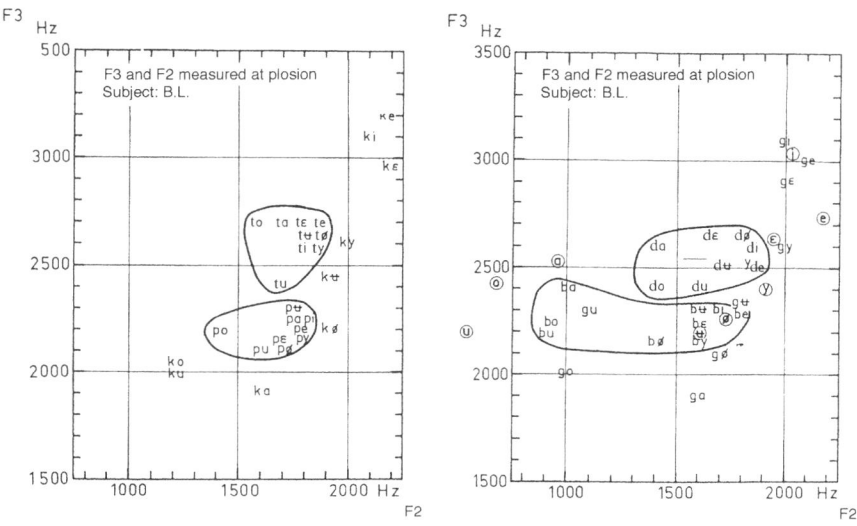

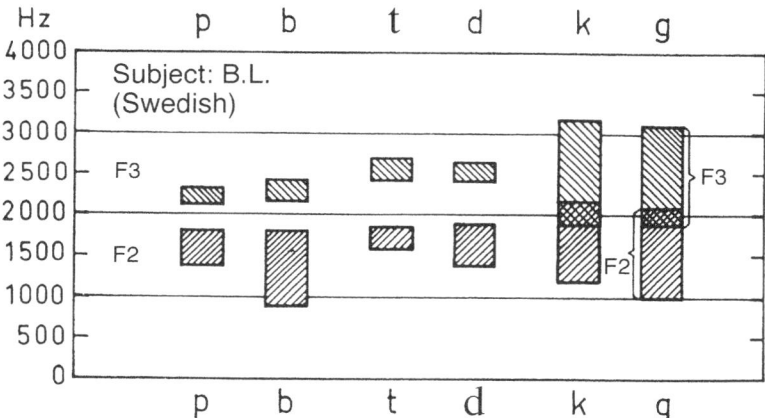

Figure 16.1 (Top) F2 × F3 values at vowel onset for Swedish CV sequences with voiced and voiceless stops of different place of articulation (/b/, /d/, /g/, /p/, /t/, /k/) and several vowels (/i/, /e/, /ɛ/, /ʉ/, /y/, /ø/, /u/, /o/, /ɑ/). (Bottom) Range of F2 and F3 values for the same data represented in the upper F2 × F3 plots (from Fant 1973).

contextual consonant), target-locus proportionality (formant transitions are scaled proportionally to the differences between the vowel targets and the consonantal loci) and exponential duration dependence and contour shapes (consonantal perturbation on a formant frequency at the vowel mid-point decays exponentially as the vowel mid-point decays). Rate of change or slope of a formant transition, i.e. frequency displacement divided by transition duration (Stevens and House 1963; van Summers 1987), can be expressed through curvature values; a comparison of curvature values before and after the vocalic mid-point provides information about asymmetries associated with syllable position and with the effect of the preceding and following consonant (Stevens, House and Paul 1966);

- loci, which have been obtained extending the CV voiced formant transition backward in time to the burst (Kewley-Port 1982) or else taking the formant frequency at the CV boundary (Krull 1989). Projected formant transitions from vowel offset back to the stop burst in figure 16.3 provide support for single loci for labials and alveolars but not so for velars. Locus equations have been investigated as a method for exploring relational invariance for stop place of articulation across vowel contexts (Sussman, McCaffrey and Matthews 1991): extremely linear regression functions (or locus equations) were found to relate F2 transition onset values to F2 mid-vowel values while showing distinct slopes and y intercepts as a function of consonantal place of articulation; moreover, velars should be assigned two locus equation prototypes depending on whether they appear before front or back vowels.

Vowel stable portion

The analysis of C-to-V coarticulatory effects may be carried out at some representative point during the most stable period of the vowel. Several criteria have been proposed in this respect: at the discontinuity between a vowel transition and the vowel stable portion following cutoff criteria such as those given above; at the vowel mid-point which may correspond to a single time frame (Kondo 1994; Koopmans-van Beinum 1994) or to an average of temporal points (e.g. three points representing a 25 ms interval in Stevens and House 1963); at a stable phase close to vowel onset/offset (Ohde and Sharf 1975); at several equidistant points along the vowel (Stålhammar, Karlsson and Fant 1973).

C-to-V effects in a given consonantal environment have been calculated by

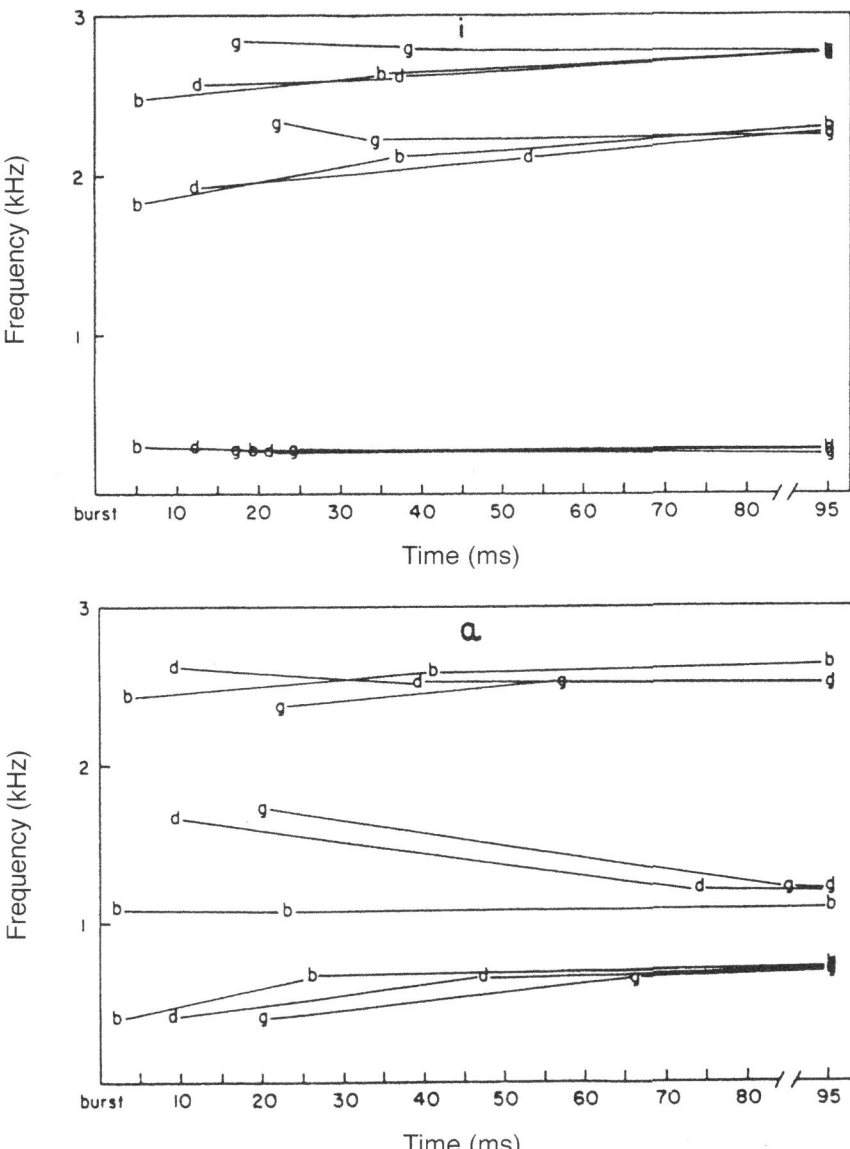

Figure 16.2   F1, F2 and F3 trajectories extending from the stop burst until 95 ms inside the vowel in American English CV sequences with the vowels /i/, /ɑ/ and /u/ and the stop consonants /b/, /d/ and /g/ (from Kewley-Port 1982).

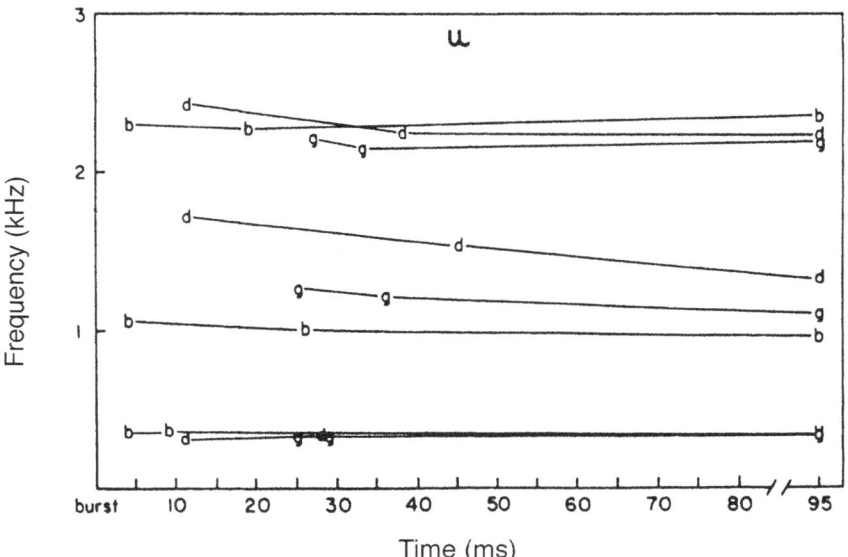

Figure 16.2 (*cont.*)

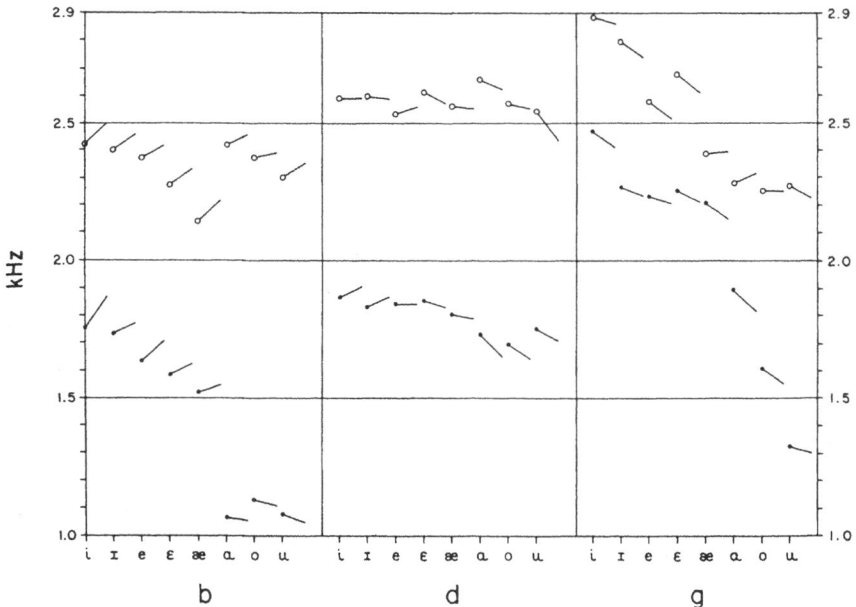

Figure 16.3   Projected CV formant transitions towards F2 loci (solid circles) and F3 loci (open circles) for different American English vowels (/i/, /ɪ/, /e/, /ɛ/, /æ/, /ɑ/, /o/, /u/) preceded by /b/, /d/ and /g/ (from Kewley-Port 1982).

subtracting the vowel formant frequencies from those for the same vowel in a 'null' context (/hVd/; Stevens and House 1963), in isolation (Ohde and Sharf 1975) or across several contextual conditions (van Bergem 1994). This calculation procedure reveals a centralizing effect of consonantal context with vowel undershoot generally increasing with the articulatory distance between the vocalic and the consonantal targets. The variance in formant frequency across consonantal environments has been taken as a measure of contextual sensitivity (Stevens and House 1963; Kondo 1994; Koopmans-van Beinum 1994). Contextual vowel reduction has been modelled using a context-dependent formula which takes into account formant frequencies for vowels in isolation and vowel duration (Stålhammar, Karlsson and Fant 1973).

Stop release

A template fitting procedure using short-term spectra has been applied to the open interval of CV syllables (i.e. the distance from the start of the explosion to vowel onset) in order to assess the existence of context-independent frequency templates for stops of different place of articulation (Blumstein and Stevens 1979; Lahiri, Gewirth and Blumstein 1984; Cohn 1988). According to this procedure, a decrease in percentage fits indicates an increase in coarticulation degree and thus a more radical departure from invariance (Cohn 1988). Templates ('diffuse-rising' for alveolars, 'diffuse-falling' for labials, 'compact' for velars) appear to work quite successfully for CV sequences but much less so for VC sequences; moreover some clear contextual effects in template identification were found, e.g. the diffuse-rising template was misidentified for initial labials and velars before specific front vowels (those realizations tended to be identified as alveolars). Figure 16.4 exemplifies the three templates mentioned above for /b/, /d/ and /g/ in different vowel contexts; it can be seen that the energy level is higher at low versus high frequency regions for /b/ and vice versa for /d/, while spectra for /g/ exhibit an energy peak in the mid-frequency range. Other studies have reported large V-to-C frequency, durational and amplitude effects at the release burst (Dorman, Studdert-Kennedy and Raphael 1977; Repp and Lin 1989). Coarticulatory trends in stop clusters also affect the frequency of occurrence and the spectral frequency components of the C1 burst (Henderson and Repp 1982; Repp 1983).

Fricative noise

Coarticulation effects at the turbulence noise for fricatives have been gathered either at different slices starting at vowel onset or offset into the noise portion (Soli 1981; Sereno *et al.* 1987; McGowan and Nittrouer 1988; Nittrouer, Studdert-Kennedy and McGowan 1988; Baum and Waldstein

1991) or else at a single slice or at one average spectrum over 25–50 ms around the centre of the noise portion (Nartey 1982; Norlin 1983; Svantesson 1983; Hoole *et al.* 1989; Hoole, Nguyen-Trong and Hardcastle 1993).

Two major frequency analysis methods have been used in the literature. The peak-picking method detects major spectral prominences within or outside the noise portion (Soli 1981; McGowan and Nittrouer 1988; Nittrouer, Studdert-Kennedy and McGowan 1988) or at a given frequency range (e.g. between 3–4.5 and 5–6.5 kHz for /s/ in Sereno *et al.* 1987); coarticulatory effects have been represented for a given peak at a given moment in time or along two time sections (e.g. F2 for /si/ versus /su/ in McGowan and Nittrouer 1988). Figure 16.5 shows spectral differences at the fricative noise of /s/ and /z/ as a function of following /i/, /a/ and /u/; indeed, a noise spectral peak between 1500 Hz and 2000 Hz before vowel onset exhibits a higher frequency when the vowel following the fricative is /i/ than when it is /a/ or /u/. According to a second method, a measure of the spectral centre of gravity is calculated from dB levels of about 22–24 critical bands obtained from FFT spectra (Norlin 1983; Svantesson 1983; Baum and Waldstein 1991; Hoole, Nguyen-Trong and Hardcastle 1993); in some of these studies, ratios or differences between centroid values have been used to study coarticulatory effects. Using a related method, Nartey (1982) multiplies log magnitude spectrum points by weighting coefficients representing a given filter's response at that frequency, and the output of the filter is calculated by summing the products and converting them to a normalized dB level; in order to study context-dependent distribution and shape of frequency peaks at all critical bands, this latter study plots centre of gravity against dispersion and intensity level for a given consonant as a function of different vowels. These studies on fricative coarticulation have reported effects from /u/ versus /i/ (in lip rounding) and from front versus back vowels, and differences in coarticulatory sensitivity across fricative consonants of different place of articulation.

Nasals, liquids and glides

Vowels have been found to affect slightly the frequency characteristics of the oral and nasal formants and antiformants at the nasal murmur, e.g. in the case of /m/ before /i/, /a/ and /u/ (Fujimura 1962; Fujimura and Lindqvist 1971; Repp 1986a). Vowel-dependent effects also occur at the spectral discontinuity at nasal release (e.g. /mi/ and /ni/ exhibit similar spectral properties at closure release) which has been quantified as the difference between the raw Fourier spectra of the two last murmur pitch pulses and the two initial vowel pitch pulses (Repp 1986a) or by dividing the energy value encompassing a given frequency range at the two events (Kurowski and

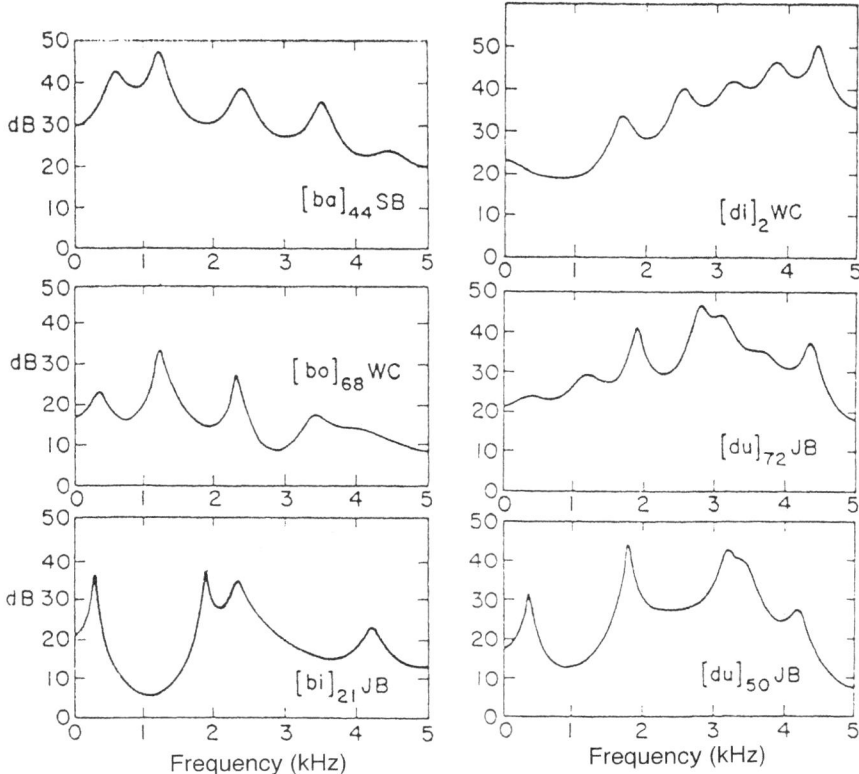

Figure 16.4   Examples of burst spectra for /b/, /d/ and /g/ in different vowel contexts exemplifying three place-dependent templates, i.e. diffuse-falling (for /bɑ/, /bo/, /bi/), diffuse-rising (for /di/, /du/) and compact (for /gɑ/, /gi/, /go/) (from Blumstein and Stevens 1979).

Blumstein 1987). In order to investigate vowel spectral changes introduced by coarticulatory nasalization, shifts in the vowel centre of gravity have been analysed using a centroid function which computes the centre frequency of an LPC spectral curve area including F1 and any close formants (Beddor 1983).

In a study on vowel-dependent effects for different positional allophones of /l/ (Bladon and Al-Bamerni 1976), coarticulation degree has been quantified in terms of the mean coarticulatory distance by which the vowel formant frequencies in a particular environment exceed or fall short of a canonical value obtained averaging all environments. Coarticulation in segmental sequences with a consonant exhibiting formant structure may be analysed through inspection of formant trajectories; thus, the F3 trajectory has been tracked for

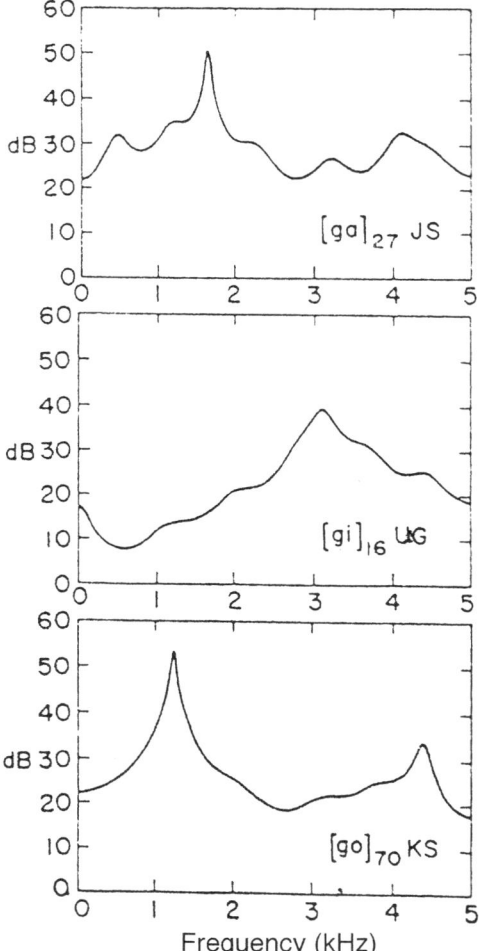

Figure 16.4 (*cont.*)

analysing the timing of the gestural onset of /r/ during a preceding vowel and during a preceding consonant (Boyce and Espy-Wilson 1997).

Voicing and tone

Literature studies (Zue 1980; Docherty 1992) reveal the existence of coarticulatory effects in the duration of VOT (i.e. the temporal interval between closure release and voicing onset) for stops as a function of vowels and adjacent consonants.

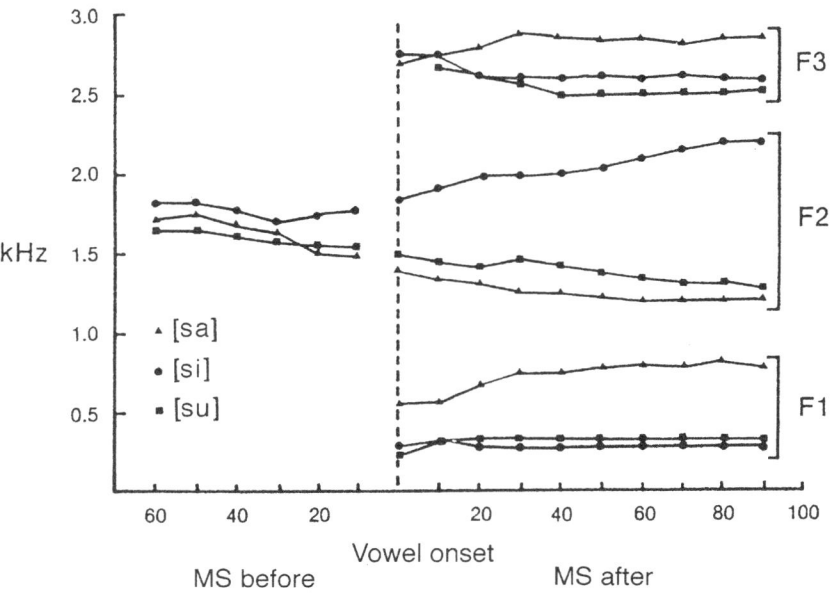

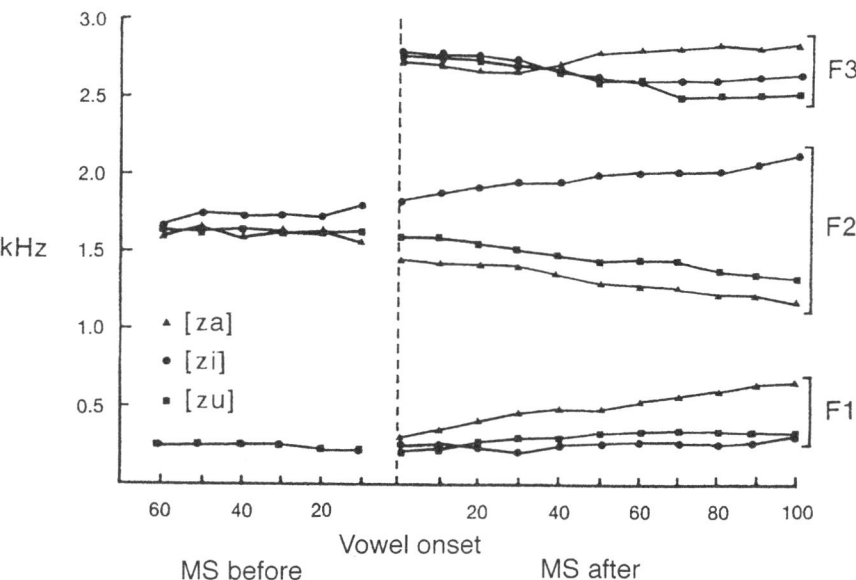

Figure 16.5   Spectral differences at the fricative noise of /s/ and /z/ as a function of following /i/, /a/ and /u/ (from Soli 1981).

Coarticulation data show changes in tonal height and slope as a function of adjacent tones; thus, a given tone may cause F_0 lowering/raising at the endpoint of the adjacent tone but further away as well (Shen 1990). F_0 contours may depend on the voicing and manner characteristics of the adjacent consonant (House and Fairbanks 1953) and on voicing and aspiration in the preceding consonant (King *et al.* 1987); vowel differences affect significant F_0 events and the duration between them (Umeda 1981).

Duration and intensity

Vowel duration may vary as a function of voicing (Peterson and Lehiste 1960; Luce and Luce 1985; Crystal and House 1988; Davis and van Summers 1989), manner (House and Fairbanks 1953) and place (Fischer-Jørgensen 1964) in the following consonant; intrasegmental cues may exhibit context-dependent durations as well (e.g. vowel transitions as a function of the consonant in CV sequences; Lehiste and Peterson 1961). Consonantal durations also exhibit coarticulatory effects, e.g. stop closure shortens in clusters versus non-clusters (Haggard 1973). Vowel intensity may also depend on the voicing and manner characteristics of the adjacent consonant (House and Fairbanks 1953).

Coarticulation involving non-adjacent phonetic segments

Long-range coarticulatory effects have been investigated as a function of two different vowels during a transconsonantal vowel in VCV sequences. Thus, for example, the presence of formant frequency differences associated with /i/ versus /a/ (often called 'changing' vowel) at transconsonantal /a/ (often called 'fixed' vowel) in the sequence pair /iCa/-/aCa/ may be taken as evidence for V-to-V coarticulatory effects. V-to-V effects across a single consonant have been measured at the edge of the formant transitions for the fixed vowel, e.g. F2 effects associated with /i/ versus /a/ in VCV sequences with several consonants in Choi and Keating (1991) and at its steady state portion as well (e.g. V-to-V effects across Swedish stops in Öhman (1966), across Russian palatalized and non-palatalized consonants in Derkach, Fant and Serpa-Leitaõ (1970) and Purcell (1979) or across bilabial /p/ in English and several African languages in Manuel (1990).

V-to-V effects may be measured more accurately in 5 or 10 ms steps along the fixed vowel. An estimate of their size (which often diminishes as temporal distance increases) may be obtained at the time point exhibiting the largest formant frequency difference associated with the changing vowel. An instance of this method of investigation is the study of V-to-V coarticulation in Japanese and American English /bVb/ sequences carried out by Magen (1984a).

Long-range vocalic coarticulatory effects have also been investigated in VCCV sequences with stop consonant clusters (e.g. C_2-dependent effects in formant frequency at V_1; Zsiga 1992) and with clusters made of fricative C1 and stop C_2 (e.g. C_1-dependent effects in formant frequency associated with /s/ versus /ʃ/ during V_2; Repp and Mann 1982).

References

Abberton, E. and Fourcin, A. 1997, Electropalatography, in Ball, M. J. and Code, C. (eds.), *Instrumental Clinical Phonetics*, London: Whurr Publications Ltd., pp. 149–93.

Abbs, J. H., Netsell, R. and Hixon, T. J. 1972, Variations in mandibular displacement, velocity, and acceleration as a function of phonetic content, *Journal of the Acoustical Society of America* 51: 89.

Abbs, J. H. and Eilenberg, G. R. 1976, Peripheral mechanisms of speech motor control, in Lass, N. J. (ed.), *Contemporary Issues in Experimental Phonetics*, New York, NY: Academic Press, pp. 139–170.

Abbs, J. H. and Gracco, V. L. 1984, Control of complex motor gestures; orofacial muscle responses to load perturbations of the lip during speech, *Journal of Neuropsychology* 51: 705–23.

Abbs, J. H., Gracco, V. L. and Cole, K. J. 1984, Control of multimovement coordination: sensorimotor mechanisms in speech motor programming, *Journal of Motor Behavior* 16: 195–231.

Abbs, J. H. and Watkin, K. L. 1976, Instrumentation for the study of speech physiology, in Lass, N. J. (ed.), *Contemporary Issues in Experimental Phonetics*, New York, NY: Academic Press, pp. 41–75.

Abelin, A., Landberg, I. and Persson, L. 1980, A study of anticipatory labial coarticulation in the speech of children, *Phonetic Experimental Research at the Institute of Linguistics, University of Stockholm* 2: 2–18.

Abercrombie, D. 1957, Direct palatography, *Zeitschrift für Phonetik* 10: 21–5.

Abramson, A. S., Nye, P. W., Henderson, J. and Marshall, C. W. 1981, Vowel height and the perception of consonantal nasality, *Journal of the Acoustical Society of America* 70: 329–39.

Abry, C. and Boë, J. L. 1980, A la recherche de corrélats géométriques discriminants pour l'opposition d'arrondissement du français, *Labialité et Phonétique*, Publications de l'Université des Langues et Lettres de Grenoble, pp. 217–37.
    1986, 'Laws' for lips, *Speech Communication* 5: 97–104.

Abry, C., Boë, J. L. and Descout, R. 1980, Voyelles arrondies et voyelles protrusés en français. Etude labiographique, *Labialité et Phonétique*, Publications de l'Université des Langues et Lettres de Grenoble, pp. 203–15.

Abry, C. and Lallouache, M. T. 1991a, Does increasing representational complexity lead to more speech variability? *Phonetic Experimental Research at the Institute of Linguistics, University of Stockholm* 14: 1–5.

1991b, Audibility and stability of articulatory movements, *Proceedings of XIIth International Congress of Phonetic Sciences, Aix-en-Provence* 1: 220–5.

1995, Le MEM: un modèle d'anticipation paramétrable par locuteur. Données sur l'arrondissement en français, *Bulletin du Laboratoire de la Communication Parlée*, 3: 85–99.

Al-Ani, S. H. 1970, *Arabic Phonology*. The Hague: Mouton.

Al-Bamerni, A. and Bladon, A. 1982, One-stage and two-stage patterns of velar coarticulation, *Journal of the Acoustical Society of America* 72: S104.

Alfonso, P. J. and Horiguchi, S. 1987, Vowel-related lingual articulation in /əCVC/ syllables as a function of stop consonants. *Proceedings of the XIth International Congress of Phonetic Sciences, Tallinn* 2: 41–4.

Alfonso, P., Neely, J. R., van Lieshout, P. H. H. M., Hulstijn, W. and Peters, H. F. M. 1993, Calibration, validation and hardware–software modifications to the Carstens EMMA system, *Forschungsberichte des Instituts für Phonetik und Sprachliche Kommunikation, München* 31: 105–20.

Ali, L., Daniloff, R. and Hammarberg, R. 1979, Intrusive stops in nasalfricative clusters: an aerodynamic and acoustic investigation, *Phonetica* 36: 85–97.

Ali, L., Gallagher, T., Goldstein, J. and Daniloff, R. 1971, Perception of coarticulated nasality, *Journal of the Acoustical Society of America* 49: S38–540.

Allen, J. S., Hunnicutt, S. and Klatt, D. H. 1987, *From Text to Speech: The MITalkSystem*, Cambridge University Press.

Allen, G. D., Lubker, J. F. and Harrison, E. Jnr 1972, New paint on electrodes for surface electromyography, *Journal of the Acoustical Society of America* 52: 124.

Allen, G. D., Lubker, J. F. and Turner, D. T. 1973, Adhesion to mucous membrane for electropalatography, *Journal of Dental Research* 52: 394.

Ananthapadmanabha, T. V. 1984, Acoustic analysis of voice source dynamics, *(STL-QPSR) Speech Transmission Laboratory, Royal Institute of Technology, Stockholm, Sweden* 2–3: 1–24.

Andrews, S., Warner, J. and Stewart, R. 1986, EMG biofeedback and relaxation in the treatment of hyperfunctional dysphasia, *British Journal of Disorders of Communication* 21: 353–69.

Archangeli, D. 1988, Aspects of underspecification theory, *Phonology* 5: 183–207.

Baer, T., Alfonso, P. and Honda, K. 1988, Electromyography of the tongue muscle during vowels in /əpVp/ environment, *Annual Bulletin 22 Research Institute Logopedics and Phoniatrics, University of Tokyo:* 7–20.

Baer, T., Löfqvist, A. and McGarr, N. S. 1983, Laryngeal vibrations: a comparison between high-speed filming and glottographic techniques, *Journal of the Acoustical Society of America* 73: 1304–8.

Baer, T., Gore, J. C., Gracco, L. C. and Nye, P. W. 1991, Analysis of vocal tract shape and dimensions using Magnetic Resonance Imaging: vowels, *Journal of the Acoustical Society of America* 90: 799–828.

Baken, R. J. 1987, *Clinical Measurement of Speech and Voice*, London: Taylor and Francis.

Baken, R. J. 1998, *Clinical Measurement of Speech and Voice* (2nd edition). San Diego, CA: Singular.

Barry, M. 1985, A palatographic study of connected speech processes, *Cambridge Papers in Phonetics and Experimental Linguistics*, 4, University of Cambridge.
1991, Temporal modelling of gestures in articulatory assimilation, *Proceedings of the XIIth International Congress of Phonetic Sciences, Aix-en-Provence* 4: 14–7.
Basmajian, J. V. 1973, Electrodes and electrode connectors, in Desmedt, J. E. (ed.), *New Developments in Electromyography and Clinical Neurophysiology* I: *New Concepts of the Motor Unit, Neuromuscular Disorders, Electromyographic Kinesiology*, Basel: Karger, pp. 502–10.
Basmajian, J. V. and De Luca, C. J. 1985, *Muscles Alive: their Functions Revealed by Electromyography (5th edition)*, Baltimore, MD: Williams and Wilkins.
Basmajian, J. V. and Stecko, G. A. 1962, A new bipolar indwelling electrode for electromyography, *Journal of Applied Psycholinguistics* 17: 849.
Baum, S. R. and Waldstein, R. S. 1991, Perseveratory coarticulation in the speech of profoundly hearing-impaired and normally hearing children, *Journal of Speech and Hearing Research* 34: 1286–92.
Båvegård, M., Fant, G., Gauffin, J. and Liljencrants, J. 1993, Vocal tract sweeptone data and model simulations of vowels, laterals and nasals, *(STL-QPSR) Speech Transmission Laboratory Quarterly Progress Status Report, Royal Institute of Technology, Stockholm, Sweden* 4: 43–76.
Beckman, M. E. 1986, *Stress and Non-Stress Accent*, Dordrecht: Foris.
1996, When is a syllable not a syllable? in Otake, T. and Cutler, A. (eds.), *Phonology in Speech: Cross-Linguistic Studies of Phonological Structure and Speech Processing*, Berlin: Walter de Gruyter, pp. 95–123.
Beckman M. E., Edwards J. and Fletcher J. 1992, Prosodic structure and tempo in a sonority model of articulatory dynamics, in Docherty, G. and Ladd, D. L. (eds.), *Papers in Laboratory Phonology* II: *Gesture, Segment, Prosody*, Cambridge University Press, pp. 66–86.
Beckman, M. and Pierrehumbert, J. 1992, Comments on chapters 14 and 15, in Docherty, G. J. and Ladd, D. R. (eds.) *Papers in Laboratory Phonology* II: *Gesture, Segment, Prosody*, Cambridge University Press, pp. 387–97.
Beddor, P. S. 1983, Phonological phonetic effects of nasalization on vowel height, *Indiana University Linguistic Club*.
1993, The perception of nasal vowels, in Huffman, M. and Krakow, R. A. (eds.), *Phonetics and Phonology: Nasals, Nasalization, and the Velum*, San Diego, CA: Academic Press, pp. 171–96.
Bell, A. 1867, Visible speech, *Universal Alphabetics or Self-Interpreting Physiological Letters for the Writing of all Languages in one Alphabet*, London: Simpkin & Marschall.
Bell-Berti, F. 1973, The velopharyageal mechanism: an electromyographic study, *Haskins Laboratories Status Report on Speech Research, Supplement*, 1–159.
1976, An electromyographic study of velopharyngeal function in speech, *Journal of Speech and Hearing Research* 19: 225–40.
1980, Velopharyngeal function: a spatial-temporal model, in Lass, N. J. (ed.) *Speech and Language: Advances in Basic Research and Practice* IV, New York, NY: Academic Press, pp. 291–316.
Bell-Berti, F., Baer, T., Harris, K. S. and Mimi, S. 1979, Coarticulatory effects of vowel quality on velar elevation, *Phonetica* 36: 187–93.

Bell-Berti, F. and Harris, K. S. 1979, Anticipatory coarticulation: some implications from a study of lip rounding, *Journal of the Acoustical Society of America* 65: 1268–70.

1981, A temporal model of speech production, *Phonetica* 38: 9–20.

1982, Temporal patterns of coarticulation: lip rounding, *Journal of the Acoustical Society of America* 71: 449–54.

Bell-Berti, F. and Hirose, H. 1975, Palatal activity in voicing distinctions: a simultaneous fiberoptic and electromyographic study, *Journal of Phonetics* 3: 69–74.

Bell-Berti, F. and Krakow R. A. 1991, Anticipatory velar lowering: a co-production account, *Journal of the Acoustical Society of America* 90: 112–23.

Benguerel, A. P. 1975, Nasal airflow patterns and velar coarticulation in French, *Proceedings of the Speech Communication Seminar, Stockholm* 2: 105–12.

Benguerel, A. P. and Adelman, S. 1976, Perception of coarticulated lip rounding, *Phonetica* 33: 113–26.

Benguerel, A. P. and Cowan, H. 1974, Coarticulation of upper lip protrusion in French, *Phonetica* 30: 41–55.

Benguerel A. P. and Lafargue, A. 1981, Perception of vowel nasalization in French *Journal of Phonetics* 9: 309–22.

Benguerel, A. P., Hirose, H., Sawashima, M. and Ushijima T. 1977a, Velar coarticulation in French: a fiberscopic study, *Journal of Phonetics* 5: 149–58.

1977b, Velar coarticulation in French: an electromyographic study, *Journal of Phonetics* 5: 159–67.

Bergem, D. R. van 1994, A model of coarticulatory effects on schwa, *Speech Communication* 14: 143–62.

Bernhardt, J. 1988, The establishment of frequency-dependent limits for electric and magnetic fields and evaluation of indirect effects, *Radiation and Environmental Biophysics* 27: 1–27.

Bickley, C. A. 1982, Acoustic analysis and perception of breathy vowels, *Speech Communication Group Working Papers I (Research Lab. of Electronics, MIT, Cambridge)*, 71–82.

Bickley, C. A. and Stevens, K. N. 1986, Effects of a vocal-tract constriction on the glottal source: experimental and modelling studies, *Journal of Phonetics* 14: 373–82.

Bjork, L. 1961, Velopharyngeal function in connected speech, *Acta Radiologica, Supplementum*, 202.

Bladon, R. A. W. and Al-Bamerni, A. 1976, Coarticulation resistance in English /l/, *Journal of Phonetics* 4: 137–50.

1982, One stage and two-stage temporal patterns of velar coarticulation, *Journal of the Acoustical Society of America* 72: S104 (abstract).

Bladon, R. A. W. and Carbonaro, E. 1978, Lateral consonants in Italian, *Journal of Italian Linguistics* 3: 43–54.

Bladon, R. A. W. and Nolan, F. 1977, A video-fluorographic investigation of tip and blade alveolars in English, *Journal of Phonetics* 5: 185–93.

Blair, C. 1986, Interdigitating muscle fibers throughout orbicularis oris inferior: preliminary observations, *Journal of Speech and Hearing Research* 29: 266–9.

Blair, C. and Muller, E. 1987, Functional identification of the perioral neuromuscular system: a signal flow diagram, *Journal of Speech and Hearing Research* 30: 60–70.

Blair, C. and Smith, A. 1986, EMG recording in human lip muscles: can single muscles be isolated? *Journal of Speech and Hearing Research* 29: 256–66.

Blumstein, S. and Stevens, K. N. 1979, Acoustic invariance in speech production: evidence from measurements of the spectral characteristics of stop consonants, *Journal of the Acoustical Society of America* 66: 1001–17.

Böe, L. J., Badin, P. and Perrier, P. 1995, From sensitivity functions to macrovariations, *Proceedings of the XIIIth International Congress of Phonetic Sciences*, ICPhS 95, Stockholm, Sweden 2: 234–7.

Bole, C. T. 1965, *Electromyographic kinesiology of the genioglossus muscles in man.* MS thesis: Ohio State University, Columbus, OH.

Bonnot, J. F., Chevrie-Muller, C., Greiner, G. and Maton, B. 1980, A propos de l'activité électromyographique labiale et vélaire durant la production de consonnes et de voyelles nasales en français, *Travaux de l'Institut de Phonétique de Strasbourg* 12: 177–224.

Borden, G. and Gay, T. 1979, Temporal aspects of articulatory movements for /s/-stop clusters, *Phonetica* 36: 21–31.

Boves, L. and de Veth, J. 1989, Pole-zero analysis of speech, Part of summary and overview of research activities in *Proceedings No. 13, Department of Language and Speech, University of Nijmegen,* 11–12.

Boyce, S. E. 1988, The influence of phonological structure on articulatory organization in Turkish and in English: vowel harmony and coarticulation, PhD dissertation, Yale University, New Haven, CT.

1990, Coarticulatory organization for lip rounding in Turkish and English, *Journal of the Acoustical Society of America* 88: 2584–95.

Boyce, S. E. and Espy-Wilson, C. 1997, Coarticulatory stability in American English /r/, *Journal of the Acoustical Society of America* 101: 3741–53.

Boyce, S., Krakow, R. and Bell-Berti, F. 1991a, Phonological underspecification and speech motor organisation, *Haskins Laboratories Status Report on Speech Research SR-105/106*, 141–52.

1991b, Phonological underspecification and speech motor organization, *Phonology* 8: 219–36.

Boyce, S. E., Krakow, R. A., Bell-Berti, F. and Gelfer, C. E. 1990, Converging sources of evidence for dissecting articulatory movements into core gestures, *Journal of Phonetics* 18: 173–88.

Branderud, P. 1985, Movetrack – a movement tracking system. *Phonetic Experimental Research at the Institute of Linguistics, University of Stockholm* 4: 20–9.

Branderud, P., McAllister, A. and Kassling. B 1993, Methodological studies of Movetrack coil placement procedures and their consequences for accuracy, *Forschungsberichte des Instituts für Phonetik and Sprachliche Kommunikation, München,* 31: 6581.

Bretonnel Cohen, K., Beckman, M. E., Edwards, J. and Fourakis, M. 1995, Modelling the articulatory dynamics of two kinds of stress contrast, *Journal of the Acoustical Society of America,* 98: S2894.

Brito, G. A. 1975, The perception of nasal vowels in Brazilian Portugese: a pilot study, *Nasalfest: Papers from a Symposium on Nasals and Nasalization. Language Universals Project*, Stanford University, CA, 45–59.

Broad, D. J. and Clermont, F. 1987, A methodology for modeling vowel formant contours in CVC context, *Journal of the Acoustical Society of America* 81: 155–65.

Broe, M. 1993, *Specification theory: the treatment of redundancy in generative phonology*, PhD dissertation, University of Edinburgh.

Broselow, E. 1994, Skeletal positions and mores, in Goldsmith, J. A. (ed.), *The Handbook of Phonological Theory*, Oxford: Basil Blackwell, pp. 174–205.

Browman, C. P. and Goldstein, L. 1986, Towards an articulatory phonology, *Phonology* 3: 219–52.

1989, Articulatory gestures as phonological units, *Phonology* 6: 201–51.

1990a, Gestural specification using dynamically defined articulatory structures, *Haskins Laboratories Status Report on Speech Research, SR-103/104,* 95–110.

1990b, Gestural specification using dynamically defined articulatory structures, *Journal of Phonetics* 18: 299–320.

1990c, Gestural structures and phonological patterns, in Mattingly, I. G. and Studdert-Kennedy, M. (eds.), *Modularity and the Motor Theory of Speech Perception*. Hillsdale, NJ: Erlbaum, pp. 313–38.

1990d, Tiers in articulatory phonology, with some implications for casual speech, in Kingston, J. and Beckman, M. E. (eds.), *Papers in Laboratory Phonology* I: *Between Grammar and the Physics of Speech*. Cambridge University Press, pp. 341–76.

1992, Articulatory phonology: an overview, *Phonetica* 49: 155–80.

1993, Dynamics and articulatory phonology, *Haskins Laboratories Status Reports on Speech Research* 113: 51–62.

Browman, C. P., Goldstein, L., Saltzman, E. and Smith, C. 1986, GEST: a computational model for speech production using dynamically defined articulatory gestures, *Journal of the Acoustical Society of America* 80: S97.

Brown, G. 1981, Consonant rounding in British English: the status of phonetic descriptions as historical data, in Asher, R. and Henderson, E. J. A. (eds.), *Towards a History of Phonetics*, Edinburgh University Press, pp. 67–76.

Brücke, E. 1856, *Grundzüge der Physiologie und Systematik der Sprachlaute für Linguisten und Taubstummenlehrer,* Vienna: Gerold.

Butcher, A. 1977, Coarticulation in intervocalic plosives and fricatives in connected speech. *Arbeitsberichte Kiel* 8: 154–213.

1989, Measuring coarticulation and variability in tongue contact patterns, *Clinical Linguistics and Phonetics* 3: 39–47.

Butcher, A. and Weiher, E. 1976, An electropalatographic investigation of coarticulation in VCV sequences, *Journal of Phonetics* 4: 59–74.

Byrd, D. 1996, Influences on articulatory timing in consonant sequences, *Journal of Phonetics* 24: 209–44.

Byrd, D. and Tan, C. C. 1996, Saying consonant clusters quickly, *Journal of Phonetics* 24: 263–82.

Byrd, D., Flemming, E., Mueller, C. A. and Tan, C. C. 1995, Using regions and indices in EPG data reduction, *Journal of Speech and Hearing Research* 38: 821–27.

Carlson, R. and Granstrom, B. 1975, A phonetically oriented programming language for rule description of speech, in Fant, G. (ed.), *Speech Communication*, II, Uppsala: Almqvist and Wiksell, pp. 245–53.

Carlson, R., Grandstrom, B. and Pauli, S. 1972, Perceptive evaluation of segmental cues, *(STL-QPSR) Speech Transmission Laboratory, Quarterly Progress and Status Report, Royal Institute of Technology, Stockholm, Sweden* 1: 18–24.

Carney, P. and Moll, K. 1971, A cinefluorographic investigation of fricative consonant–vowel coarticulation, *Phonetica* 23: 193–202.

Castelli, E. 1993, Glottis-constriction co-ordination for fricatives. Deliverable 3, Annex A, WP1.3, *Grenoble Review Meeting, Esprit/Basic Research Action No 6975: SPEECH MAPS*, II.

Catford, J. C. 1977, *Fundamental Problems in Phonetics*, Edinburgh University Press.

Chan, D. S. F. and Brookes, D. M. 1989, Variability of excitation parameters derived from robust closed phase glottal inverse filtering, *Proceedings of European Conference on Speech Communication and Technology, Paris*, Paper 33.1.

Cheney, D. L. and Seyfarth, R. M. 1990, *How Monkeys See the World: Inside the Mind of Another Species*, Chicago, IL: University of Chicago Press.

Chiu, W. S. C., Shadle, C. H. and Carter, J. N. 1995, Quantitative measures of the palate using enhanced electropalatography, *European Journal of Disorders of Communication* 30: 149–60.

Choi, J. D. 1992, Phonetic underspecification and target interpolation: an acoustic study of Marshallese vowel allophony, University of California, Los Angeles, CA, PhD disseration. Published in *UCLA Working Papers in Phonetics* 82.

1995, An acoustic–phonetic underspecification account of Marshallese vowel allophony, *Journal of Phonetics* 23: 323–47.

Choi, J. D. and Keating, P. 1991, Vowel-to-vowel coarticulation in three Slavic languages, *UCLA Working Papers in Phonetics* 78: 78–86.

Chomsky, N. and Halle, M. 1968, *The Sound Pattern of English*, New York, NY: Harper and Row.

Clark, J. E., Palethorpe, S. and Hardcastle, W. J. 1982, Analysis of English lingual fricatives: multi-modal data using stepwise regression methods, *Working Papers of the Speech and Laguage Research Centre, Maquarie University* 3: 1–90.

Clarke, W. M. and Mackiewicz-Krassowska, H. 1977, Variations in the oral and nasal sound pressure levels of vowels in changing phonetic contexts, *Journal of Phonetics* 5: 195–203.

Clements, G. N. and Hume, E. V. 1994, The internal organization of speech sounds, in Goldsmith, J. A. (ed.), *The Handbook of Phonological Theory*, Oxford: Basil Blackwell, pp. 245–306.

Clements, G. N. and Keyser, S. J. 1983, *CV Phonology*, Cambridge, MA: MIT Press.

Clumeck, H. 1976, Patterns of soft palate movement in six languages, *Journal of Phonetics* 4: 337–51.

Cohen, K. B. 1994, Vocal tract evolution and vowel production, *Working Papers in Linguistics*, Ohio State University 45: 11–35.

Cohn, A. C. 1988, Quantitative characterization of degrees of coarticulation in CV tokens, *UCLA Working Papers in Phonetics* 69: 51–9.

1990, Phonetic and phonological rules of nasalization, University of California, Los Angeles, CA, PhD dissertation. Published in *UCLA Working Papers in Phonetics* 76.

1992, The consequences of dissimilation in Sundanese, *Phonology* 9: 199–220.

Cole, D. T. 1955, *An Introduction to Tswana Grammar*, London: Longmans, Green.

Coleman, J. 1992, Synthesis-by-rule without segments or rewrite rules, in Bailly, G. and Benoit, C. (eds.), *Talking Machines: Theories, Model, and Applications*, Amsterdam: Elsevier, pp. 43–60.

Connell, B. 1992, Tongue contact, active articulators and coarticulation, in Ohala, J. J., Nearey, T. M., Derwing, B. L., Hodge, M. M. and Wiebe, G. E. (eds.), *Proceedings of the 1992 International Conference on Spoken Language Processing* I, University of Alberta, Edmonton, pp. 1075–8.

Cooper, A. M. 1991, Laryngeal and oral gestures in English /p, t, k/, *Proceedings of XIIth International Congress of Phonetic Sciences*, Aix-en-Provence, 2: 50–3.

Cooper, F. S. 1965, Research techniques and instrumentation: EMG, *Proceedings of the Conference on Communicative Problems of Cleft Palate*. *ASHA Reports* 1: 153–68.

Cranen, B. and Boves, L. 1985, Pressure measurements during speech production using semiconductor miniature pressure transducers: impact on models for speech production, *Journal of the Acoustical Society of America* 77: 1543–51.

Croft, C. B., Shprintzen, R. B. and Rakoff, S. J. 1981, Patterns of velopharyngeal valving in normal and cleft palate subjects, *Laryngoscope* 91: 265–71.

Crowther, C. S. 1994, Inferring degree of coarticulation and relational invariance of stop place in CVs using locus equations, *Journal of the Acoustical Society of America* 95: 2922.

Crystal, T. H. and House, A. S. 1988, Segmental durations in connected-speech signals: current results, *Journal of the Acoustical Society of America* 83: 1553–73.

Curtiss, J. F. 1968, Acoustics of speech production and nasalization, in Spriesterbach, D. C. and Sherman, D. (eds.), *Cleft Palate and Communication*, New York, NY: Academic Press, pp. 27–60.

Cutler, A. 1994, Segmentation problems: rhythmic solutions, *Glossa* 92: 81–104.

Cutler, A. and Norris, D. G. 1988, The role of strong syllables in segmentation for lexical access, *Journal of Experimental Psychology: Human Perception and Performance* 14: 113–21.

Dagenais, P. A., Critz-Crosby, P. and Adams, J. B. 1994, Defining and remediating persistent lateral lisps in children using electropalatography: preliminary findings, *American Journal of Speech Language Pathology* September: 67–76.

Dagenais, P. A., Lorendo, L. C. and McCutcheon, M. J. 1994, A study of voicing and context effects upon consonant linguapalatal contact patterns, *Journal of Phonetics* 22: 225–38.

Dalston, R. M. 1989, Using simultaneous photodetection and nasometry to monitor velopharyngeal reaction times in normal speakers, *Cleft Palate Journal* 25: 205–9.

Dalston, R. M., Warren, D. W. and Dalston, E. T. 1993, Use of nasometry as a diagnostic tool for identifying patients with velopharyngeal impairment, *Cleft Palate–Craniofacial Journal* 28: 184–9.

Daniel, B. and Guitar, B. 1978, EMG feedback and recovery of facial and speech gestures following neural anastomosis, *Journal of Speech and Hearing Disorders* 43: 9–20.

Daniloff, R. and Hammarberg, R. 1973, On defining coarticulation, *Journal of Phonetics* 1: 239–48.

Daniloff, R. and Moll, K. 1968, Coarticulation of lip rounding, *Journal of Speech and Hearing Research* 11: 707–21.

Dart, S. 1991, Articulatory and acoustic properties of apical and laminal articulations, *UCLA Working Papers in Phonetics* 79.

Davis, K. 1990, The acquisition of VOT: is it language-dependent? *Papers and Reports on Child Language Development* 29: 28–37.

Davis, S. and van Summers, W. 1989, Vowel length and closure duration in word-medial VC sequences, *Journal of Phonetics* 17: 339–53.

Delattre, P. C. 1951, A l'usage des étudiants anglo-americains, 2nd edn. *Principles de phonétique française*, Middlebury College, Middlebury, VT.

1954, Les attributes acoustiques de la nasalisé vocalique et consonantique, *Studia Linguistica* 8: 103–9.

Dent, H. 1984, Coarticulated devoicing in English laterals, *Reading Working Papers* 4: 111–34.

Derkach, M., Fant, G. and Serpa-Leitaõ, A. 1970, Phoneme coarticulation in Russian hard and soft VCV-utterances with voiceless fricatives, *(STL-QPSR) Speech Transmission Laboratory Quarterly Progress Status Report, Royal Institute of Technology, Stockholm, Sweden* 2–3: 1–7.

Descout, R., Boë, L. J. and Abry, C. 1980, Labialité vocalique et labialité consonantique, *Labialité et Phonétique*, Publications de l'Université des Langues et Lettres de Grenoble, pp. 111–26.

Dickson, D. R. 1961, An acoustic and radiographic study of nasality, PhD dissertation, North Western University, Evanston, IL.

Dickson, D. R. and Maue-Dickson, W. R. 1980, Velopharyngeal structure and function, in Lass, N. J. (ed.), *Speech and Language: Advances in Basic Research and Practice* III, New York, NY: Academic Press, pp. 167–222.

Diehl, R. L. 1986, Coproduction and direct perception of phonetic segments: a critique, *Journal of Phonetics* 14: 61–6.

Disner, S. F. 1983, Vowel quality. The relation between universal and language specific factors, *UCLA Working Papers in Phonetics* 58.

Dixit, R. P. 1989, Glottal gestures in Hindi plosives, *Journal of Phonetics* 17: 213–37.

1990, Linguotectal contact patterns in the dental and retroflex stops of Hindi, *Journal of Phonetics* 18: 189–203.

Dixit, R. P. and Flege, J. E. 1991, Vowel context, rate and loudness effects of linguopalatal contact patterns in Hindi retroflex /t/, *Journal of Phonetics* 19: 213–30.

Dixit, R. P. and MacNeilage, P. F. 1972, Coarticulation of nasality: evidence from Hindi, *Journal of the Acoustical Society of America* 52: 131.

Docherty, G. J. 1992, *The Timing of Voicing in British English Obstruents*, Berlin: Foris.

Doke, C. M. 1954, *The South Bantu Languages*, London: Oxford University Press.

Dorman, M. F., Studdert-Kennedy, M. and Raphael, L. J. 1977, Stop-consonant recognition: release burst and formant transitions as functionally equivalent, context-dependent cues, *Perception and Psychophysics* 22: 109–22.

Duez, D. 1992, Second formant locus–nucleus patterns: an investigation of spontaneous French speech, *Speech Communication* 11: 417–27.

1995, On spontaneous French speech: aspects of the reduction and contextual assimilation of voiced stops, *Journal of Phonetics* 23: 407–27.

Dunn, M. H. 1993, The phonetics and phonology of geminate consonants: a production study, PhD dissertation, Yale University, New Haven, CT.

Eblen, R. E. Jnr 1963, Limitations on use of surface electromyography in studies of speech breathing, *Journal of Speech Research* 6: 3–18.

Edmonds, T. D., Lilly, D. J. and Hardy, J. C. 1971, Dynamic characteristics of air-pressure measuring systems used in speech research, *Journal of the Acoustical Society of America* 50: 1051–7.

Edwards, J. 1985, Contextual effects on lingual–mandibular coordination, *Journal of the Acoustical Society of America* 78: 1944–8.

Edwards, J., Beckman, M. and Fletcher J. 1991, The articulatory kinematics final lengthening, *Journal of the Acoustical Society of America* 89: 369–82.

Eek, A. 1973, Observations in Estonian palatalization. An articulatory study, *Estonian Papers in Phonetics*, 18–36.

Emanuel, F. and Counihan, D. 1970, Some characteristics of oral and nasal airflow during plosive consonant production, *Cleft Palate Journal* 7: 249–60.

Engelke, W. D. and Schönle, P. W. 1991, Elektromagnetische Artikulographie: Eine neue Methode zur Untersuchung von Bewegungsfunktionen des Gaumensegels, *Folia Phoniatrica* 43: 147–52.

Engstrand, O. 1981, Acoustic constraints or invariant input representation? An experimental study of selected articulatory movements and targets, *Reports from Uppsala University Department of Linguistics* 7: 67–95.

1983, Articulatory coordination in selected VCV utterances: a means–end view, *Reports from Uppsala University Department of Linguistics* 10: 1–145.

1988, Articulatory correlates of stress and speaking rate in Swedish VCV utterances, *Journal of the Acoustical Society of America* 83: 1863–75.

1989, Towards an electropalatographic specification of consonant articulation in Swedish, *Phonetic Experimental Research at the Institute of Linguistics, University of Stockholm* 10: 115–56.

Espy-Wilson, C. Y. 1992, Acoustic measurements for linguistic features distinguishing the semivowels /w j r l/ in American English, *Journal of the Acoustical Society of America* 92: 736–57.

Ewen, C. J. 1982 The internal structure of complex segments, in van der Hulst, H. and Smith, N. (eds.), *The Structure of Phonological Representations*, Part II, Dordrecht, Foris, pp. 27–67.

Faber, A. 1989, Lip protrusion in sibilants, *Journal of the Acoustical Society of America* 86: S1, TT4.

1990, The time-course of labial gestures for sibilant articulations, *Journal of the Acoustical Society of America* 88: S1, S120.

Fant, G. 1960, *Acoustic Theory of Speech Production*, The Hague: Mouton.

1968, Analysis and synthesis of speech processes, in Malmberg, B. (ed.), *Manual of Phonetics*, Amsterdam: North-Holland, pp. 173–277.

1972, Subglottal formants, *(STL-QPSR) Speech Transmission Laboratory, Quarterly Progress and Status Report, Royal Institute of Technology, Stockholm, Sweden* 1: 1–12.

1973, *Speech Sounds and Features*, Cambridge, MA: MIT Press.

1979, Vocal source analysis – a progress report, *(STL-QPSR) Speech Transmission Laboratory, Royal Institute of Technology, Stockholm, Sweden* 3–4: 31–54.

1980, Voice source dynamics, *(STL-QPSR) Speech Transmission Laboratory, Royal Institute of Technology, Stockholm, Sweden* 2–3: 17–37.

1981, The source filter concept in voice production, *(STL-QPSR) Speech Transmission Laboratory, Royal Institute of Technology, Stockholm, Sweden* 1: 21–37.

1982a, Preliminaries to analysis of the human voice source, *(STL-QPSR) Speech Transmission Laboratory, Royal Institute of Technology, Stockholm, Sweden* 4: 1–27.

1982b, The voice source–acoustic modeling, *(STL-QPSR) Speech Transmission Laboratory, Royal Institute of Technology, Stockholm, Sweden* 4: 28–48.

1988, Glottal flow parameters from the frequency domain. *Paper presented at 2nd Symposium on Advanced Man–Machine Interface through Spoken Language*, Hawaii.

1993, Some problems in voice source analysis, *Speech Communication* 13: 7–22.

Fant, G, and Lin, Q. 1988, Frequency domain interpretation and derivation of glottal flow parameters, *(STL-QPSR) Speech Transmission Laboratory Quarterly Progress and Status Report, Royal Institute of Technology, Stockholm, Sweden* 2–3: 1–21.

Fant, G. and Liljencrants, J. 1994, Data reduction of LF voice source parameters. *Working Papers* 43, *Lund University, Department of Linguistics.* 62–5.

Fant, G., Liljencrants, J. and Lin, Q. 1985, A four-parameter model of glottal flow, *(STL-QPSR) Speech Transmission Laboratory, Royal Institute of Technology, Stockholm, Sweden* 4: 1–13.

Fant, G., Kruckenberg, A., Liljencrants, J. and Bavegard, M. 1994, Voice source parameters in connected speech. Transformation of LF-parameters, *Proceedings of the International Conference on Spoken Language Processing*, Yokohama.

Farnetani, E. 1986a, A pilot study of the articulation of /n/ in Italian using electropalatography and airflow measurements, *Journées d'Etudes sur la Parole*, Aix-en-Provence, pp. 23–6.

1986b, Lingual and velar coarticulatory movements in the production of /n/ in Italian: some preliminary data, *Quaderni del Centro di Studio per le Ricerche di Fonetica, Padova, Consiglo nazionale delle richerche* 5: 285–307.

1988, Asymmetry of lingual movements: EPG data on Italian, *Quaderni del Centro di Studio per le Ricerche di Fonetica, Padova, Consiglio nazionale delle richerche* 7: 211–28.

1989, An articulatory study of voicing in Italian by means of dynamic palatography, *Speech Research* 89, *Budapest*, 395–8.

1990, V-C-V lingual coarticulation and its spatio-temporal domain, in Hardcastle, W. J. and Marchal A. (eds.), *Speech Production and Speech Modelling*, Netherlands: Kluwer Academic, pp. 93–110.

1991, Coarticulation and reduction in consonants: comparing isolated words and continuous speech, *Phonetic Experimental Research at the Institute of Linguistics, Royal Institute of Technology, Stockholm, Sweden* 14: 11–16.

1997, Coarticulation and connected speech processes, in Hardcastle, W. J. and Laver, J. (eds.), *A Handbook of Phonetic Science*, Oxford: Blackwell, pp. 371–404.

in preparation, A pilot study on the coordination of lingual and labial gestures in the production of high vowels in Italian.

Farnetani, E. and Busà, M. G. 1994, Italian clusters in continuous speech, *Proceedings ICSLP 94, Yokohama* 1: 359–362.

Farnetani, E. and Faber, A. 1991, Vowel production in isolated words and in connected speech: an investigation of the linguo–mandibular subsystem, *Proceedings of the ESCA Workshop, Barcelona.*

1992, Tongue jaw coordination in vowel production: isolated words versus connected speech, *Speech Communication* 11: 401–410.

Farnetani, E. and Provaglio, A. 1991, Assessing variability of lingual consonants in Italian, *Quaderni del Centro di Studio per le Ricerche di Fonetica* 10: 117–45.

Farnetani, E. and Recasens, D. 1993, Anticipatory consonant-to-vowel coarticulation in the production of VCV sequences in Italian, *Language and Speech* 36: 279–302.

Farnetani, E., Hardcastle, W. J. and Marchal, A. 1989, Cross-language investigation of lingual coarticulatory processes using EPG, in Tubach, J. P. and Mariani, J. J. (eds.), *Euro-speech 1989. European Conference on Speech Communication and Technology* 429–32.

Farnetani, E., Vagges, K. and Magno-Caldognetto, E. 1985, Coarticulation in Italian /VtV/ sequences: a palatographic study, *Phonetica* 42: 78–99.

Feng, G. 1986, Modelisation acoustique et traitement du signal de parole: le cas des voyelles nasalés et la simulation des poles et des zeros, Thèse de Docteur Ingenieur, University of Grenoble.

Ferguson, C. A. 1986, Discovering sound units and constructing sound systems: it's child's play, in Perkell, J. S. and Klatt, D. H. (eds.), *Invariance and Variability of Speech Processes*, Hillsdale, NJ: Lawrence Erlbaum, pp. 36–51.

Firth, J. R. 1948, Sounds and prosodies, *Transactions of the Philological Society*, 127–52.

Fischer-Jørgensen, E. 1964, Sound duration and place of articulation, *Zeitschrift für Phonetik und Kommunikationsforschung* 17: 175–207.

1967, Phonetic analysis of breathy (murmured) vowels in Gujarati, *Indian Linguistics* 28: 71–139.

1979, Temporal relations in consonant–vowel syllables with stop consonants based on Danish material, in Lindblom, B. and Öhman, S. (eds.), *Frontiers of Speech Communication Research*, London: Academic Press, pp. 51–68.

Flege, J. 1988, Anticipatory and carryover nasal coarticulation in the speech of children and adults, *Journal of Speech and Hearing Research* 31: 525–36.

Fletcher, J. and Vatikiotis-Bateson, E. 1991, Articulation of prosodic contrasts in French, *Proceedings of the XIIth International Congress of Phonetic Sciences*, Aix-en-Provence 4: 16–21.

1994, Prosody and intra-syllabic timing in French, *Ohio State University Working Papers* 43: 41–6.

Fletcher, S. G. 1970, Theory and instrumentation for quantitative measurement of nasality, *Cleft Palate Journal* 7: 601–9.

1983, New prospects for speech by the hearing impaired, in Lass, N. J. (ed) *Speech and Language: Advances in Basic Research and Practice*, New York, NY: Academic Press, pp. 1–42

1985, Speech production and oral motor skill in an adult with an unrepaired palatal cleft, *Journal of Speech and Hearing Disorders* 50: 254–61.

1988, Speech production following partial glossectomy, *Journal of Speech and Hearing Disorders* 53: 232–8.

Fletcher, S. G., McCutcheon, M. J. and Wolf, M. B. 1975, Dynamic palatometry, *Journal of Speech and Hearing Research* 18: 812–19.

Folkins, J. and Linville, R. N. 1983, The effects of varying lower-lip displacement on upper lip movements: implications in the coordination of speech movements, *Journal of Speech and Hearing Research* 26: 209–17.

Folkins, J. W., Linville, R. N., Garrett, J. D. and Brown, C. K. 1988, Interactions in the labial musculature during speech, *Journal of Speech and Hearing Research* 31: 253–64.

Fontdevila, J., Pallarès, M. D. and Recasens, D. 1994, The contact index method of electropalatographic data reduction, *Journal of Phonetics* 22: 141–54.

Forrest, K., Weismer, G. and Adams, S. 1990, Statistical comparison of movement amplitudes from groupings of normal geriatric speakers, *Journal of Speech and Hearing Research* 33: 386–9.

Fourakis, M. 1991, Tempo, stress, and vowel reduction in American English, *Journal of the Acoustical Society of America* 90: 1816–27.

Fowler, C. A. 1977, *Timing Control in Speech Production*, Bloomington, IN: Indiana University Linguistics Club.

1980, Coarticulation and theories of extrinsic timing, *Journal of Phonetics* 8: 113–33.

1981a, A relationship between coarticulatory and compensatory shortening, *Phonetica* 38: 35–50.

1981b, Production and perception of coarticulation among stressed and unstressed vowels, *Journal of Speech and Hearing Research* 24: 127–39.

1983a, Converging sources of evidence on spoken and perceived rhythms of speech: cyclic production of vowels in monosyllabic feet, *Journal of Experimental Psychology: General* 112: 386–412.

1983b, Realism and unrealism: a reply, *Journal of Phonetics* 11: 303–22.

1984, Segmentation of coarticulated speech in perception, *Perception and Psychophysics* 36: 359–68.

1985, Current perspective on language and speech production: a critical overview, in Daniloff, R. (ed.), *Speech Science*, London: Taylor and Francis, pp. 193–278.

1986, An event approach to the study of speech perception from a direct-realist perspective, *Journal of Phonetics* 14: 3–28.

1990, Some regularities in speech are not consequences of formal rules: comments on Keating's paper, in Beckman, M. and Kingston, J. (eds.), *Papers in Laboratory Phonology* I: *Between the Grammar and Physics of Speech*, Cambridge University Press, pp. 476–89.

1992, Phonological and articulatory characteristics of spoken language, *Haskins Laboratories Status Report on Speech Research* SR-109/110, 1–12.

1993, Phonological and articulatory characteristics of spoken language, in Blasken, G., Dittman, J., Grimm, H., Marshall, J. and Wallesch, C.-W. (eds.), *Linguistic Disorders and Pathologies: An International Handbook*, Berlin: Walter de Grutyer, pp. 34–46.

1995, Speech production, in Miller, J. and Eimas, P. (eds.), *Handbook of Perception and Cognition: Speech, Language, and Communication* (vol. XI), New York, NY: Academic Press.

Fowler C. A. and Rosenblum L. D. 1989, The perception of phonetic gestures, *Haskins Laboratories Status Report on Speech Research*, SR-99/100, 102–17.

Fowler, C. A. and Saltzman, E. 1993, Coordination and coarticulation in speech production, *Language and Speech* 36: 171–95.

Fowler, C. A. and Smith, M. R. 1986, Speech perception as 'vector analysis': an approach to the problems of invariance and segmentation, in Perkell, J. S. and Klatt, D. H. (eds.), *Invariance and Variability in Speech Processes*, Hillsdale, NJ: Lawrence Erlbaum Associates, pp. 123–39.

Fowler, C. A., Rubin, P., Remez, R. and Turvey, M. 1980, Implications for speech production of a general theory of action, in Butterworth, B. (ed.), *Language Production* I, London: Academic Press, pp. 371–420.

Fritzell, B. 1969, The velopharyngeal muscles in speech: an electromyographic and cineradiographic study, *Acta Otolaryngologica* Supplementum 250: 81.

Frøkjær-Jensen, B. 1967, A photo-electric glottograph, *Annual Report of the Institute of Phonetics of the University of Copenhagen* 2: 5–19.

Frøkjær-Jensen, B., Ludvigsen, C. and Rischel, J. 1971, A glottographic study of some Danish consonants, in Hammerich, L., Jakobson, R. and Zwirner, E. (eds.), *Form and Substance*, Copenhagen: Akademisk Forlag, pp. 123–40.

Fromkin, V. 1964, Lip position in American English vowels, *Language and Speech* 7: 215–25.

Fromkin, V. and Ladefoged, P. 1966, Electromyography in speech research, *Phonetica* 15: 219–42.

Fujimura, O. 1961a, Analysis of nasalized vowels, *Quarterly Progress Report-MIT* 62: 191–2.

1961b, Bilabial stops and nasal consonants: a motion picture study and its acoustical implications, *Journal of Speech and Hearing Research* 4: 233–47.

1962, Analysis of nasal consonants, *Journal of the Acoustical Society of America* 34: 1865–75.

1977, Recent findings on articulatory processes: velum and tongue movements as syllable features, in Carre, R., Descout, R. and Wajskop, M. (eds.), *Articulatory Modeling and Phonetics*, Grenoble: GALF, pp. 115–26.

Fujimura, O. and Lindqvist, J. 1971, Sweep-tone measurements of vocal-tract characteristics, *Journal of the Acoustical Society of America* 49: 541–57.

Fujimura, O. and Lovins, J. B. 1978, Syllables as concatenative phonetic units, in Bell, A. and Hooper, J. B. (eds.), *Syllables and Segments*, Amsterdam: North-Holland, pp. 107–20.

Fujimura, O., Baer, T. and Niimi, A. 1979, A stereoscopic fiberscope with magnetic interlens bridge for laryngeal observation, *Journal of the Acoustical Society of America* 65: 478–80.

Fujimura, O., Tatsumi, I. F. and Kagaya, R. 1973, Computational processing of palatographic patterns, *Journal of Phonetics* 1: 47–54.

Fujisaki, H. and Ljungqvist, M. 1987, Estimation of voice source and vocal tract parameters based on ARMA analysis and a model for the glottal source waveform, *Proceedings of the International Conference on Acoustics, Speech, and Signal Processing*, Tokyo, 15.4.1–15.4.4.

Gandour, J., Potisuk, S. and Dechongkit, S. 1994, Tonal coarticulation in Thai, *Journal of Phonetics* 22: 477–92.

Gandour, J., Petty, S. H., Dardarananda, R., Dechongkit, S. and Mulcnogen, S. 1986, The acquisition of the voicing contrast in Thai: a study of voice onset time in word-initial stop consonants, *Journal of Child Language* 13: 561–72.

Gay, T. J. 1974, A cinefluorographic study of vowel production, *Journal of Phonetics* 2: 255–66.

1977, Articulatory movements in VCV sequences, *Journal of the Acoustical Society of America* 62: 183–93.

1978a, Articulatory units: segments or syllables? in Bell, A. and Hooper, J. (eds.), *Syllables and Segments*, Amsterdam: North-Holland, pp. 121–31.

1978b, Effect of speaking rate on vowel formant movements, *Journal of the Acoustical Society of America* 63: 223–30.

1979, Coarticulation in some consonant–vowel and consonant cluster–vowel syllables, in Lindblom, B. and Öhman, S. (eds.), *Frontiers of Speech Communication Research*, London: Academic Press, pp. 69–76.

1981, Mechanisms in the control of speech rate, *Phonetica* 38: 148–58.

Gay, T. J. and Harris, K. 1971, Some recent developments in the use of electromyography in speech research, *Journal of Speech and Hearing Research* 14: 241–6.

Gay, T. J. and Hirose, H. 1973, Effects of speaking rate on labial consonant production: a combined electromyographic high speed motion picture study, *Phonetica* 22: 44–56.

Gay, T. J., Lindblom, B., and Lubker, J. 1981, Production of bite-block vowels: acoustic equivalence by selective compensation, *Journal of the Acoustical Society of America* 69: 802–10.

Gay, T. J., Ushijima, T., Hirose, H. and Cooper, F. S. 1974, Effect of speaking rate on labial consonant–vowel coarticulation, *Journal of Phonetics* 2: 47–63.

Geddes, L. A. 1972, *Electrodes and the Measurement of Bioelectric Events*, New York, NY: Wiley.

Gelfer, C., Bell-Berti, F. and Harris, K. 1989, Determining the extent of coarticulation: effects of experimental design, *Journal of the Acoustical Society* 6: 2443–5.

Gentil, M. and Boë, L. J. 1980, Les lèvres et la parole, *Labialité et Phonétique*, Publications de l'Université des Langues et Lettres de Grenoble, 11–106.

Ghazeli, S. 1977, Back consonants and backing coarticulation in Arabic, PhD dissertation, University of Texas at Austin.

Gibbon, F. 1990, Lingual activity in two speech disordered children's attempts to produce velar/alveolar stop contrasts: evidence from electropalatographic (EPG) data, *British Journal of Disorders of Communication* 25: 329–40.

Gibbon, F., Hardcastle, W. J. and Nicolaidis, K. 1993, Temporal and spatial aspects of lingual coarticulation in /kl/ sequences: a cross-linguistic investigation, *Language and Speech* 36: 261–277.

Giet, G. van der 1977, Computer-controlled method for measuring articulatory activities, *Journal of the Acoustical Society of America* 61: 1072–6.

Giles, S. and Moll, K. 1975, Cinefluorographic study of selected allophones of English /l/, *Phonetica* 31: 206–27.

Gleason, H. A. 1961, *An Introduction to Descriptive Linguistics*, revised edition, New York, NY: Holt, Rinehart, and Winston.

Gobl, C. 1985, Rostkallans variation i tal, MSc thesis, Royal Intitute of Technology, Stockholm.

1988, Voice source dynamics in connected speech, *(STL-QPSR) Speech Transmission Laboratory, Royal Institute of Technology, Stockholm*, 1: 123–59.

Gobl, C. and Ní Chasaide, A. 1988, The effects of adjacent voice/voiceless consonants on the vowel voice source: a cross language study, *(STL-QPSR) Speech Transmission Laboratory, Royal Institute of Technology, Stockholm, Sweden*, 2–3: 23–59.

1992, Acoustic characteristics of voice quality, *Speech Communication* 11: 481–90.

Goldsmith, J. 1990, *Autosegmental and Metrical Phonology*, Oxford: Basil Blackwell.

Goldstein, L. 1989, On the domain of quantal theory, *Journal of Phonetics* 17: 91–7.

1990, On articulatory binding: comments on Kingston's paper, in Kingston, J. and Beckman, M. E. (eds.), *Papers in Laboratory Phonology* 1, *Between the Grammar and Physics of Speech*, Cambridge University Press, pp. 445–50.

1994, Do acoustic landmarks constrain the coordination of articulatory events? in Keating, P. A. (ed.), *Papers in Laboratory Phonology* III, *Phonological Structure and Phonetic Form,* Cambridge University Press, pp. 234–41.

Goldstein, L. M. and Browman, C. P. 1986, Representation of voicing contrasts using articulatory gestures, *Journal of Phonetics* 14: 339–42.

Gracco, V. L. 1988, Timing factors in the co-ordination of speech movements, *Journal of Neuroscience* 8: 4628–39.

1993, Some organisational characteristics of speech movement control, *Journal of Speech and Hearing Research* 37: 4–27.

1995, Electromagnetic articulography: a brief overview, *Proceedings of XIIth International Conference of Phonetic Science, Stockholm*, 4: 58–61.

Gracco, V. L and Nye, P. W. 1993, Magnetometry in speech articulation research: some misadventures on the road to enlightenment, *Forschungsberichte des Instituts für Phonetik und Sprachliche Kommunikation, München*, 31: 91–104.

Gubrynowicz, R. 1983, La détection des consonnes nasalés dans le système de recon-naissance de la parole continué KEAL, *Recherches Acoustique* 7: 93–107.

Guenther, F. H. 1994, Skill acquisition, coarticulation, and rate effects in a neural network model of speech production, *Journal of the Acoustical Society of America* 95: 2924.

1995, Speech sound acquisition, coarticulation and rate effects in a neural network model of speech production, *Psychological Review* 102: 594–621.

Guérin, B. and Mrayati, M. 1977, Nasal vowels study: sensitivity functions, in Carré, R., Descout, R. and Wajskop, M. (eds), *Modèles articulatoires et phonetique,*

Actes du symposium de Grenoble, 10–12 juillet 1977: GALF Groupe de la Communication parlée, pp. 137–46.

Hadding, K., Hirose, H. and Harris, K. S. 1976, Facial muscle activity in the production of Swedish vowels: an electromyographic study, *Journal of Phonetics* 4: 233–45.

Haggard, M. 1973, Abbreviation of consonants in English pre- and post-vocalic clusters, *Journal of Phonetics*, 1: 9–24.

Halle, M. 1959, *The Sound Pattern of Russian*, The Hague: Mouton.

Halle, M. and Stevens, K. N. 1964, Speech recognition: a model and program for research, in Fodor, J. A. and Katz, J. J. (eds.), *The Structure of Language: Readings in the Philosophy of Language*, Englewood Cliffs, NJ: Prentice-Hall, pp. 604–12.

Halwes, T. and Jenkins, J. 1971, Problem of serial order in behavior is not resolved by context-sensitive associative memory models, *Psychological Review* 78: 122–9.

Hamlet, S. L. 1981, Ultrasound assessment of phonatory function, in Ludlow, C. L. and O'Connell Hart, M. (eds.), *Proceedings of the Conference on the Assessment of Vocal Pathology* (ASHA reports 11): 128–40.

Hammarberg, R. 1976, The metaphysics of coarticulation, *Journal of Phonetics* 4: 353–63.

1982, On redefining coarticulation, *Journal of Phonetics* 10: 123–37.

Haraguchi, S. 1977, *The Tone Pattern of Japanese: an Autosegmental Theory of Tonology*, Tokyo: Kaitakusha.

Hardcastle, W. J. 1981, Experimental studies in lingual coarticulation, in Asher, R. and Henderson, E. (eds.), *Towards a History of Phonetics*, Edinburgh University Press, pp. 50–66.

1985, Some phonetic and syntactic constraints on lingual coarticulation during /kl/ sequences, *Speech Communication* 4: 247–63.

Hardcastle, W. J. and Clark, J. E. 1981, Articulatory, aerodynamic and acoustic properties of lingual fricatives in English, *Phonetics Laboratory University of Reading Work in Progress* 3: 51–78.

Hardcastle, W. J. and Roach, P. J. 1979, An instrumental investigation of coarticulation in stop consonant sequences, in Hollien, H. and Hollien, P. (eds.), *Current Issues in the Phonetic Sciences*, Amsterdam: John Benjamins, pp. 531–40.

Hardcastle, W. J., Gibbon, F. E. and Jones, W. 1991, Visual display of tongue–palate contact: electropalatography in the assessment and remediation of speech disorders, *British Journal of Disorders of Communication* 26: 41–74.

Hardcastle, W. J., Gibbon, F. and Nicolaidis K. 1991, EPG data reduction methods and their implications for studies of lingual coarticulation, *Journal of Phonetics* 19: 251–66.

Hardcastle, W. J., Gibbon, F., Dent, H. and Nixon, F. 1991, Modelling lingual articulation in normal and deviant sibilant production, Paper presented at the XIIth International Congress of Phonetic Science, Aix-en-Provence, France.

Hardcastle, W. J., Jones, W., Knight, C., Trudgeon, A. and Calder, G. 1989, New developments in electropalatography: a state-of-the-art report, *Clinical Linguistics and Phonetics* 3: 1–38.

Harrington, J., Fletcher, J. and Beckman, M. E. in press, Manner and place conflicts in the articulation of accent in Australian English, in Broe, M. (ed.), *Papers in Laboratory Phonology* V: *Language Acquisition and the Lexicon*, Cambridge University Press.

Harrington, J., Fletcher, J. and Roberts, C. 1995, Coarticulation and the accented/unaccented distinction: evidence from jaw movement data, *Journal of Phonetics* 23: 305–22.

Harrington, J., Beckman, M., Fletcher, J. and Palethorpe, S. 1997, Kinematic and spectral measures of supralaryngeal correlates of the accent contrast in Australian English high vowels, *Journal of the Acoustical Society of America* 105: S3205.

Harrington, R. 1944, A study of the mechanics of velopharyngeal closure, *Journal of Speech and Hearing Disorders* 9: 325–45.

Harris, K. S. 1971, Vowel stress and articulatory reorganization, *Haskins Laboratories Status Report Speech Research* 28: 167–78.

    1981, Electromyography as a technique for laryngeal investigation, in Ludlow, C. L. and O'Connell Hart, M. (eds.), *Proceedings of the Conference on the Assessment of Vocal Pathology, ASHA Reports* 11: 70–87.

Harris, K., Rosov, R., Cooper, F. and Lysaught, G. 1964, A multiple suction electrode system, *Journal of EEG Clinical Neurophysiology* 17: 698–700.

Harris, K. S., Schvey, M. and Lysaught, G. F. 1962, Component gestures in the production of oral and nasal stops, *Journal of the Acoustical Society of America* 34: 743(A).

Hasegawa, A., Christensen, J. M., McCutcheon, M. J. and Fletcher, S. G. 1979, Articulatory properties of /s/ in selected consonant clusters, 97th ASA Meeting, MIT, *Haskins Laboratories Status Report on Speech Research*, 45/46: 197–204.

Hattori, S., Yamamoto, K. and Fujimura, O. 1958, Nasalization of vowels in relation to nasals, *Journal of the Acoustical Society of America* 30: 267–74.

Hawkins, S. 1979, Temporal coordination in the speech of children: further data, *Journal of Phonetics* 7: 235–67.

Hawkins, S. and Stevens, K. N. 1985, Acoustic and perceptual correlates of the non-nasal–nasal distinction for vowels, *Journal of the Acoustical Society of America* 77: 1560–75.

Hayes, B. 1989, Compensatory lengthening in moraic phonology, *Linguistic Inquiry* 20: 253–306.

Hayes, K. J. 1960, Wave analysis of tissue noise and muscle action potentials, *Journal of Applied Physiology* 15: 749–52.

Hedelin, P. 1984, A glottal LPC-vocoder, *Proceedings of IEEE International Conference on Acoustics, Speech, and Signal Processing, San Diego*, 1.6.1–1.6.4.

    1986, High quality glottal LPC-vocoder, *Proceedings of IEEE International Conference on Acoustics, Speech, and Signal Processing, Tokyo*, 9.9.1–9.9.4.

Hedrick, W., Hykes, D. and Starchman, D. 1995, *Ultrasound Physics and Instrumentation*, St. Louis, MO: Mosby Inc. Publ.

Henderson, J. B. 1984, Velopharyngealfunction in oral and nasal vowels: a cross-language study, PhD dissertation, University of Connecticut, Storrs, CT.

Henderson, J. B. and Repp, B. H. 1982, Is a stop consonant released when followed by another stop consonant? *Phonetica* 39: 71–82.

Henke, W. L. 1966, Dynamic articulatory model of speech production using computer simulation, Unpublished doctoral dissertation, MIT Cambridge, MA.

Herberts, P. 1969, Myoelectric signals in control of prostheses, *Acta Orthopaedica Scandinavia* Supplement 124.

Hertrich, I. and Ackermann, H. 1997, Articulatory control of phonological vowel length contrasts: kinematic analysis of labial gestures, *Journal of the Acoustical Society of America* 102: 523–36.

Hertz, S. R. 1982, From text to speech with SRS, *Journal of the Acoustical Society of America* 72: 1151–70.

Hiki, S. and Itoh, H. 1986, Influence of palate shape on lingual articulation, *Speech Communication* 5: 141–58.

Hirano, M. 1981, *Clinical Examination of Voice,* Vienna and New York, NY: Springer Verlag.

Hirano, M. and Ohala, J. 1969, Use of hooked-wire electrodes for electromyography of the intrinsic laryngeal muscles, *Journal of Speech and Hearing Research* 12: 362–73.

Hirose, H. 1971, Electromyography of the articulatory muscles: current instrumentation and technique, *Haskins Laboratories Status Report on Speech Research* 25/26: 73–86.

   1975, The posterior cricoarytenoid as a speech muscle, *Annual Bulletin of the Research Institute of Logopedics and Phoniatrics, University of Tokyo* 9: 47–66.

   1977, Electromyography of the larynx and other speech organs, in Sawashima, M. and Cooper, F. S. (eds.), *Dynamic Aspects of Speech Production*, University of Tokyo Press, pp. 49–67.

   1979, Laryngeal EMG, *Annual Bulletin of the Research Institute of Logopedics and Phoniatrics, University of Tokyo* 13: 13–22.

   1986, Pathophysiology of motor speech disorders (dysarthria), *Folia Phoniatrica* 38: 61–88.

Hirose, H. and Gay, T. 1972, The activity of the intrinsic laryngeal muscles in voicing control – an electromyographic study, *Phonetica* 25: 140–64.

Hirose, H. and Niimi, S. 1987, The relationship between glottal opening and the transglottal pressure differences during consonant production, in Baer, T., Sasaki, C. and Harris, K. S. (eds.), *Laryngeal Function in Phonation and Respiration*, Boston, MA: College Hill, pp. 381–90.

Hirose, H. and Ushijima, T. 1978, Laryngeal control for voicing distinction in Japanese consonant production, *Phonetica* 35: 1–10.

Hixon, T. 1971, An electromagnetic method for transducing jaw movements during speech, *Journal of the Acoustical Society of America* 49: 603–6.

Hixon, T., Goldman, M. and Mead, J. 1973, Kinematics of the chest wall during speech production: volume displacements of the rib cage, abdomen and lung, *Journal of Speech and Hearing Research* 16: 78–115.

Hockett, C. F. 1960, Logical considerations in the study of animal communication, in Lanyon W. E. and Tavolga, W. N. (eds.), *Animal Sounds and Communication*, American Institute of Biological Sciences Publication no. 7, pp. 392–430. [Reprinted in Hockett, C. F. 1977, *The View From Language*, Athens, GA: The University of Georgia Press, pp. 124–62.]

Höhne, J., Schönle, P., Conrad, B., Veldscholten, H., Wenig, P., Fakhouri, H., Sandner, N. and Hong, G. 1987, Direct measurement of vocal tract shape – articulography, in Laver, J. and Jack, M. (eds.), *Proceedings of the European Conference on Speech Technology, Edinburgh* 2: 230–2.

Holmberg, E. B., Hillman, R. E. and Perkell, J. S. 1988, Glottal air flow and pressure measurements for loudness variation by male and female speakers, *Journal of the Acoustical Society of America* 84: 511–29.

Holmes, J. N. 1975, Low-frequency phase distortion of speech recordings, *Journal of the Acoustical Society of America* 58: 747–9.

Holmes, J. N., Mattingly, I. G. and Shearme, J. N. 1964, Speech synthesis by rule, *Language and Speech* 7: 127–43.

Holst T. and Nolan F. 1995, The influence of syntactic structure on [s] to [ʃ] assimilation, in Connell, B. and Arvaniti, A. (eds.), *Papers in Laboratory Phonology IV: Phonology and Phonetic Evidence,* Cambridge University Press, pp. 315–33.

Holst, T., Warren, P. and Nolan, F. 1995, Categorising [s], [ʃ] and intermediate electropalatographic patterns: neural networks and other approaches, *European Journal of Disorders of Communication* 30: 161–74.

Honda, K. 1983, Electrical characteristics and preparation technique of hooked-wire electrodes for EMG recording, *Annual Bulletin of the Research Institute of Logopedics and Phoniatric, University of Tokyo* 17: 13–22.

Honda, M. and Kaburagi, T. 1993, Comparison of electromagnetic and ultrasonic techniques for monitoring tongue motion, *Forschungsberichte des Institutes für Phonetik und Sprachliche Kommunikation, München,* 31: 121–36.

Honda, K., Kusukawa, N. and Kakita, Y. 1992, An EMG analysis of sequential control cycles of articulatory activity during /əpVp/ utterances, *Journal of Phonetics* 20: 53–63.

Honda, K., Kiritani, S., Hnagawa, H. and Hirose, H. 1987, High-speed digital recording of vocal fold vibration using a solid-state image sensor, in Baer, T., Sasaki, C. and Harris, K. S. (eds.), *Laryngeal Function in Phonation and Respiration,* Boston, MA: College Hill, pp. 485–91.

Honda, K., Kurita, T., Kakita, Y. and Maeda, S. 1995, Physiology of the lips and modeling of lip gestures, *Journal of Phonetics* 23: 243–54.

Hoole, P. 1987, Velar and glottal activity in a speaker of Icelandic, *Proceedings of the XIth International Congress of Phonetic Sciences, Tallinn,* 3: 31–4.

1989, Velar movement: a method of registration and its application to ataxic subjects, *Folia Phoniatrica* 41: 176(A).

1993a, Instrumentelle Untersuchungen in der artikulatorischen Phonetik: Überlegungen zu ihrem Stellenwert als Grundlage für Entwicklung und Einsatz eines Systems zur Analyse der räumlichen und zeitlichen Strukturierung von Sprachbewegungen. PhD dissertation, University of Munich.

1993b, Methodological considerations in the use of electromagnetic articulography in phonetic research, *Forschungsberichte des Instituts für Phonetik und Sprachliche Kommunikation, München,* 31: 43–64.

1996, Issues in the acquisition, processing, reduction and parameterization of articulographic data, *Forschungsberichte des Instituts für Phonetik und Sprachliche Kommunikation, München,* 34: 158–73.

Hoole, P. and Kühnert, B. 1995, Patterns of lingual variability in German vowel production, *Proceedings XIIIth International Conference of Phonetic Science, Stockholm*, 2: 442–5.

Hoole, P., Gfroerer, S. and Tillmann, H.G. 1990, Electromagnetic articulography as a tool in the study of lingual coarticulation, *Forschungsberichte des Institus für Phonetik und Sprachliche Kommunikation der Universität München* 28: 107–22.

Hoole, P., Nguyen-Trong, N. and Hardcastle, W. 1993, A comparative investigation of coarticulation in fricatives: electropalatographic, electromagnetic and acoustic data, *Language and Speech* 36: 235–60.

Hoole, P., Pompino-Marschall, B. and Dames, M. 1984, Glottal timing in German voiceless occlusives, in Van den Broecke, M. P. R. and Cohen, A. (eds.), *Proceedings of the Xth International Congress of Phonetic Sciences*, Dordrecht: Foris, pp. 399–403.

Hoole, P., Schröter-Morasch, H. and Ziegler, W. 1997, Patterns of laryngeal apraxia in two patients with Broca's aphasia syndrome, *Clinical Linguistics and Phonetics* 11: 429–42.

Hoole, P., Ziegler, W., Hartmann, E. and Hardcastle, W. J. 1989, Parallel electropalatographic and acoustic measures for fricatives, *Clinical Linguistics and Phonetics* 3: 59–69.

Horiguchi, S. and Bell-Berti, F. 1987, The Velotrace: a device for monitoring velar position, *Cleft Palate Journal* 24: 104–11.

Horii, Y. 1983, An accelerometric measure as a physical correlate of perceived hypernasality in speech, *Journal of Speech and Hearing Research* 26: 476–80.

House, A. S. and Fairbanks, G. 1953, The influence of consonant environment upon the secondary characteristics of vowels, *Journal of the Acoustical Society of America* 25: 105–13.

House, A. S. and Stevens, K. N. 1956, Analog studies of the nasalization of vowels, *Journal of Speech and Hearing Disorders* 21: 218–22.

Huffman, M. K. 1986, Patterns of coarticulation in English, *UCLA Working Papers in Phonetics* 63: 26–47.

1987a, Measures of phonation type in Hmong, *Journal of the Acoustical Society of America* 81: 495–504.

1987b, Timing of contextual nasalization in two languages, *Journal of the Acoustical Society of America*, Supplement 1 82: S115.

1990, Implementation of Nasal: timing and articulatory landmarks, PhD dissertation, University of California, Los Angeles, published in *UCLA Working Papers in Phonetics* 75.

Hunt, M. J. 1978, Automatic correction of low-frequency phase distortion in analogue magnetic recordings, *Acoustic Letters* 2: 6–10.

1987, Studies of glottal excitation using inverse filtering and an electroglottograph, *Proceedings of the XIth International Congress of Phonetic Sciences, Tallinn* 3: 23–6.

Hunt, M. J., Bridle J. S., and Holmes, J. N. 1978, Interactive digital inverse filtering and its relation to linear prediction methods, *Proceedings of the IEEE International Conference on Acoustics, Speech, and Signal Processing, Tulsa OK*: 15–18.

Hussein, L. 1990, VCV coarticulation in Arabic, *Ohio State University Working Papers in Linguistics* 38: 88–104.

Hutters, B. 1976, Problems in the use of the photoelectric glottograph, *Annual Bulletin of the Research Institute of Logopedics and Phoniatrics, University of Tokyo* 10: 274–312.

1984, Vocal fold adjustments in Danish voiceless obstruent production, *Annual Report of the Institute of Phonetics of the University of Copenhagen* 18: 293–385.

1985, Vocal fold adjustments in aspirated and unaspirated stops in Danish, *Phonetica* 42: 1–24.

Hyman, L. M. 1975, Nasal states and nasal processes, in Ferguson, C. A., Hyman, L. M. and Ohala, J. J. (eds.), *Nasalfest. Papers from a Symposium on Nasals and Nasalization* 249–64. Language Universals Project, Stanford University.

International Radiation Protection Association 1990, Interim guidelines on limits of exposure to 50/60Hz electric and magnetic fields, *Health Physics* 58: 113–22.

Itô, J. 1990, Prosodic minimality in Japanese. Parasession on the syllable in phonetics and phonology, *26th Meeting of the Chicago Linguistics Society*, 213–39.

Jackson, M., Ladefoged, P., Huffman, M. K. and Antoñanzas-Barroso, N. 1985, Measures of spectral tilt, *UCLA Working Papers in Phonetics* 61: 72–8.

Jakobson, R., Fant, G. and Halle, M. 1952, *Preliminaries to Speech Analysis: the Distinctive Features and their Correlates*, Cambridge, MA: MIT Press.

Jessen, M. 1995, Glottal opening in German obstruents, *Proceedings of the XIIIth International Congress of Phonetic Sciences, Stockholm* 3: 428–31.

Johnson, K. 1994, Phonetic arbitrariness and the input problem: comments on Coleman's paper, in Keating, P. A. (ed.), *Papers in Laboratory Phonology* III: *Phonological Structure and Phonetic Form,* Cambridge University Press, pp. 325–30.

Johnson, K., Ladefoged, P. and Lindau, M. 1993, Individual differences in vowel production, *Journal of the Acoustical Society of America* 94: 701–14.

Jones, D. 1932, *Outline of English Phonetics*, Cambridge University Press (3rd edn).

Jones, L. G. 1959, The contextual variants of the Russian vowels, in Halle, M. *The Sound Pattern of Russian,* The Hague: Mouton, pp. 157–67.

Jones, W. J. and Hardcastle, W. J. 1995, New developments in EPG3 software, *European Journal of Disorders of Communication* 30: 183–92.

Jong, K. J. de 1991, An articulatory study of consonant-induced vowel duration changes in English, *Phonetica* 48: 1–17.

1995a, On the status of redundant features: the case of backness and rounding in American English, in Connell, B. and Arvaniti, A. (eds.), *Papers in Laboratory Phonology* IV: *Phonology and Phonetic Evidence,* Cambridge University Press, pp. 68–86.

1995b, The supraglottal articulation of prominence in English: linguistic stress as localized hyperarticulation, *Journal of the Acoustical Society of America* 97: 491–504.

Jong, K. de, Beckman, M. E. and Edwards, J. 1993, The interplay between prosodic structure and coarticulation, *Language and Speech* 36: 197–212.

Jordan, M. I. 1991, Motor learning and the degrees of freedom problem, in Jeannerod, M. (ed.), *Attention and Performance* XIII, Hillsdale, NJ: Erlbaum, pp. 796–836.

1997, Serial order: a parallel distributed processing approach, in Donahoe, J. and Dorsel, V. P. (eds.), *Neural Network Models of Cognition: Bio-behavioral Foundations*, North-Holland: Elsevier Science Publishers, pp. 471–95,

Kane, P. and Ní Chasaide, A. 1992, A comparison of the dysphonic and normal voice source, *Journal of Clinical Speech and Language Studies* 2: 1–16.

Karlsson, I. 1990, Voice source dynamics for female speakers, *Proceedings of the 1990 International Conference on Spoken Language Processing, Kobe*: 225–31.

1992, Modelling voice source variations in female speech, *Speech Communication* 11: 1–5.

Karnell, M. P., Linville, R. N. and Edwards, B. A. 1988, Variations in velar position overtime: a nasal videoendoscopic study, *Journal of Speech and Hearing Research* 31: 417–24.

Katz, W., Kripke, C. and Tallal, P. 1991, Anticipatory coarticulation in the speech of adults and young children: acoustic, perceptual and video data, *Journal of Speech and Hearing Research* 34: 1222–32.

Katz, W., Machetanz, J., Orth, U. and Schönle, P. 1990, A kinematic analysis of anticipatory coarticulation in the speech of anterior aphasic subjects using electromagnetic articulography, *Brain and Language* 3: 555–75.

Kawasaki, H. 1986, Phonetic explanation for phonological universals: the case of distinctive vowel nasalization, in Ohala, J. J. and Jaeger, J. J. (eds.), *Experimental Phonology*, New York, NY: Academic Press, pp. 81–103.

Keating, P. A. 1985a, CV phonology, experimental phonetics, and coarticulation, *UCLA Working Papers in Phonetics* 62: 1–13.

1985b, Universal phonetics and the organization of grammars, in Fromkin, V. (ed.), *Phonetic Linguistics: Essays in Honor of Peter Ladefoged*, Orlando, FL: Academic Press, pp. 115–32.

1988a The window model of coarticulation: articulatory evidence, *UCLA Working Papers in Phonetics* 69: 3–29.

1988b, Underspecification in phonetics, *Phonology* 5: 275–92.

1990a, Phonetic representations in a generative grammar, *Journal of Phonetics* 18: 321–34.

1990b, The window model of coarticulation: articulatory evidence, in Kingston, J. and Beckman M. E. (eds.), *Papers in Laboratory Phonetics* I: *Between the Grammar and the Physics of Speech*, Cambridge University Press, pp. 451–70.

1991, Phonetics in the next ten years, *Proceedings of the XIIth International Congress of Phonetic Sciences, Aix-en-Provence* 1: 112–19.

Keating, P. A. and Huffman, M. 1984, Vowel variation in Japanese, *Phonetica* 41: 191–207.

Keating, P., Lindblom, B., Lubker, J. and Kreiman, J. 1994, Variability in jaw height for segments in English and Swedish VCVs, *Journal of Phonetics* 22: 407–22.

Keller, E. and Ostry, D. J. 1983, Computerized measurement of tongue-dorsum movement with pulsed-echo ultrasound, *Journal of the Acoustical Society of America* 73: 1309–15.

Kelsey, C. A., Woodhouse, R. J. and Minifie, F. D. 1969, Coarticulation in the pharynx, *Journal of the Acoustical Society of America* 46: 1016–18.

Kelso, J. A. S., Saltzman, E. L. and Tuller, B. 1986, The dynamical perspective on speech production: data and theory, *Journal of Phonetics* 14: 29–59.

Kelso, J. A. S., Tuller, B., Vatikiotis-Bateson, E. and Fowler, C. A. 1984, Functionally specific articulatory cooperation following jaw perturbations during speech: evidence for coordinate structures, *Journal of Experimental Psychology: Human Perception and Performance* 10: 812–32.

Kelso, J. A. S., Vatikiotis-Bateson, E., Saltzman, E. L. and Kay, B. 1985, A qualitative dynamic analysis of reiterant speech production: phase portraits, kinematics and dynamic modelling, *Journal of the Acoustical Society of America* 77: 266–80.

Kennedy, J. G. III and Abbs, J. H. 1979, Anatomical studies of the periorial motor system: foundations for studies in speech physiology, in Lass, N. J. (ed.), *Speech and Language: Advances in Basic Research and Practice*, I, New York, NY: Academic Press, pp. 212–270.

Kenstowicz, M. 1994, *Phonology in Generative Grammar*, Oxford: Basil Blackwell.

Kent, R. 1983, The segmental organization of speech, in MacNeilage, P. (ed.), *The Production of Speech*, New York, NY: Springer, pp. 57–89.

1986, Is a paradigm change needed? *Journal of Phonetics* 14: 111–15.

Kent, R. and Forner, L. 1980, Speech segment durations in sentence recitations by children and adults, *Journal of Phonetics* 8: 157–68.

Kent, R. and Minifie, F. 1977, Coarticulation in recent speech production models, *Journal of Phonetics* 5: 115–33.

Kent, R. D. and Moll K. L. 1969, Vocal-tract characteristics of the stop cognates, *Journal of the Acoustical Society of America* 46: 1549–55.

1972a, Cinefluorographic analyses of selected lingual consonants, *Journal of Speech and Hearing Research* 15: 453–73.

1972b, Tongue body articulation during vowel and diphthong gestures, *Folia Phoniatrica* 24: 278–300.

1975, Articulatory timing in selected consonant sequences, *Brain and Language* 2: 304–23.

Kent, R. D. and Netsell, R. 1971, Effects of stress contrasts on certain articulatory parameters, *Phonetica* 24: 23–44.

Kent, R. D., Carney, P. and Severeid, L. D. 1974, Velar movement and timing: evaluation of a model for binary control, *Journal of Speech and Hearing Research* 17: 470–88.

Kewley-Port, D. 1977, EMG signal processing for speech research, *Haskins Laboratories Status Report on Speech Research*, 123–46.

1982, Measurement of formant transitions in naturally produced stop consonant–vowel syllables, *Journal of the Acoustical Society of America* 72: 379–89.

Kim, C.-W. 1965, On the autonomy of the tensity feature in stop classification (with special reference to Korean stops), *Word* 21: 339–59.

King, L., Ramming, H., Schiefer, L. and Tillmann, H. G. 1987, Initial F0–contours in Shangai CV-syllables – an interactive function of tone, vowel height, and place and manner of stop articulation, *Proceedings of the XIth International Congress of Phonetic Sciences, Tallinn*, 1: 154–7.

Kingston, J. 1990, Articulatory binding, in Kingston, J. and Beckman, M. E. (eds.), *Papers in Laboratory Phonology* 1: *Between the Grammar and Physics of Speech*, Cambridge University Press, pp. 406–34.

Kingston, J. and Cohen, A. H. 1992, Extending articulatory phonology, *Phonetica* 49: 194–204.

Kingston, J. C. and Diehl, R. 1994, Phonetic knowledge, *Language* 70: 419–54.

Kiparsky, P. 1982, Lexical morphology and phonology, in Yang, I.-S. (ed.), *Linguistics in the Morning Calm*, Seoul: Hanshin, pp. 3–91.

1985, Some consequences of lexical phonology, *Phonology Yearbook* 2: 85–138.

Kiritani, S. 1971, X-ray monitoring of the position of the fiberscope by means of computer-controlled radiography, *Annual Bulletin of the Research Institute of Logopedics and Phoniatrics, University of Tokyo* 5: 35–9.

Kiritani, S. and Sawashima, M. 1987, The temporal relationship between articulations of consonants and adjacent vowels, in Channon, R. and Shockley, L. (eds.), *In Honor of Ilse Lehiste*, Netherlands Phonetic Archives VI. Dordrecht: Foris, 139–49.

Kiritani S., Imagawa, H. and Hirose, H. 1992, Vocal-cord vibration during consonants – high-speed digital imaging using a fiberscope, *Proceedings of 1992 International Conference on Spoken Language Processing* 1: 1661–4.

Kiritani, S., Itoh, K. and Fujimura, O. 1975, Tongue-pellet tracking by a computer-controlled X-ray microbeam system, *Journal of the Acoustical Society of America* 57: 1516–20.

Kiritani, S., Itoh, K., Hirose, H. and Sawashima, M. 1977, Coordination of the consonant and vowel articulations – X-ray microbeam study on Japanese and English, *Annual Bulletin of the Research Institute of Logopedics and Phoniatrics, University of Tokyo* 11: 31–7.

Kiritani, S., Tanaka, T., Hashimoto, K., Masaki, S. and Shirai, K. 1983, Contextual variation of the jaw movement for the intervocalic consonant in VCV utterances, *Annual Bulletin of the Research Institute for Logopedics and Phoniatrics* 17: 45–53.

Kirk, P., Ladefoged, P. and Ladefoged, J. 1984, Using a spectrograph for measures of phonation types in a natural language, *UCLA Working Papers in Phonetics* 59: 102–13.

Kitzing, P. and Löfqvist, A. 1975, Subglottal and oral pressure during phonation – preliminary investigation using a miniature transducer system, *Medical and Biological Engineering* 13: 644–8.

Klatt, D. H. 1973, Duration of pre-stress word-initial consonant clusters in English, *MIT Research Lab. of Electronics Quarterly Progress Report* 108: 253–60.

1974, The duration of [s] in English words, *Journal of Speech and Hearing Research* 17: 51–63.

Kohler, K. J. 1990, Segmental reduction in connected speech in German: phonological facts and phonetic explanation, in Hardcastle, W. J. and Marchal, A. (eds.), *Speech Production and Speech Modelling*, Dordrecht: Kluwer, pp. 69–92.

1991, The phonetics/phonology issue in the study of articulatory reduction, *Phonetica* 48: 180–92.

Kollia, H. B., Gracco, V. L. and Harris, K. S. 1994, Articulatory organization of mandibular, labial and velar movements during speech, *Haskins Laboratories Status Report on Speech Research* 117/118: 49–65.

Kondo, Y. 1994, Phonetic underspecification in schwa, International Conference on Spoken Language Processing, 1, Yokohama, *The Acoustical Society of Japan*: 311–14.

Koopmans-van Beinum, F. J. 1994, What's in a schwa? Durational and spectral analysis of natural continuous speech and diphones in Dutch, *Phonetica* 51: 68–79.

Kozhevnikov, V. and Chistovich, L. 1965, *Speech: Articulation and Perception*, Translation 30, 543, Washington, DC: Joint Publications Research Service.

Krakow, R. A. 1986, Prosodic effects on velic movements, Paper presented at the meeting of the Linguistic Society of America, New York.

   1993, Nonsegmental influences on velum movement patterns: syllables, sentences, stress and speaking rate, in Huffman, M. K. and Krakow, R. A. (eds.), *Phonetics and Phonology, Nasals, Nasalization and the Velum* V, San Diego, CA: Academic Press, pp. 87–116.

Krakow, R. A. and Beddor, P. S. 1991, Coarticulation and the perception of nasality, *Proceedings of the XIIth International Congress of Phonetic Sciences, Aix-en-Provence*, 5: 38–52.

Krakow, R. A. and Huffman, M. K. 1993, Instruments and techniques for investigating nasalization and velopharyngeal function in the laboratory: an introduction, in Huffman, M. K. and Krakow, R. A. (eds.), *Phonetics and Phonology, Nasals, Nasalization and the Velum* V, San Diego, CA: Academic Press, pp. 3–59.

Krakow, R. A., Beddor, P. S. Goldstein, L. M. and Fowler, C. 1988, Coarticulatory influences on the perceived height of nasal vowels, *Journal of the Acoustical Society of America* 83: 1146–58.

Kröger, B. J. 1993, A gestural production model and its application to reduction in German, *Phonetica* 50: 213–33.

Kroos, C., Hoole, P., Kühnert, B. and Tillmann, H. 1996, Phonetic evidence for the phonological status, *Journal of the Acoustical Society of America* 100: 2691.

Krull, D. 1987, Second formant locus patterns as a measure of consonant–vowel coarticulation, *Phonetic Experimental Research at the Institute of Linguistics, University of Stockholm, Sweden* V: 43–61.

   1989, Consonant–vowel coarticulation in spontaneous speech and in reference words, *(STL-QPSR) Speech Transmission Laboratory Quarterly Progress Status Report, Royal Institute of Technology, Stockholm, Sweden* 1: 101–5.

Kuehn, D. P. and Moll, K. L. 1972, Perceptual effects of forward coarticulation, *Journal of Speech and Hearing Research* 15: 654–64.

   1976, A cineradiographic study of VC and CV articulatory velocities, *Journal of Phonetics* 4: 303–20.

Kuehn, D. P. and Moon, J. B. 1994, Levator veli palatini muscle activity in relation to intraoral air pressure variation, *Journal of Speech and Hearing Research* 37: 1260–70.

Kuenzel, H. J. 1977, Photoelektrische Untersuchung zur Velumhohe bei Vokalen: erste Anwendungen des Velographen, *Phonetica* 34: 352–70.

   1979, Some observations on velar movement in plosives, *Phonetica* 36: 384–404.

Kühnert, B. 1993, Some kinematic aspects of alveolar–velar assimilations, *Forschungsberichte des Instituts für Phonetik und Sprachliche Kommunikation, München*, 31: 263–72.

Kühnert, B., Ledl, C., Hoole, P. and Tillmann, H. G. 1991, Tongue–jaw interactions in lingual activity, *Phonetic Experimental Research at the Institute of Linguistics, University of Stockholm* 14: 21–5.

Kurowski, K. and Blumstein, S. E. 1987, Acoustic properties for place of articulation in nasal consonants, *Journal of the Acoustical Society of America* 81: 1917–27.

Kuwahara, H. and Sakai, H. 1972, Perception of vowels and C-V syllables segmented from connected speech, *Journal of the Acoustical Society of Japan* 28: 225–34.

Kuznetsov, V. B. and Ott, A. 1987, Spectral properties of Russian stressed vowels in the context of palatalized and nonpalatalized consonants, *Proceedings of XIth International Congress of Phonetic Sciences, Tallinn* 3: 117–20.

Lacerda, A. de and Head, B. F. 1963, *Analise de sons nasais e sons nasalizados do Portugues*, Rev. Lab. Fonetica, University of Coimbra, Portugal.

Ladefoged P. 1964, *A Phonetic Study of West African Language*, Cambridge University Press.

1967a, Linguistic phonetics, *UCLA Working Papers in Phonetics* 6 (monograph).

1967b, *Three Areas of Experimental Phonetics*, Oxford University Press.

1975, *A Course in Phonetics*, New York, NY: Harcourt Brace Jovanovich.

1983a, The limits of biological explanation in phonetics, *UCLA Working Papers in Phonetics* 57: 1–10.

1983b, The linguistic use of different phonation types, in Bless, D. and Abbs, J. (eds.), *Vocal Fold Physiology. Contemporary Research and Clinical Issues,* San Diego, CA: College Hill Press, pp. 351–60.

Ladefoged, P. and Maddieson, I. 1990, Vowels of the world's languages, *Journal of Phonetics* 18: 93–122.

Lahiri, A., Gewirth, L. and Blumstein, S. 1984, A reconsideration of acoustic invariance for place of articulation in diffuse stop consonants, *Journal of the Acoustical Society of America* 76: 391–414.

Lallouache, M. T. and Abry, C. 1992, Une autre vision des modèles d'anticipation, *19e Journees d'Etudes sur la Parole, Bruxelles*, 47–52.

Larkey, L. S., Wald, J. and Strange, W. 1978, Perception of synthetic nasal consonants in initial and final syllable position, *Perception and Psychophysics* 23: 299–312.

Leanderson, R., Persson, A. and Öhman, S. 1971, Electromyographic studies of facial muscles activity in speech, *Acta Otolaryngologica* 72: 361–9.

Lehiste, I. and Peterson, G. E. 1959, Vowel amplitude and phonemic stress in American English, *Journal of the Acoustical Society of America* 31: 428–35.

1961, Transitions, glides and diphthongs, *Journal of the Acoustical Society of America* 33: 268–77.

Liberman, A. M., Delattre, P. C., Cooper F. S. and Gerstman, L. J. 1954, The role of consonant–vowel transitions in the perception of the stop and nasal consonants, *Psychological Monographs* 68: 1–13.

Lindblom, B. 1963a, *On Vowel Reduction, Report no. 29*, The Royal Institute of Technology, Speech Transmission Laboratory, Stockholm.

1963b, Spectrographic study of vowel reduction, *Journal of the Acoustical Society of America* 35: 1773–81.

1966, Studies of labial articulation, *(STL-QPSR) Speech Transmission Laboratory, Royal Institute of Technology, Stockholm, Sweden* 7–9.

1967, Vowel duration and a model of lip-mandible coordination, *(STL-QPSR) Speech Transmission Laboratory, Royal Institute of Technology, Stockholm, Sweden* 4: 1–29.

1983, Economy of speech gestures, in MacNeilage, P. F. *The Production of Speech*, New York, NY: Springer-Verlag, pp. 217–45.

1989, Phonetic invariance and the adaptive nature of speech, in Elsendoom, B. A. G. and Bouma, H. (eds.) *Working Models of Human Perception*, London: Academic Press, pp. 139–73.

1990, Explaining phonetic variation: a sketch of the H&H theory, in Hardcastle, W. J. and Marchal, A. (eds.), *Speech Production and Speech Modelling*, Dordrecht: Kluwer Academic Publishers, pp. 403–39.

Lindblom, B. and Engstrand, O. 1989, In what sense is speech quantal? *Journal of Phonetics* 17: 107–21.

Lindblom, B. and Lindgren, R. 1985, Speaker–listener interaction and phonetic variation, *Phonetic Experimental Research at the Institute of Linguistics, University of Stockholm, Sweden* 4: 77–85.

Lindblom, B. and MacNeilage, P. 1986, Action theory: problems and alternative aproaches, *Journal of Phonetics* 14: 117–32.

Lindblom, B. and Sundberg, J. 1971, Acoustical consequences of lip, tongue, jaw and larynx movement, (*STL-QPSR*) *Speech Transmission Laboratory Quarterly Progress and Status Report, Royal Institute of Technology, Stockholm, Sweden* 2: 1–21.

Lindblom, B., Lubker, J. and Gay, T. 1979, Formant frequencies of some fixed-mandible vowels and a model of speech motor programming by predictive simulation, *Journal of Phonetics* 7: 147–61.

Lindblom, B., Pauli, S. and Sundberg, J. 1975, Modeling coarticulation in apical stops, in Fant, G. (ed.), *Speech Communication*, II, Uppsala: Almqvist and Wiksell, pp. 87–94.

Lindblom, B., Brownlee, S., Davis, B. and Moon, S. J. 1992, Speech transforms, *Speech Communication* 11: 357–68.

Lindqvist-Gauffin, J. and Sundberg J. 1976, Acoustic properties of the nasal tract, *Phonetica* 33: 161–8.

Linker, W. 1982, Articulatory and acoustic correlates of labial activity in vowels: a cross-linguistic study, *UCLA Working Papers in Phonetics*, 56 (monograph).

Lisker, L. and Abramson, A. 1964, A cross-language study of voicing in initial stops: acoustic measurements, *Word* 20: 384–422.

Lisker L., Abramson, A. S., Cooper, F. S. and Schvey, M. 1969, Transillumination of the larynx in running speech, *Journal of the Acoustical Society of America* 45: 1544–6.

Ljungqvist, M. and Fujisaki, H. 1985a, A comparative study of glottal waveform models, *Technical Report of the Institute of Electronics and Communications Engineers*, Japan, EA85–58: 23–9.

1985b, A method for simultaneous estimation of voice source and vocal tract parameters based on linear predictive analysis, *Transactions of the Committee on Speech Research, Acoustical Society of Japan*, S85–21: 153–60.

1985c, Correction of low frequency distortion in speech recordings and its effect on the glottal wave shape, *Proceedings of the Spring Meeting of Acoustical Society of Japan*, 161–2.

Local, J. 1992, Modeling assimilation in nonsegmental, rule-free synthesis, in Docherty, G. J. and Ladd, D. R. (eds.), *Papers in Laboratory Phonology* II: *Gesture, Segment, Prosody*, Cambridge University Press, pp. 190–223.

Löfqvist, A. 1980, Interarticulatory programming in stop production, *Journal of Phonetics* 8: 475–90.

1990, Speech as audible gestures, in Hardcastle, W. J. and Marchal, A. (eds.), *Speech Production and Speech Modelling*, Dordrecht: Kluwer Academic Publishers, pp. 289–322.

Löfqvist, A. and Gracco, V. 1995, Articulatory kinematics in stop consonants, *Proceedings of the XIIIth International Congress of Phonetic Sciences, Stockholm, Sweden* 3: 572–5.

Löfqvist, A. and McGarr, N. 1987, Laryngeal dynamics in voiceless consonant production, in Baer, T., Sasaki, C. and Harris, K. S. (eds.), *Laryngeal Function in Phonation and Respiration*, Boston, MA: College Hill, pp. 391–402.

Löfqvist, A. and McGowan, R. S. 1988, Voice source variations during consonant–vowel transitions, *Journal of the Acoustical Society of America* 84: S85(A).

Löfqvist, A. and Yoshioka, H. 1980a, Laryngeal activity in Icelandic obstruent production, *Haskins Laboratories Status Report on Speech Research* 63: 275–92.

1980b, Laryngeal activity in Swedish obstruent clusters, *Journal of the Acoustical Society of America* 63: 792–801.

1984, Intrasegmental timing: laryngeal-oral coordination in voiceless consonant production, *Speech Communication* 3: 279–89.

Lonchamp, F. 1978, *Recherches sur les indices perceptifs des voyelles vales et nasales du français, Thèse de 3ème cycle*, University of Nancy.

Lotz, W. K., Shaughnessy, A. L. and Netsell, R. 1981, Velopharyngeal and nasal cavity resistance during speech production, Paper presented at the Convention of the American Speech and Hearing Association.

Lubker, J. F. 1968, An electromyographic–cineradiographic investigation of velar function during normal speech production, *Cleft Palate Journal* 5: 1–18.

1970, Aerodynamic and ultrasonic assessment techniques in speech dento-facial research, *Proceedings of the Workshop and the Dento-facial Complex: the State of the Art, ASHA Report 5*, Washington DC.

1981, Temporal aspects of speech production: anticipatory labial coarticulation, *Phonetica* 38: 51–65.

Lubker, J. F. and Gay, T. 1982, Anticipatory labial coarticulation: experimental, biological, and linguistic variables, *Journal of the Acoustical Society of America* 71: 437–48.

Lubker, J. F. and Moll, K. L. 1965, Simultaneous oral–nasal airflow measurements and cinefluorographic observations during speech production, *Cleft Palate Journal* 2: 257–72.

Lubker, J.F., Lindgren, R. and Gibson, A. 1984, Cross-language effects of coarticulation in Italian, *Abstracts of the Xth International Congress of Phonetic Sciences*, Dordrecht: Foris, p. 514.

Lubker, J. F., McAllister, B. and Carlson, J. 1975, Labial co-articulation in Swedish: a preliminary report, in Fant, G. (ed.), *Speech Communication*, II, Stockholm: Almqvist and Wiksell, pp. 55–63.

Luce, P. A. and Luce, J.-C. 1985, Contextual effects on vowel duration, closure duration, and the consonant/vowel ratio in speech production, *Journal of the Acoustical Society of America* 78: 1949–57.

Macchi, M. 1988, Labial articulation patterns associated with segmental features and syllable structure in English, *Phonetica* 45: 109–21.

Mack, M. and Blumstein, S. 1983, Further evidence of acoustic invariance in speech production: the stop–glide contrast, *Journal of the Acoustical Society of America* 73: 1739–50.

Macken, M. 1980, Aspects of the acquisition of stop systems: a cross-linguistic perspective, in Yeni-Komshian, G., Kavanagh, J. and Ferguson, C. (eds.), *Child Phonology*, I, London: Academic Press pp. 143–68.

MacLean, I. C. 1980, Neuromuscular junction, in Johnson, E. W. (ed.), *Practical Electromyography*, Baltimore, MD: Williams and Wilkins, pp. 73–90.

MacNeilage, P. 1963, Electromyographic and acoustic study of the production of certain final clusters, *Journal of the Acoustical Society of America* 35: 461–3.

1970, Motor control and serial ordering of speech. *Psychological Review* 77: 182–96.

MacNeilage, P. F. and DeClerk, J. L. 1969, On the motor control of coarticulation in CVC monosyllables, *Journal of the Acoustical Society of America* 45: 1217–33.

MacNeilage, D. F., Sussman, H. M. and Powers, R. K. 1977, Discharge patterns accompanying sustained activation of motor units in speech musculature, *Journal of Phonetics* 5: 135–48.

Maddieson, I. and Ladefoged, P. 1985, 'Tense' and 'lax' in four minority languages of China, *UCLA Working Papers in Phonetics* 60: 59–83.

Maeda, S. 1982, The role of the sinus cavities in the production of nasal vowels, *Proceedings of the International Conference on Acoustics, Speech and Signal Processing 82, Paris*, 2: 911–14.

1984, Une paire de pies spectraux comme corrélat acoustique de la nasalisation des voyelles, *13èmes Journées d'Etudes sur la Parole*, Bruxelles: GALF, pp. 223–4.

1993, Acoustics of vowel nasalization and articulatory shifts in French nasal vowels, in Huffman, M. K. and Krakow, R. A. (eds.), *Nasals, Nasalization, and the Velum*, London: Academic Press, pp. 147–67.

Maeda, S. and Honda, K. 1995, Articulatory co-ordination and its neurobiological aspects: an essay, *Proceedings of the XIIIth International Congress of Phonetic Sciences, Stockholm, Sweden* 2: 76–83.

Magen, H. 1984a, Vowel-to-vowel coarticulation in English and Japanese, *Journal of the Acoustical Society of America, Supplement* 1, 75: S41.

1984b, Vowel-to-vowel coarticulation in English and Japanese, Paper presented at the 107th meeting of the Acoustical Society of America, Norfolk, Virginia.

1989, An acoustic study of vowel-to-vowel coarticulation in English, PhD dissertation, Yale University, New Haven, CT.

1997, The extent of vowel-to-vowel coarticulation in English, *Journal of Phonetics* 25: 187–206.

Magno-Caldognetto, E., Vagges, K., Ferrigno, G. and Busà, M. G. 1992, Lip rounding coarticulation in Italian, *Proceedings of the International Conference on Spoken Language Processing 92* 1: 41–64.

Malécot, A. 1960, Vowel nasality as a distinctive feature in American English, *Language* 36: 222–9.

Malécot, A. and Peebles, K. 1965, An optical device for recording glottal abduction–adduction during normal speech, *Zeitschrift für Phonetik*, 18: 545–50.

Mann, V. A. and Repp, B. H. 1980, Influence of vocalic context on perception of /ʃ/–/s/ distinction, *Perception and Psychophysics* 28: 213–28.

Mansell, P. 1973, Coarticulation of muscle activity for lip-sounding, *Forschugsberichte des Institut für Phonetik und Sprachliche Kommunikation der Universität München* 2: 33–157.

Mantakas, M., Schwarz, J. L. and Escudier, P. 1988, An acoustic-perceptual study of the rounding opposition in French front vowels, *Bulletin du Laboratoire de la Communication Parlée, Université de Grenoble* 2: 95–130.

Manuel S. 1986, Perception of coarticulatory variation in Shona, *Journal of the Acoustical Society of America* 79: Supplement 1, S27(A).

1987, Acoustic and perceptual consequences of vowel-to-vowel coarticulation in three Bantu languages, PhD dissertation, Yale University, New Haven, CT.

1990, The role of contrast in limiting vowel-to-vowel coarticulation in different languages, *Journal of the Acoustical Society of America* 88: 1286–98.

1995, Speakers nasalize /ð/ after /n/, but listeners still hear /ð/', *Journal of Phonetics* 23: 453–76.

Manuel S. and Krakow, R. 1984, Universal and language particular aspects of vowel-to-vowel coarticulation, *Haskins Laboratories Status Report on Speech Research* SR-77/78: 69–78.

Manuel, S. Y., Shattuck-Hufnagel, S., Huffman, M., Stevens, K. N., Carlson, R. and Hunnicutt, S. 1992, Studies of vowel and consonant reduction, in Ohala, J. J., Nearey, T. M., Derwing, B. L., Hodge, M. M. and Wiebe, G. E. (eds.), *Proceedings of the 1992 International Conference on Spoken Langauge Processing,* Edmonton, University of Alberta: 943–6.

Marchal, A. 1985, Description articulatoire et acoustique des groupes d'occlusives, *Travaux de l'Institut de Phonétique d'Aix* 10: 13–61.

Marchal, M. and Espesser, R. 1987, *L'asymétrie des appuis linguo-palatins. Communication aux 16èmes Journées d'Études sur la Parole,* Hammamet.

Marchal, A. and Hardcastle, W. J. 1993, ACCOR: instrumentation and database for the cross-language study of coarticulation, *Language and Speech* 36: 137–53.

Martin, J. G. and Bunnell, H. T. 1981, Perception of anticipatory coarticulation effects, *Journal of the Acoustical Society of America* 69: 559–67.

Martinet, A. 1952, Function, structure, and sound change, *Word* 8: 1–32. Reprinted in Baldi, P. and Werth, R. (eds.), 1978, *Readings in Historical Phonology: Chapters in the Theory of Sound Change,* University Park, PA: The Pennsylvania State University Press, pp. 121–59.

1957, Phonetics and linguistic evolution, in Malmberg, M. (ed.), *Manual of Phonetics,* Amsterdam: North Holland, pp. 252–72.

Matsuno, K. 1989, An electropalatographic study of Japanese palatal sounds, *The Bulletin, The Phonetic Society of Japan* 190: 8–17.

Mattingly, I. G. 1981, Phonetic representations and speech synthesis by rule, in Myers, T., Laver, J. and Anderson, J. (eds.), *The Cognitive Representation of Speech,* Amsterdam: North-Holland, pp. 415–25.

Maturi, P. 1991, The perception of consonantal nasality in Italian: conditioning factors, *Proceedings of the XIIth International Congress of Phonetic Sciences, Aix-en-Provence* 5: 50–3.

McAllister, R. 1978, Temporal asymmetry in labial co-articulation, *Papers from the Institute of Linguistics, University of Stockholm* 35: 1–29.

1980, Some phonetic correlates of the tense–lax feature in Swedish rounded vowels, *Journal of Phonetics* 8: 39–51.

McAllister, R., Lubker, J. and Carlson, J. 1974, An EMG study of some characteristics of the Swedish rounded vowels, *Journal of Phonetics* 2: 267–78.

McCarthy, J. 1983, Consonantal morphology in the Chaha verb, in Barlow, M., Flickinger, D. and Wescoat, M. (eds.), *Proceedings of the Second West Coast Conference on Formal Linguistics*, Stanford: Stanford Linguistic Association, 176–88.

McCarthy, J. and Prince, A. 1990a, Foot and word in prosodic morphology: the Arabic broken plural, *Natural Language and Linguistic Theory* 8: 209–83.

1990b, Prosodic morphology and templatic morphology, in Eid, M. and McCarthy, J. (eds.), *Perspectives in Arabic Linguistics 2: Papers from the Second Annual Symposium on Arabic Linguistics*, Amsterdam: John Benjamins, pp. 1–54.

McClean, M. 1973, Forward coarticulation of velar movement at marked junctural boundaries, *Journal of Speech and Hearing Research* 16: 286–96.

McGarr, N. and Löfqvist, A. 1988, Laryngeal kinematics of voiceless obstruents produced by hearing-impaired speakers, *Journal of Speech and Hearing Research* 31: 234–9.

McGowan, R. and Nittrouer, S. 1988, Differences in fricative production between children and adults: evidence from an acoustic analysis of /ʃ/ and /s/, *Journal of the Acoustical Society of America* 83: 229–36.

McLeod, W. D. 1973, EMG instrumentation in biomechanical studies: amplifiers, recorders and integrators, in Desmedt, J. E. (ed.), *New Developments in Electromyography and Clinical Neuropsychology* I, Basal: Karger, pp. 511–18.

Menzerath, P. and de Lacerda, A. 1933, *Koartikulation, Steuerung und Lautabgrenzung*, Berlin and Bonn: Fred. Dummlers.

Mermelstein, P. 1977, On detecting nasals in continuous speech, *Journal of the Acoustical Society of America* 61: 581–7.

Miller, R. A. 1967, *The Japanese Language*, University of Chicago Press.

Miyawaki, K. 1972, A preliminary study of American English /r/ by use of dynamic palatography, *Annual Bulletin of the Research Institute of Logopedics and Phoniatrics, University of Tokyo* 6: 19–24.

Molis, M. R., Lindblom, B., Castelman, W. and Carre, R. 1994, Cross-language analysis of VCV coarticulation, *Journal of the Acoustical Society of America* 95: 2925.

Moll, K. 1962, Velopharyngeal closure in vowels, *Journal of Speech and Hearing Research* 5: 30–7.

Moll, K. and Daniloff, R. 1971, Investigation of the timing of velar movements during speech, *Journal of the Acoustical Society of America* 50: 678–84.

Moll, K. L. and Shriner, T. H. 1967, Preliminary investigation of a new concept of velar activity during speech, *Cleft Palate Journal* 4: 58–69.

Monsen, R. B. and Engebretson, A. M. 1977, Study of variations in the male and female glottal wave, *Journal of the Acoustical Society of America* 62: 981–93.

Moon, S. J. and Lindblom, B. 1994, Interaction between duration, context, and speaking style in English stressed vowels, *Journal of the Acoustical Society of America* 96: 40–55.

Mooshammer, C. and Hoole, P. 1993, Articulation and coarticulation in velar consonants, *Institut für Phonetik und Sprachliche Kommunikation, München*, 31: 249–62.

Mooshammer, C., Hoole, P. and Kühnert, B. 1995, On loops, *Journal of Phonetics* 23: 3–21.

Munhall, K., Fowler, C. A., Hawkins, S. and Saltzman, E. 1992, Compensatory shortening in monosyllables of spoken English, *Journal of Phonetics* 20: 225–39.

Munhall, K. and Löfqvist, A. 1992, Gestural aggregation in speech: laryngeal gestures, *Journal of Phonetics* 20: 111–26.

Munhall, K. G., and Ostry, D. J. 1985, Ultrasonic measurements of laryngeal kinematics, in Titze, I. and Scherer, R. (eds.), *Vocal Fold Physiology: Biomechanics, Acoustics and Phonatory Control*, Denver Center for the Performing Arts, pp. 145–62.

Munhall, K. G., Ostry, D. J. and Parush, A. 1985, Characteristics of velocity profiles of speech movements, *Journal of Experimental Psychology, Human Perception and Performance* 11: 457–74.

Nartey, J. N. A. 1982, On fricative phones and phonemes, *UCLA Working Papers in Phonetics* 55.

Nguyen, N. 1995, EPG bidimensional data reduction, *European Journal of Disorders of Communication* 30: 175–82.

Nguyen, N. and Marchal, A. 1993, Assessment of an electromagnetic system for the investigation of articulatory movements in speech production, *Journal of the Acoustical Society of America* 94: 1152–5.

Ní Chasaide, A. 1985, Preaspiration in phonological stop contrasts, PhD thesis, University College of North Wales, Bangor.

  1986, The perception of preaspirated stops, *Journal of the Acoustical Society of America* 79: S7(A).

Ní Chasaide, A. and Fealey, G. 1991, Articulatory and acoustic measurements of coarticulation in Irish (Gaelic) stops, *Proceedings of the XIIIth International Congress of Phonetic Science, Stockholm, Sweden* 5: 30–3.

Ní Chasaide, A. and Fitzpatrick, L. 1995, Assimilation of Irish palatalized and velarized stops, *Proceedings of the XIIIth International Congress of Phonetic Science, Stockholm, Sweden* 2: 334–7.

Ní Chasaide, A. and Gobl, C. 1993, Contextual variation of the vowel voice source as a function of adjacent consonants, *Language and Speech* 36: 303–30.

Ní Chasaide, A., Gobl, C. and Monahan, P. 1992, A technique for analysing voice quality in pathological and normal speech, *Journal of Clinical Speech and Language Studies* 2: 1–16.

Nicolaidis, K., Hardcastle, W. and Gibbon, F. 1993, Bibliography of electropalatographic studies in English (1957–1992), Part I (full list of references), Part II (clinical references) and Part III (abstracts of selected articles), *Speech Research Laboratory Work in Progress, University of Reading* 7: 26–106.

Nittrouer, S. and Whalen, D. 1989, The perceptual effects of child–adult differences in fricative vowel coarticulation, *Journal of the Acoustical Society of America* 86: 1266–76.

Nittrouer, S., Studdert-Kennedy, M. and McGowan, R. 1989, The emergence of phonetic segments: evidence from the spectral structure of fricative-vowel syllables spoken by children and adults, *Journal of Speech and Hearing Research*
32: 120–32.

Nolan, F. 1982, The role of Action Theory in the description of speech production,
Linguistics 20: 287–308.

1983, *The Phonetic Bases of Speaker Recognition*, Cambridge University Press.

1985, Idiosyncrasy in coarticulatory strategies, *Cambridge Papers in Phonetics and
Experimental Linguistics* 4: 1–9.

1992, The descriptive role of segments: evidence from assimilation, in Docherty,
G. J. and Ladd, D. R. (eds.), *Papers in Laboratory Phonology* II: *Gesture,
Segment, Prosody*, Cambridge University Press, pp. 261–80.

1994, Phonetic correlates of syllable affiliation, in Keating, P. A. (ed.), *Papers in
Laboratory Phonology* III: *Phonological Structure and Phonetic Form*,
Cambridge University Press, pp. 160–7.

Nolan, F., Holst, T. and Kühnert B. 1996, Modelling [s] to [ʃ] accommodation in
English, *Journal of Phonetics* 24: 113–38.

Nord, L. 1974, Vowel reduction–centralization or contextual assimilation? in Fant,
G. (ed.), *Speech Communication* II, Stockholm: Almwvist & Wiksell, pp.
149–54.

1986, Acoustic studies of vowel reduction in Swedish, *Quarterly Progress and
Status Report, Dept. of Speech Communication, KTH, Stockholm, Sweden:* 4:
19–36.

Norlin, K. 1983, Acoustic analysis of fricatives in Cairo Arabic, *Lund University
Department of Linguistics Working Papers* 25: 113–37.

O'Dwyer, N., Quinn, P., Guitar, B., Andrews, G. and Neilson, P. 1981, Procedures
for verification of electrode placement in EMG studies of orofacial and mandibular muscles, *Journal of Speech and Hearing Research* 24: 273–88.

Ogata, K. and Sonoda, Y. 1994, A study of sensor arrangements for detecting movements and inclinations of tongue point during speech, *Proceedings of the 1994
International Conference Spoken Language Processing* 2: 659–62.

Ogden, R. 1995, 'Where' is timing? Comments on C. L. Smith '*Prosodic Patterns in
the Coordination of Vowel Gestures*', in Connell, B. and Arvaniti, A. (eds.),
Papers in Laboratory Phonology IV: *Phonology and Phonetic Evidence*,
Cambridge Univeristy Press, pp. 223–34.

Ohala, J. J. 1966, A new photoelectric glottograph, *UCLA Working Papers in Phonetics*
4: 40–54.

1971, Monitoring soft palate movements in speech, *Linguistic Analysis* 2: 13–27.

1974, Experimental historical phonology, in Anderson, J. M. and Jones C. (eds.),
Historical Linguistics, II *Theory and Description in Phonology*, Amsterdam:
North Holland, pp. 353–89. [*Proceedings of the First Internationall Conference
on Historical Linguistics*, Edinburgh, 2–7 September 1973.]: pp. 353–87.

1975, Phonetic explanations for nasal sound patterns, in Ferguson, C. A., Hyman,
L. M. and Ohala, J. J. (eds.), *Nasalfest, Papers from a Symposium on Nasals and
Nasalization*, Language Universal Project, Stanford, CA, pp. 289–316.

1986, Against the direct realist view of speech perception, *Journal of Phonetics* 14:
75–82.

1990a, The phonetics and phonology of aspects of assimilation, in Kingston, J. and Beckman, M. E. (eds.), *Papers in Laboratory Phonology* 1: *Between the Grammar and the Physics of Speech*, Cambridge University Press, pp. 258–75.

1990b, There is no interface between phonology and phonetics, *Journal of Phonetics* 18: 153–71.

1993a, Coarticulation and phonology, *Language and Speech* 36: 155–71.

1993b, Sound change as nature's speech perception experiment, *Speech Communication* 13: 155–61.

Ohala, M. 1996, Connected speech in Hindi, *Arbeitsberichte, Institut für Phonetic und Digitale Sprachverarbeitung, Universität Kiel* 31: 75–82.

Ohala, J. J. and Busá, M. G. 1995, Nasal loss before voiceless fricatives: a perceptually based sound change, in Fowler, C. A. (ed.), *Rivista di Linguistica (Special issue on the phonetic basis of sound change)* 7: 125–44.

Ohala, J. J. and Feder, D. 1994, Listener's normalization of vowel quality is influenced by 'restored' consonantal context, *Phonetica* 51: 111–18.

Ohala, J. and Kawasaki, H. 1979, The articulation of [i]'s. *Paper presented at the 98th Acoustical Society of America Meeting,* Salt Lake City, UT.

1984, Prosodic phonology and phonetics, *Phonology Yearbook* 1: 113–28.

Ohala, J. J. and Ohala, M. 1991, Nasal epenthesis in Hindi, *Phonetica* 48: 207–20.

1993, The phonetics of nasal phonology: theorems and data, in Huffman, M. K. and Krakow, R. A. (eds.), *Nasals, Nasalization, and the Velum*, San Diego, CA: Academic Press, pp. 225–49.

Ohde, R. N. and Sharf, D. J. 1975, Coarticulatory effects of voiced stops on the reduction of acoustic targets, *Journal of the Acoustical Society of America* 58: 923–7.

Öhman, S. 1966, Coarticulation in VCV utterances: spectrographic measurements, *Journal of the Acoustical Society of America* 39: 151–68.

1967, Numerical model of coarticulation, *Journal of the Acoustical Society of America* 41: 310–20.

1968, Peripheral motor commands in labial articulation, (STL-QPSR) *Speech Transmission Laboratory Quarterly Progress and Status Report, Royal Institute of Technology, Stockholm, Sweden* 30–63.

Ostreicher, H. J. and Sharf, D. J. 1976, Effects of coarticulation on the identification of deleted consonant and vowel sounds, *Journal of Phonetics* 4: 285–301.

Ostry, D., Gribble, P. and Gracco, V. 1996, Is coarticulation in speech kinematics centrally planned? *Journal of Neuroscience* 16: 1570–9.

Ostry, D. and Munhall, G. 1994, Control of jaw orientation and position in mastication and speech, *Journal of Neurophysiology* 71: 1515–32.

Otake, T., Hatano, G., Cutler, A. and Mehler, J. 1993, Mora or syllable? speech segmentation in Japanese, *Journal of Memory and Language* 32: 358–78.

Panagos, G. and Strube, H. W. 1987, Two magnetic methods for articulatory measurements, *Phonetica* 44: 197–209.

Parker, F. and Walsh, T. 1985, Mentalism vs physicalism: a comment on Hammarberg and Fowler, *Journal of Phonetics* 13: 147–53.

Parush, A., Ostry, D. and Munhall, G. 1983, A kinematic study of lingual coarticulation in VCV sequences, *Journal of the Acoustical Society of America* 74: 1115–25.

Paul, H. 1898, *Prinzipien der Sprachgeschichte* (3rd edn), Halle: Niemeyer.

Peng, S. 1993, Cross-language influence on the production of Mandarin /f/ and /x/ and Taiwanese /h/ by native speakers of Taiwanese Amoy, *Phonetica* 50: 245–60.

Perkell, J. S. 1969, *Physiology of Speech Production: Results and Implications of a Quantitative Cineradiographic Study*, Cambridge, MA: The MIT Press.

1986, Coarticulation strategies: preliminary implications of a detailed analysis of lower lip protrusion movements, *Speech Communication* 5: 47–86.

1990, Testing theories of speech production: implications of some detailed analyses of variable articulatory data, in Hardcastle, W. J. and Marchal, A. (eds.), *Speech Production and Speech Modelling*, Dordrecht: Kluwer Publications, pp. 263–88.

Perkell, J. S. and Chiang, C.-M. 1986, Preliminary support for a 'hybrid model' of anticipatory coarticulation, *Proceedings of the XIIth International Congress of Acoustics*, Toronto: Canadian Acoustical Association, A3–6.

Perkell, J. S. and Cohen, M. H. 1986, An alternating magnetic field system for tracking multiple speech articulatory movements in the midsaggital plane, *Technical Report no.* 512 Research Laboratory of Electronics, Massachusetts Institute of Techology.

1989, An indirect test of the quantal nature of speech in the production of the vowels /i/, /a/ and /u/, *Journal of Phonetics* 17: 123–33.

Perkell, J. S. and Matthies, M. 1992, Temporal measures of anticipatory labial coarticulation for the vowel /u/: within- and cross-subject variability, *Journal of the Acoustical Society of America* 91: 2911–25.

Perkell, J. S. and Nelson, W. L. 1985, Variability in production of the vowels /i/ and /a/, *Journal of the Acoustical Society of America* 77: 1889–95.

Perkell, J. S., Boyce, S. E. and Stevens, K. N. 1979, Articulatory and acoustic correlates of the [s-ʃ] distinction, in Wolf, J. J. and Klatt, D. H. (eds.), *Speech Communication Papers, 97th Acoustical Society of America Meeting*, MIT, Cambridge, MA, pp. 109–13.

Perkell, J. S., Matthies, M. L., Svirsky, M. N and Jordan, M. I. 1993, Trading relations between tongue–body raising and lip rounding in production of vowel /u/: a pilot 'motor equivalence' study, *Journal of the Acoustical Society of America* 93: 2948–61.

Perkell, J. S., Cohen, M., Svirsky, M., Matthies, M., Garabieta, I. and Jackson, M. 1992, Electro-magnetic midsaggittal articulometer (EMMA) systems for transducing speech articulatory movements, *Journal of the Acoustical Society of America* 92: 3078–96.

Peterson, G. E. and Barney, B. L. 1952, Control method used in a study of the vowels, *Journal of the Acoustical Society of America* 24: 175–84.

Peterson, G. E. and Lehiste, I. 1960, Duration of syllable nuclei in English, *Journal of the Acoustical Society of America* 32: 693–703.

Pétursson, M. 1977, Timing of glottal events in the production of aspiration after [s], *Journal of Phonetics* 5: 205–12.

Picheny, M. A., Durlach, N. I. and Braida, L. D. 1985, Speaking clearly for the hard of hearing, I: Intelligibility differences between clear and conversational speech, *Journal of Speech and Hearing Research* 28: 96–103.

Picheny, M. A., Durlach, N. I. and Braida, L. D. 1986, Speaking clearly for the hard of hearing, II: Acoustic characteristics of clear and conversational speech, *Journal of Speech and Hearing Research* 29: 434–46.

Pierrehumbert, J. B. 1989, A preliminary study of the consequences of intonation for the voice source, *(STL-QPSR) Speech Transmission Laboratory, Royal Institute of Technology, Stockholm, Sweden* 4: 23–36.

1990, Phonological and phonetic representation, *Journal of Phonetics* 18: 375–94.

1994, Knowledge of variation. Parasession on Variation and Linguistic Theory, *30th Meeting of the Chicago Linguistics Society.*

Pierrehumbert, J. B. and Beckman, M. E. 1988, *Japanese Tone Structure*, Cambridge, MA: MIT Press.

Pierrehumbert, J. B. and Pierrehumbert, R. T. 1990, On attributing grammars to dynamical systems, *Journal of Phonetics* 18: 465–77.

Pols, L. C. W. 1977, *Spectral Analysis and Identification of Dutch Vowels in Monosyllabic Words,* Soesterberg: Institute for Perception TNO.

Poser, W. 1990, Evidence for foot structure in Japanese, *Language* 66: 78–105.

Purcell, E. T. 1979, Formant frequency patterns in Russian VCV utterances, *Journal of the Acoustical Society of America* 66: 1691–702.

Rabiner, L. R. and Schafer, R. W. 1978, *Digital Processing of Speech*, London: Prentice-Hall.

Recasens, D. 1983, Place cues for nasal consonants with special reference to Catalan, *Journal of the Acoustical Society of America* 73: 1346–53.

1984a, Timing constraints and coarticulation: alveolo-palatals and sequences of alveolar + /j/ in Catalan, *Phonetica* 41: 125–39.

1984b, Vowel-to-vowel coarticulation in Catalan VCV sequences, *Journal of the Acoustical Society of America* 76: 1624–35.

1985, Coarticulatory patterns and degrees of coarticulatory resistance in Catalan CV sequences, *Language and Speech* 28: 97–114.

1986, *Estudis de Fonètica Experimental del Català Oriental Central,* Barcelona: Publications de l'Abadia de Montserrat.

1987, An acoustic analysis of V-to-C and V-to-V coarticulatory effects in Catalan and Spanish VCV sequences, *Journal of Phonetics* 15: 299–312.

1989, Long range effects for tongue dorsum contact in VCVCV sequences, *Speech Communication* 8: 293–307.

1990, The articulatory characteristics of palatal consonants, *Journal of Phonetics* 18: 267–80.

1991a, An electropalatographic and acoustic study of consonant-to-vowel coarticulation, *Journal of Phonetics* 19: 177–92.

1991b, On the production characteristics of apicoalveolar taps and trills, *Journal of Phonetics* 19: 267–80.

1995, An EMMA investigation of lingual assimilation and coarticulation in a selected set of Catalan consonant clusters, *Proceedings of the XIIIth International Congress of Phonetic Science, Stockholm, Sweden* 2: 582–5.

Recasens, D. and Farnetani, E. 1990, Articulatory and acoustic properties of different allophones of /l/ in American English, Catalan and Italian, *Proceedings of the 1990 International Conference on Spoken Language Processing, Kobe* 961–4.

1992, Timing in phonology. Evidence from velarized and non velarized allophones of /l/, *Quaderni del Centro di Studio per le Ricerche di Fonetica* 11: 236–51.

Recasens, D., Fontdevila, J. and Pallarès, M. D. 1992, Alveolar-palatal correlations for a subset of Catalan consonants, *Bulletin de la Communication Parlée*, Grenoble.

1993, An electropalatographic study of stop consonant clusters, *Speech Communication* 12: 335–55.

1995a, Linguopalatal coarticulation and alveolar-palatal correlations for velarized and non velarized [l], *Journal of Phonetics* 24: 165–85.

1995b, Velarization degree and coarticulatory resistance for [l] in Catalan and German, *Journal of Phonetics* 23: 37–52.

Recasens, D., Pallarès, M. D. and Fontdevila, J. 1997, A model of lingual coarticulation based on articulatory constraints, *Journal of the Acoustical Society of America* 102: 544–61.

Recasens, D., Farnetani, E., Fontdevila, J. and Pallarès, M. D. 1993, An electropalatographic study of alveolar and palatal consonants in Catalan and Italian, *Language and Speech* 36: 213–34.

Repp, B. H. 1983, Coarticulation in sequences of two nonhomorganic stop consonants: perceptual and acoustic evidence, *Journal of the Acoustical Society of America* 74: 420–7.

1986a, Perception of the [m]–[n] distinction in CV syllables, *Journal of the Acoustical Society of America* 79: 1987–99.

1986b, Some observations in the development of anticipatory coarticulation, *Journal of the Acoustical Society of America* 79: 1616–19.

Repp, B. and Lin, H. B. 1989, Acoustic properties and perception of stop consonant release transients, *Journal of the Acoustical Society of America* 85: 379–96.

Repp, B. H. and Mann, V. A. 1982, Fricative-stop coarticulation: acoustic and perceptual evidence, *Journal of the Acoustical Society of America* 71: 1562–7.

Rialland, A. 1994, The phonology and phonetics of extrasyllabicity in French, in Keating, P. A. (ed.), *Papers in Laboratory Phonology* III: *Phonological Structure and Phonetic Form*, Cambridge University Press, pp.136–59.

Rischel, J. and Hutters, B. 1980, Filtering of EMG signals, *Annual Report of the Institute of Phonetics of the University of Copenhagen* 14: 285–316.

Rochet, A. P. and Rochet, B. L. 1991, The effect of vowel height on patterns of assimilation nasality in French and English, *Proceedings of the XIIth International Congress of Phonetic Sciences, Aix-en-Provence* 3: 54–7.

Romero, J. 1996, Articulatory blending of lingual gestures, *Journal of Phonetics* 24: 99–111.

Rothenberg, M. 1973, A new inverse filtering technique for deriving the glottal air flow waveform during voicing, *Journal of the Acoustical Society of America* 53: 1632–45.

Rouco, A. and Recasens, D. 1996, Reliability of electromagnetic midsaggital articulometry and electropalatography data acquired simultaneously, *Journal of the Acoustical Society of America* 100: 3384–90.

Rousselot, P.-J. 1897–1901, *Principes de Phonétique Experimentale*, I-II. Paris: H. Welter.

Rubach, J. 1994, Representations and the organization of rules in Slavic phonology, in Goldsmith, J. A. (ed.), *The Handbook of Phonological Theory*, Oxford: Basil Blackwell, pp. 848–66.

Saltzman, E. L. 1991, The task dynamic model in speech production, in Peters, H. F.

M., Hulstijin, W. and Starkweather, C. W. (eds.), *Speech Motor Control and Stuttering*, Amsterdam: Excerpta Medical, pp. 37–52.

Saltzman, E. L. and Munhall, K. 1989, A dynamic approach to gestural patterning in speech production, *Ecological Psychology* 1: 333–82.

Saltzman, E. L., Löfqvist, A. and Mitra, S. in press, 'Glue and clocks' – intergestural cohesion and global timing, in Broe, M. (ed.), *Papers in Laboratory Phonology V: Language Acquisition and the Lexicon*, Cambridge University Press.

Saltzman, E. L., Goldstein, L., Browman, C. P. and Rubin, P. 1988, Dynamics of gestural blending during speech production, *Neural Networks* 1 (Supplement 1): 316.

Sawashima, M. and Hirose, H. 1968, A new laryngoscopic technique by means of fiberoptics, *Journal of the Acoustical Society of America* 43: 168–9.

1983, Laryngeal gestures in speech production, in MacNeilage, P. F. (ed.), *The Production of Speech*, New York, NY: Springer, pp. 11–38.

Sawashima, M. and Miyazaki, S. 1974, Stereo-fiberscopic measurement of the larynx: a preliminary experiment by use of ordinary laryngeal fiberscopes, *Annual Bulletin of the Research Institute of Logopedics and Phoniatrics, University of Tokyo* 8: 7–12.

Sawashima, M. and Ushijima, T. 1971, Use of the fiberscope in speech research, *Annual Bulletin of the Research Institute of Logopedics and Phoniatrics, University of Tokyo* 5: 25–34.

Sawashima, M., Abramson, A. S., Cooper, F. S. and Lisker, L. 1970, Observing laryngeal adjustments during running speech by use of a fiberoptics system, *Phonetica* 22: 193–201.

Schönle, P. 1988, *Elektromagnetische Artikulographie*, Berlin: Springer.

Schönle, P., Müller, C. and Wenig, P. 1989, Echtzeitanalyse von orofacialen Bewegungen mit Hilfe der electromagnetischen Artikulographie, *Biomedizinische Technik* 34: 126–30.

Schönle, P., Grabe, K., Wenig, P., Hohne, J., Schrader, J. and Conrad, B. 1987, Electromagnetic articulography: use of alternating magnetic fields for tracking movements of multiple points inside and outside the vocal tract, *Brain and Language* 31: 26–35.

Schouten, M. E. H. and Pols, L. C. W. 1979a, Vowel segments in consonantal contexts: a spectral study of coarticulation – Part 1, *Journal of Phonetics* 7: 1–23.

1979b, CV- and VC- transitions: a spectral study of coarticulation – Part II, *Journal of Phonetics* 7: 205–24.

Schulman, R. 1989, Articulatory dynamics of loud and normal speech, *Journal of the Acoustical Society of America* 85: 295–312.

Scripture, E. 1902, *The Elements of Experimental Phonetics*, New York, NY: Charles Scribner's Sons.

Scully, C., Grabe-Georges, E. and Badin, P. 1991, Movement paths: different phonetic contexts and different speaking styles, *Phonetic Experimental Research at the Institute of Linguistics, University of Stockholm* 14: 69–74.

Sereno, J. A. and Lieberman, P. 1987, Developmental aspects of lingual coarticulation, *Journal of Phonetics* 15: 247–57.

Sereno, J. A., Baum, A. R., Cameron Marean, G. and Lieberman, P. 1987, Acoustic analyses and perceptual data on anticipatory labial coarticulation in adults and children, *Journal of the Acoustical Society of America* 81: 512–19.

Shaffer, L. 1984, Motor programming in language-production – a tutorial review, in Bouma, H. and Bouwhuis, D. (eds.), *Attention and Performance X: Control of Language Processes*, London: Lawrence Erlbaum Associates, pp. 17–41.

Shaiman, S. 1989, Kinematic and electromyographic responses to the perturbation of the jaw, *Journal of the Acoustical Society of America* 86: 78–88.

Sharf, D. J. and Ohde, R. N. 1981, Physiologic, acoustic and perceptual aspects of coarticulation: implications for the remediation of articulatory disorders, in Lass, N. J. (ed.), *Speech and Language: Advances in Basic Research and Practice* V, New York, NY: Academic Press, pp. 153–247.

Sharf, D. J. and Ostreicher, H. J. 1973, Effect of forward and backward coarticulation on the identification of speech sounds, *Language and Speech* 16: 196–206.

Sharkey, S. and Folkins, J. 1985, Variability of lip and jaw movements in children and adults: implications for the development of speech motor control, *Journal of Speech and Hearing Research* 28: 3–15.

Shen, X.-N. S. 1990, Tonal coarticulation in Mandarin, *Journal of Phonetics* 18: 281–95.

Shibata, S. 1968, A study of dynamic palatography, *Annual Bulletin of the Research Institute of Logopedics and Phoniatrics, University of Tokyo* 2: 28–36.

Shipp, T. 1982, Aspects of voice production and motor control, in Grillner, S., Lindblom, B., Lubker, J. and Persson, A. (eds.), *Speech Motor Control*, Oxford: Pergamon, pp. 105–12.

Shipp, T., Fishman, B. V. and Morrisey, P. 1970, Method and control of laryngeal EMG electrode placement in man, *Journal of Acoustical Society of America* 48: 429–30.

Shuken, C. R. 1980, An instrumental investigation of some Scottish Gaelic consonants, PhD thesis, University of Edinburgh.

Sievers, E. 1876, *Grundzuge der Lautphysiologie zur Einfuhrung in das Studium der Lautlehre der Indogermanischen Sprachen.* Leipzig: Breitkopf and Hartel.

Skolnick, M. L., McCall, G. N. and Barnes, M. 1973, The sphincteric mechanism of velopharyngeal closure, *Cleft Palate Journal* 10: 286–305.

Skolnick, M. L., Shprintzen, R. J. and McCall, G. N. 1975, Patterns of velopharyngeal closure in subjects with repaired cleft palate and normal speech: a multiview videofluoroscopic analysis, *Cleft Palate Journal* 12: 369–76.

Smith, A. C. S., Moore, D. H., McFarland, D. H. and Weber, C. M. 1985, Reflex responses of human lip muscles to mechanical stimulation during speech, *Journal of Motor Behaviour* 17: 131–47.

Smith, C. L. 1992, The timing of vowel and consonant gestures, PhD dissertation, Yale University, New Haven, CT.

  1995, Prosodic patterns in the coordination of vowel and consonant gestures, in Connell, B. and Arvaniti, A. (eds.), *Papers in Laboratory Phonology* IV: *Phonology and Phonetic Evidence*, Cambridge University Press, pp. 205–22.

Södersten, M. 1994, Vocal fold closure during phonation, PhD thesis, *Studies in Logopedics and Phoniatrics* 3, Stockholm: Huddinge University Hospital.

Solé, M.-J. 1992, Phonetic and phonological processes: the cases of nasalization, *Language and Speech* 35: 29–43.

1995, Spatio-temporal patterns of velopharyngeal action in phonetic and phonological nasalization, *Language and Speech* 38: 1–23.

Solé, M.-J. and Ohala, J. J. 1991, Differentiating between phonetic and phonological processes: the case of nasalization, *Proceedings of the XIIth International Congress of Phonetic Sciences, Aix-en-Provence* 2: 110–13.

Soli, S. D. 1981, Second formants in fricatives: acoustic consequences of fricative–vowel coarticulation, *Journal of the Acoustical Society of America* 70: 976–84.

Sondhi, M. M. 1975, Measurement of the glottal waveform, *Journal of the Acoustical Society of America* 57: 228–32.

Sonesson, B. 1960, On the anatomy and vibratory pattern of the vocal folds, *Acta Otolarynologica*, Supplement, 156: 1–80.

Sonoda, Y. and Ogata, K. 1992, Improvements of magnetometer sensing system for monitoring tongue point movements during speech, *Proceedings of 1992 International Conference on Spoken Language Processing* 2: 843–6.

Speculand, B., Butcher, G. and Stephens, C. 1988, Three-dimensional measurement: the accuracy and precision of the Reflex microscope, *Journal of Oral and Maxillofacial Surgery* 26: 276–83.

Sproat, R. and Fujimura, O. 1993, Allophone variation in English /l/ and its implications for phonetic implementation, *Journal of Phonetics* 21: 291–312.

Stålhammar, U., Karlsson, I. and Fant, G. 1973, Contextual effects on vowel nuclei, *(STL-QPSR) Speech Transmission Laboratory Quarterly Progress Status Report, Royal Institute of Technology, Stockholm, Sweden* 4: 1–18.

Stemple, J. C., Weiler, E., Whitehead, W. and Komray, R. 1980, Electromyographic biofeedback training with patients exhibiting a hyperfunctional voice disorder, *Laryngoscope* 90: 471–6.

Steriade, D. 1990, Gestures and autosegments: comments on Browman and Goldstein's paper, in Kingston, J. and Beckman, M. E. (eds.), *Papers in Laboratory Phonology* I: *Between the Grammar and the Physics of Speech*, Cambridge University Press, pp. 382–97.

1994, Underspecification and markedness, in Goldsmith, J. A. (ed.), *The Handbook of Phonological Theory*, Oxford: Basil Blackwell, pp. 114–74.

Stetson, R. 1951, *Motor Phonetics: a Study of Speech Movements in Action* (2nd edn), Amsterdam: North Holland.

Stetson, R. H. and Hudgens, C. V. 1930, Functions of breathing movements in the mechanism of speech, *Archives Nérlandaises de Phonetique Experimental* 5: 1–30.

Stevens, K. N. 1989, On the quantal nature of speech, *Journal of Phonetics* 17: 3–45.

1994, Phonetic evidence for hierarchies of features, in Keating, P. A. (ed.), *Papers in Laboratory Phonology* III: *Phonological Structure and Phonetic Form*, Cambridge University Press, pp. 242–58.

Stevens, K. N. and House, A. S. 1963, Perturbations of vowel articulations by consonantal context: an acoustical study, *Journal of Speech and Hearing Research* 6: 111–28.

Stevens, K. N., House, A. S. and Paul, A. P. 1966, Acoustical description of syllabic nuclei: an interpretation in terms of a dynamic model of articulation, *Journal of the Acoustical Society of America* 40: 123–32.

Stevens, K. N., Kalikow, D. N. and Willemain, T. R. 1975, A miniature accelerometer for detecting glottal waveforms and nasalization, *Journal of Speech and Hearing Research* 18: 594–9.

Stevens, K. N., Keyser, S. J. and Kawasaki, H. 1986, Toward a phonetic and phonological theory of redundant features, in Perkell, J. S. and Klatt, D. (eds.), *Invariance and Variability in Speech Processes*, Hillsdale, NJ: Lawrence Erlbaum, pp. 426–63.

Stone, M. 1996, Instrumentation for the study of speech pathology, in Lass, N. J. (ed.), *Principles of Experimental Phonetics*, St Louis, MO: Mosley, pp. 495–524.

Stone, M. and Davis, E. P. 1995, A head and transducer support system for making ultrasound images of tongue/jaw movement, *Journal of the Acoustical Society of America* 98: 3107–12.

Stone, M., and Lundberg, A. 1994, Tongue–palate interactions in consonants versus vowels, *Proceedings of the International Conference on Spoken Language Processing, Yokohama* 1: 49–52.

1996, Three-dimensional tongue surface shapes of English consonants and vowels, *Journal of Acoustical Society of America* 99: 3728–37.

Stone, M. and Vatikiotis-Bateson, E. 1995, Trade-offs in tongue, jaw and palate contributions to speech production, *Journal of Phonetics* 23: 81–100.

Stone, M., Faber, A. and Cordaro, M. 1991, Cross-sectional tongue movement and tongue–palate movement patterns in [s] and [ʃ] syllables, *Proceedings of the XIIth International Conference on Phonetic Sciences, Aix-en-Provence*, 354–8.

Stone, M., Faber, A., Raphael, L. J. and Shawker, T. H. 1992, Cross-sectional tongue and linguopalatal contact patterns in [s], [ʃ] and [l], *Journal of Phonetics* 20: 253–70.

Stone, M., Shawker, T., Talbot, T. and Rich, A. 1988, Cross-sectional tongue shape during the production of vowels, *Journal of the Acoustical Society of America* 83: 1586–96.

Su, L. S., Daniloff, R. and Hammarberg, R. 1975, Variation in lingual coarticulation at certain juncture boundaries, *Phonetica* 32: 254–63.

Su, L. S., Li, K. P. and Fu, K. S. 1974, Identification of speakers by use of nasal coarticulation, *Journal of the Acoustical Society of America* 56: 1876–82.

Sudo, M. M, Kiritani, S and Sawashima, M. 1983, The articulation of Japanese intervocalic /d/ and /r/: an electropalatographic study, *Annual Bulletin Research Institute of Logopedics and Phoniatrics, University of Tokyo* 17: 55–9.

Sudo, M. M., Kiritani, S. and Yoshioka, H. 1982, An electropalatographic study of Japanese intervocalic /r/, *Annual Bulletin Research Institute of Logopedics and Phonetics, University of Tokyo* 16: 21–5.

Summers, W. van 1987, Effects of stress and final-consonant voicing on vowel production: articulatory and acoustic analysis, *Journal of the Acoustical Society of America*, 82, 847–63.

Suomi, K. 1980, *Voicing in English and Finnish Stops, Publications of the Department of Finnish and General Linguistics of the University of Turku*, 10.

1983, Palatal vowel harmony: a perceptually motivated phenomenon? *Nordic Journal of Linguistics* 6: 1–35.

Sussman, H. M. and Westbury, J. 1981, The effects of antagonistic gestures on temporal and amplitude parameters of anticipatory labial coarticulation, *Journal of Speech and Hearing Research* 24: 16–24.

Sussman, H. M., Hoemeke, K and McCaffrey, H. 1992, Locus equations as an index of coarticulation and place of articulation distinctions in children, *Journal of Speech and Hearing Research* 35: 769–81.

Sussman, H. M., MacNeilage, P. and Hanson, R. 1973, Labial and mandibular movement dynamics during the production of bilabial stop consonants, *Journal of Speech and Hearing Research* 16: 397–420.

Sussman, H. M., McCaffrey, H. A. and Matthews, S. A. 1991, An investigation of locus equations as a source of relational invariance for stop place categorization, *Journal of the Acoustical Society of America* 90: 1309–25.

Svantesson, J.-O. 1983, Acoustic analysis of Chinese fricatives and affricates, *Lund University Department of Linguistics Working Papers* 25: 195–211.

Tatham, M. A. A. 1984, Towards a cognitive phonetics, *Journal of Phonetics* 12: 37–47.

Teston, B. 1984 Un système de mesure des parametres aerodynamiques de la parole: le polyphonomètre modèle III, *Travaux de l'Institut de Phonetique d' Aix* 9: 373–83.

Thompson, A. and Hixon, T. 1979, Nasal air flow during normal speech production, *Cleft Palate Journal* 16: 412–20.

Tillmann, H.-G. 1994, Phonetics, early modern, especially instrumental work, in Asher, R. (ed.), *The Encyclopedia of Language and Linguistics* VI, Oxford: Pergamon, 3082–94.

Tillmann, H.-G. and Mansell, P. 1980, *Phonetik*, Stuttgart: Klett-Cotta.

Trager, F. H. 1971, The phonology of Picuris, *International Journal of American Linguistics* 37: 29–33.

Tuller, B., Harris, K. S. and Gross, B. 1981, Electromyographic study of jaw muscles during speech, *Journal of Phonetics* 9: 175–88.

Tuller, B., Harris, K. S. and Kelso, J. A. S. 1982, Stress and rate: differential transformations of articulation, *Journal of the Acoustical Society of America* 71: 1534–43.

Tuller, B., Shao, S. and Kelso, J. A. S. 1990, An evaluation of an alternating magnetic field device for monitoring tongue movements, *Journal of the Acoustical Society of America* 88: 674–9.

Umeda N. 1975, Vowel duration in American English, *Journal of the Acoustical Society of America* 58: 434–45.

1981, Influence of segmental factors on fundamental frequency in fluent speech, *Journal of the Acoustical Society of America* 70: 350–5.

Unser, M. and Stone, M. 1992, Automated detection of the tongue surface in sequences of ultrasound images, *Journal of the Acoustical Society of America* 91: 3001–7.

Ushijima, T. and Hirose, H. 1974, Electromyographic study of the velum during speech, *Journal of Phonetics* 2: 315–26.

Ushijima, T. and Sawashima, M. 1972, Fiberscopic observation of velar movements during speech, *Annual Bulletin Research Institute of Logopedics and Phoniatrics, University of Tokyo* 6: 25–38.

Vaissière, J. 1988, Prediction of velum movement from phonological specifications, *Phonetica* 45: 122–39.

Vatikiotis-Bateson, E. and Ostry, D. J. 1995, An analysis of the dimensionality of jaw movement in speech, *Journal of Phonetics* 23: 101–17.

Vayra, M., Fowler, C. A. and Avesani, C. 1987, Word-level coarticulation and shortening in Italian and English speech, *Studi di Grammatica Italiana, XIII*, Firenze: Accademia della Crusca, pp. 249–69.

Vihman, M. M. and Velleman, S. 1989, Phonological reorganization: a case study, *Language and Speech* 32: 149–70.

Wada, T., Yasumoto, M., Iteoka, N., Fujiki, Y. and Yoshinaga, R. 1970, An approach for the cinefluorographic study of articulatory movements, *Cleft Palate Journal* 7: 506–22.

Warren, D. W. 1967, Nasal emission of air and velopharyngeal function, *Cleft Palate Journal* 4: 148–56.

  1976, Aerodynamics of speech production, in Lass, N. J. (ed.), *Contemporary Issues in Experimental Sciences*, New York, NY: Academic Press, pp. 105–37.

  1996, Regulation of speech aerodynamics, in Lass, N. J. (ed.), *Principles of Experimental Phonetics*, St Louis, MO: Mosby, pp. 46–92.

Warren, D. W., Dalston, R. M. and Mayo, R. 1993, Aerodynamics of nasalization, in Huffman, M. K. and Krakow, R. A. (eds.), *Phonetics and Phonology, Nasals, Nasalization and the Velum Volume* V, San Diego, CA: Academic Press, pp 119–44.

Warren, D. and Devereux, J. L. 1966, An analog study of cleft palate speech, *Cleft Palate Journal* 3: 103–14.

Weeks, R. 1893, A method of recording the soft palate movements in speech, *Studies and Notes in Philology and Literature* II: 213.

Weismer, G. 1980, Control of the voicing distinction for intervocalic stops and fricatives: some data and theoretical considerations, *Journal of Phonetics* 8: 427–38.

Westbury, J. 1979, Aspects of the temporal control of voicing in consonant clusters in English, unpublished dissertation, University of Texas at Austin.

  1988, Mandible and hyoid bone movements during speech, *Journal of Speech and Hearing Research* 31: 405–16.

  1994, *X-ray Microbeam Speech Production Database User's Handbook,* University of Wisconsin, Madison, WI: Waisman Center on Mental Retardation and Human Development.

Westbury, J. and Moy, G. 1996, Descriptive characterization of kinematic effects of changes in speaking rate, *Journal of the Acoustical Society of America* 100: 2850.

Whalen, D. 1981, Effects of vocal formant transitions and vowel quality on the English [s]–[ʃ] boundary, *Journal of the Acoustical Society of America* 69: 275–82.

  1989, Vowel and consonant judgments are not independent when cued by the same information, *Perception and Psychophysics* 46: 284–92.

Wickelgren, W. 1969, Context-sensitive coding, associative memory, and serial order in (speech) behaviour, *Psychological Review* 76: 1–15.

1972, Discussion paper on speech perception, in Gilbert, J. (ed.), *Speech and Cortical Functioning*. New York, NY: Academic Press, pp. 237–62.

Wieneke, G., Janssen, P. and Belderbos, I. 1987, The influence of speaking rate on the duration of jaw movements, *Journal of Phonetics* 15: 111–26.

Wohlert, A. B. and Goffman, L. 1994, Human perioral muscle activation patterns, *Journal of Speech and Hearing Research* 37: 1032–40.

Wood, S. 1979, A radiographic analysis of constriction locations for vowels, *Journal of Phonetics* 7: 25–43.

Wright, J. T. 1986, The behavior of nasalized vowels in the perceptual vowel space, in Ohala, J. J. and Jaeger, J. J. (eds.), *Experimental Phonology*, Orlando, FL: Academic Press, pp. 45–67.

Xu, Y. 1989, Distribution of vowel information in prevocalic fricative noise, Unpublished manuscript, University of Connecticutt, Storrs, CT.

1994, Production and perception of coarticulated tones, *Journal of the Acoustical Society of America* 95: 2240–53.

Yeou, M. 1995, An investigation of locus equations as a source of information for consonantal place, *Proceedings of Eurospeech '95* 3: 1901–4.

Yoshioka, H. 1984 Glottal area variation and supraglottal pressure change in voicing control, *Annual Bulletin of the Research Institute of Logopedics and Phoniatrics, University of Tokyo* 18: 45–9.

Yoshioka, H., Löfqvist, A. and Collier, R. 1982, Laryngeal adjustments in Dutch voiceless obstruent production, *Annual Bulletin of the Research Institute of Logopedics and Phoniatrics, University of Tokyo* 16, 27–35.

Yoshioka, H., Löfqvist, A. and Hirose, H. 1980, Laryngeal adjustments in Japanese voiceless sound production, *Haskins Laboratories Status Report on Speech Research* 63: 293–308.

1981, Laryngeal adjustments in the production of consonant clusters and geminates in American English, *Journal of the Acoustical Society of America* 70: 1615–23.

Zagzebski, J. A. 1975, Ultrasonic measurement of lateral pharyngeal wall motion at two levels in the vocal tract, *Journal of Speech and Hearing Research* 18: 308–18.

Zawadzki, P. A. and Kuehn, D. P. 1980, A cineradiographic study of static and dynamic aspects of American English /l/, *Phonetica* 37: 253–66.

Zee, E. 1981, Effect of vowel quality on perception of post-vocalic nasal consonant in noise, *Journal of Phonetics* 9: 35–48.

Zerling, J.-P. 1981, Particularités articulatoires et acoustiques de l'occlusive [g], *12èmes Journees d'Etude sur la Parole, Université de Montreal*, 328–38.

1992, Frontal lip shape for French and English vowels, *Journal of Phonetics* 20: 3–14.

Zierdt, A. 1993, Problems of electromagnetic position transduction for a three-dimensional articulographic measurement system, *Forschungsberichte des Instituts für Phonetic und sprachliche Kommunikation, Münich* 31: 137–41.

Zimmerman, G., Dalston, R. M., Brown, C., Folkins, J. W., Linville, R. N. and Seaver, E. J. 1987, Comparison of cineradiographic and photodetector techniques for assessing velopharyngeal function during speech, *Journal of Speech and Hearing Research* 30: 564–9.

Zsiga, E. 1992, Acoustic evidence for gestural overlap in consonant sequences, *Haskins Laboratories Status Report on Speech Research* 111/112: 43–62.

Zsiga, L. 1995, An acoustic and electropalatographic study of lexical and post-lexical palatalization, in Connell, B. and Arvaniti, A. (eds.), *Papers in Laboratory Phonology* IV: *American English, Phonology and Phonetic Evidence,* Cambridge University Press, pp. 282–302.

Zue, V. W. 1980, Acoustic characteristics of stop consonants: a controlled study, *Indiana University Linguistics Club.*

Index

acoustic analysis, 38, 80, 124, 189, 265, 288, 322
  FFT (Fast Fourier Transform), 323, 331
  formant transitions, 104, 202, 324, 325–7, 335
  intensity, 335
  loci, 327
  LPC analysis (Linear Predictive Coding), 304, 322–3, 332
  of duration, 335
  of fricative noise, 330
  of stop release, 330
  of tone, 334
  of voicing, 333
  segmentation, 230, 323–5
  spectrograms, 169, 322–3, 324
Action Theory, 15
adaptation, 13
adaptive variability, theory of, 33–4, 35
allophone, 15, 44, 70, 102, 199, 201, 202, 207, 215, 222, 332
  context-sensitive, 14, 18
  extrinsic allophones, 18–9
Articulatory Phonology, 15, 16, 29, 50–1, 120, 175, 191, 192–3, 194, 217
assimilation, 13–4, 15, 16, 21, 24, 40, 45, 47, 48, 53, 75, 103, 189, 195, 199, 209–10, 211, 212, 215

coarticulation (*see also* labial coarticulation; lingual coarticulation; laryngeal coarticulation; lip and jaw coarticulation; velopharyngeal coarticulation)
  anticipatory, 19, 27, 30 n.1, 33, 41–3, 52, 58, 59, 60, 105, 154, 164–5, 167, 168, 185, 186, 188, 241
  carryover, 30 n.1, 41, 52, 105, 164, 165, 167, 168, 241
  consonant-vowel, 34, 193
    vowel duration, 34

cross-language (cross-linguistic) differences in, 47–8, 49, 50, 53, 149, 180, 222, 294
  laryngeal coarticulation, 125, 127, 133, 141
  see also coarticulation, cross-language study; coarticulation, interlanguage differences
cross-language study, 58, 79, 179, 288
cross-linguistic difference in, 180, 222
  velar coarticulation, 182–3
  see also interlanguage differences
effects of speech rate on, 32, 49, 59, 63, 75, 78, 117, 183, 290, 292
influence of contrast on, 162, 166, 172, 174, 180–91, 197n.13, 203, 206–7, 209–10
  output constraints, 180–1, 184, 185, 186, 190-1, 201
interlanguage differences, 32, 44, 47, 48, 208; *see also* cross-language (cross-linguistic) differences
models of
  coarticulation resistance (CR), 18–19, 22, 33, 44, 49, 53, 56, 57, 189, 221
  degree of articulatory constraint (DAC), 98
  feature-based, 20, 62
  feature-spreading account, 20–1, 24, 28, 40–1, 42, 45, 51, 105, 153, 154
  frame, 24, 27, 58
  hybrid, 24–5, 59–60, 61, 156–7, 158, 159, 163
  look-ahead, 20–1, 24, 26, 27, 41–3, 58, 59, 60, 61, 62, 63, 153–6, 158, 161, 163, 195
  movement expansion, 60–1
  target undershoot, 16, 34–5, 64, 171
  time-locked, 24, 25, 26, 58, 59, 60, 73, 98, 105, 153–6, 158
  see also frame model
  window, 22, 44–6, 47, 48, 49, 61, 148, 153–5, 187, 190–1, 197n.13
  see also adaptive variability, theory of
  see also coproduction

coarticulation (*cont.*)
  ontogenetic origin of, 25
  output constraints, 23, 50, 57
  perception of, 9, 33, 225 n.1, 285, 288
  temporal domain, 32, 166; *see also* gestures
  vowel-consonant-vowel (VCV), 12, 17–18, 19,
      20, 37–8, 40, 43, 46, 48, 49, 63, 87, 97,
      98, 99, 100, 101, 103, 162, 165, 167,
      168, 169, 193, 194, 197 n.9, 207, 238,
      239, 241, 335
  vowel-to-vowel (V-to-V), 13, 17, 19, 38–40,
      46, 49, 79, 97, 99, 100, 101, 154, 158,
      161, 162, 182, 184–8, 192, 193–4, 196
      n.4, 197 n.6, 197 n.8, 208, 212, 215, 335
coordinative structures, 15, 23–4, 52
coproduction, 15, 16, 28, 81, 107, 115, 153, 154,
      161, 163, 169, 172, 173, 175, 183, 191,
      195, 223
  accentual prominence, 169, 173
  blending, 174
  dissimilation, 169
  hyperarticulation, 173
  sound changes, 173
  sonority expansion,173
  theory of, 22–4, 50, 58, 81, 169, 172, 173
  truncation, 169, 172, 174

devoicing, 105–6, 107–21, 173, 294, 296, 297, 299
  blending of gestures, 107, 116, 118, 119,
      120–1, 295
  fricative dominance, 119–20
  gestural dominance, 113
  glottalization, 119
  interarticulator coordination, 105–6, 107,
      112
  manner of articulation, 108–9, 122, 141
  place of articulation, 109–12, 113
  voiceless clusters, 113, 114, 115–21
  VOT (voice onset time), 110–14
distinctive feature, 20–2, 180, 187, 206, 207–8,
      214,
double articulation, 91, 93, 235

electromagnetic articulography (EMMA), 164,
      260, 284, 293
  combination of other equipment, 264–5
  description, 260
  environmental conditions, 264
  error sources, 261–3
  illustration of use, 267
  interference with articulation, 265
  measurement principle, 261
  safety, 265–7
  systems' accuracy, 263–4
electromyography, 70, 73, 74, 80, 149, 164, 270,
      273, 284, 286–7, 295, 299
  action potentials, 271, 274
  amplification, 270, 279,

hooked–wire electrodes, 274–7, 278, 279, 280,
      299
  limitations of, 282–3
  measurements, 281
  needle electrodes, 274, 278, 279, 280, 299
  signal processing, 279–80
  surface electrodes, 276–9, 280
  technique, 273–4
electropalatography (EPG), 54, 80, 83, 161, 169,
      229, 256, 258, 285
  artificial palate, 230–2
  centre of gravity indices, 238–9
  coarticulation index, 239–41
  contact distribution indices, 239
  contact indices, 238
  contact profile displays, 238
  data reduction methods 236–7
  EPG raw data, 233–6
  multi-channel approach, 241–5
  place of articulation measures, 237–8
  spatial coarticulatory effects, 236
  zoning schemes, 232–3
extrinsic timing theories, 22

fleshpoint, 260, 261, 264, 267
  tracking systems, 260, 261, 290
  issues, 261

gestures, 61, 78, 80, 81, 83, 84, 104, 148, 154,
      165, 166, 168, 169, 171, 172, 173, 174,
      175, 179, 180, 181, 182, 183, 188, 192,
      193, 196, 196 n.2, 196 n.3, 200, 206,
      208, 212, 213, 222, 223, 238, 243
  and hybrid model, 59–60
  and movement expansion model, 61
  as underlying units, 23–4, 51–6, 64, 191, 216
  bilabial gesture, 114
  blending strength, 56, 65 n.5
  devoicing gesture, 121
  duration of, 58
  gestural conflict, 32, 33, 54, 64
  hidden, 16, 114
  in children's productions, 25
  in VCV syllables, 39
  labial gesture, 164
  laryngeal gesture, 106, 113, 117, 119, 123,
      140, 173
  lingual gesture, 83, 94, 95, 154, 164
  lip gesture, 144, 145, 151, 156, 161
  perception of, 33
  spatio-temporal organization of, 53
  temporal overlap of, 23, 25, 53, 54, 169, 191
  velar gesture, 232, 285, 286, 290

imaging techniques
  applications to coarticulatory questions,
      255–9
  cinefluorography, 164, 289

cineradiography, 44, 70, 73, 80, 286, 289, 290, 291, 292, 293
computed tomography (CT), 247, 248–9, 293
endoscopy, 70, 73, 283, 284, 287, 290–1, 292, 320
lateral X-ray, 247–8
magnetic resonance imaging (MRI), 247, 249–52, 293, 294
ultrasound, 82, 108, 243, 246, 247, 248, 252–5, 256, 258, 259, 264, 265, 284, 292–3, 295, 299–300
videofluography, 19, 289–90, 293, 299–300

Koarticulation, 11, 12, 14
kymography, 11
   kymogram, 12, 14, 70

labial coarticulation, 16, 41, 42, 60, 61, 62, 213
   anticipatory, 16, 17, 20, 24, 58, 148, 152, 153, 155, 158, 162
   anticipatory lip rounding, 26, 28, 151, 153, 154, 155, 157, 158, 159, 160, 161, 162, 183, 188, 213
   articulatory specification, 148
   blending, 152, 161, 162
   carryover, 161–2
   cross-language study of, 145, 146, 147, 155, 158, 162, 213
   labialization, 146–8, 163
   liprounding, 144–6, 149–50, 151, 152, 155, 156, 158, 162
   motor commands, 149
   movement expansion model of, 159–61, 163
   perception of, 150
   phonological neutrality, 148
   spatial effects of, 152
   speech rate, role of, 156, 157, 158–9, 161
laryngeal articulation, techniques for investigating
   acoustic analysis, 294, 300
   electromyography, 299
   fibreoptic endoscopy, 295–6
   glottal airflow, 302, 307, 309, 310, 311, 312
   inverse filtering, 124, 300, 301–9, 310, 312, 314, 315
   miniature pressure transducers, 311–13
   model matching, 301, 313–16
   Sondhi Tube, 309–11
   spectral measurements, 319
   time domain source parameters, 319–20
   transillumination, 295, 296–8, 299
   voice source parameters, 300, 304, 309, 315, 316, 317
laryngeal coarticulation
   anticipatory effects: fricatives, 131–3, 140
   anticipatory effects: stops, 125–31, 133, 139, 140
   carryover effects: stops, 133–9, 140
   glottal abduction gesture, 109, 123, 127, 133, 139, 140, 142

laryngeal abduction, 108, 116, 139, 140
lingual coarticulation, 13, 42, 43, 57, 222, 229, 233, 245
   anticipatory, 26, 90, 94, 98–102, 103
   articulatory compatability, 83
   articulatory constraints, 57
   articulatory control, 80, 83, 104
   articulatory model of, 19, 94
   articulatory repositioning, 85
   blending, 87–8
   carryover, 95–6, 98–102, 103
   coarticulatory resistance, 85
   coarticulatory sensitivity, 80, 84, 90, 93, 94, 102, 103
   coproduction, 81
   coupling effects, 90, 93
   duration: influence of, 103
   gestural compatibility, 100, 101
   gestural conflict, 101
   gestural overlap, 81, 103
   speech rate: influence of, 99, 103
   stress: influence of, 99, 102–3
   syllable position: influence of, 102
   temporal overlap, 87
   undershoot, 94, 103
lip and jaw coarticulation, 144, 162, 175, 281, 283
   dynamic perturbation, 168
   static perturbation, 168

motor equivalence, 33, 165, 255, 256, 259
muscle activity
   neuromuscular features of, 149–50, 270–3

nasalization, 46, 48, 50, 59, 69, 70, 72, 75, 76, 78, 79, 179, 183, 191, 284, 288, 289, 291
   nasalized vowels, 48, 72–3, 76, 181, 286, 287, 288, 323, 332
   see also nasal coarticulation; velopharyngeal coarticulation
nasal coarticulation, 26–7, 73–4, 77, 78, 79, 284, 285, 286
   acoustic evidence, 70–1, 75
   acoustics, 77
   anticipatory, 73–4, 75, 76, 78, 79, 288, 289
   carryover, 73, 74–5, 76, 78
   connected speech, 78
   nasalance, 75
   nasility in Italian, 77
   perceptual evidence, 71–3, 76
   spontaneous speech, 77–8
   suprasegmentals, 78–9
   see also velopharyngeal coarticulation

phonological theory, implications for, 200, 201, 222
   alphabetic model, 199, 202, 206, 208, 216–17, 218, 220–1, 222, 224

phonological theory, implications for, (*cont.*)
  phonetic representation, 40, 42, 45, 199–201,
      206, 213
  phonological representation, 24, 45, 48, 107,
      200–1, 208, 219, 222, 224–5
  phonological underspecification, 45, 48, 49,
      148, 187, 208
  segmentation, 15, 29, 199, 205, 206, 208, 209
  vervet monkeys, 203–4

speech production, unit of
  syllable, 13, 15, 17, 21, 25
  syntagma, 17
Steuerung, 11, 14

Task Dynamics, 15, 51, 113–14, 169, 174, 191
temporal coarticulation, 10, 235
trough, 20–1, 22, 195, 241

velar coarticulation, 24, 41, 42, 50, 59, 61, 63,
      105, 159, 182, 183, 285

anticipatory, 156
velopharyngeal coarticulation
  acoustics, 287–9
  aerometry, 284–6
  articulatory modelling, 288
  nasograph, 291
  nasometer, 288
  observation techniques
      direct, 289–93
      indirect, 284–9
      recent, 292–3
  photoelectric devices: drawbacks, 291
  pneumotachograph, 285
  radiographic technique: drawbacks, 289, 290
  spectographic method, 286, 287
  velograph, 291
  velotrace, 291–2
  see also nasal coarticulation

.